Gettysburg Surgeons

Facing a Common Enemy in the Civil War's Deadliest Battle

Barbara Franco

STACKPOLE BOOKS

Essex, Connecticut
Blue Ridge Summit, Pennsylvania

STACKPOLE BOOKS

The Globe Pequot Publishing Group, Inc.
64 South Main Street
Essex, CT 06426
www.globepequot.com

Distributed by NATIONAL BOOK NETWORK

Copyright © 2025 by Barbara Franco

Maps by The Globe Pequot Publishing Group, Inc.

British Library Cataloguing in Publication Information available

Library of Congress Cataloging-in-Publication Data available
ISBN 978-0-8117-7648-6 (cloth: alk paper)
ISBN 978-0-8117-7649-3 (electronic)

♾™ The paper used in this publication meets the minimum requirements of American National Standard for Information Sciences—Permanence of Paper for Printed Library Materials, ANSI/ NISO Z39.48-1992.

Dedicated to Captain Alexander Franco, MD, and the medical staff of all wars who have fought a common enemy of death and disease

CONTENTS

CONTENTS

Preface

The idea for this book began with a list of names and a modest project to identify the surgeons who cared for the wounded at the Lutheran Seminary hospital in Gettysburg in 1863. The project was precipitated by the opening of a new museum in the historic Seminary building—the Seminary Ridge Museum and Education Center—commemorating the 150th anniversary of the battle on July 1, 2013. The museum's exhibits on the care of the wounded adopted a personal approach that identified the names of patients treated in the hospital, the surgeons who attended them, and the nurses and volunteers who provided care. We knew little about the surgeons who were listed in the Seminary register or those who were mentioned in contemporary accounts, beyond their name, regiment, and rank. The list included both Union and Confederate surgeons as well as civilian physicians who volunteered or served as contract surgeons.

It soon became clear that the Seminary hospital did not stand alone but was part of a complex system of doctors and caretakers both during and after the battle. Although no comprehensive listing of surgeons at Gettysburg had been compiled, previous research provided important parts of the story. Gregory Coco's *A Vast Sea of Misery*, Roland Maust's *Grappling with Death: The Union Second Corps Hospital at Gettysburg*, Kent Masterson Brown's *Retreat from Gettysburg*, and Ronald D. Kirkwood's *"Too Much for Human Endurance"* all provided important documentation to identify individual surgeons. Regimental histories sometimes mention surgeons, usually only if they were very good and beloved or very bad and disliked. The *Medical and Surgical History of the War of the Rebellion* includes case studies that provide surgeons' names, but many of the cases are based on the better-documented work of hospital physicians rather than regimental staff in the field.

Why Gettysburg? The 1,200 surgeons who worked in some capacity during and after the battle of Gettysburg represent a significant sampling of all Civil War physicians, estimated at 17,000. Because 1863 is midway through the war, Gettysburg represents a period when both medical corps were better organized and fully staffed with doctors who had been examined and tested by medical examining boards. Although many of the characters are the same, the story of care at Gettysburg is different than First Bull Run in 1861, the Peninsular campaign of 1862, or even Antietam in September 1862. Looking at this particular group of surgeons at a specific moment in time, the study includes not only a few well-documented and prominent physicians or those who left written accounts in diaries and letters but also lesser-known surgeons whose stories have not been told.

At first the idea of identifying the surgeons at Gettysburg seemed an impossible task. Jonathan Letterman, medical director of the U.S. Army of the Potomac, reported that there were 650 Union medical personnel at the battle; there was no corresponding report for the Confederate surgeons, but based on the number of regiments, each with a surgeon and one assistant surgeon, about 450 might be expected. The first step was to create a methodology and a structure for organizing the amount of data collected for a large number of individuals. The obvious structure was based on the order of battle and organized by the participating regiments. The next task was to find and verify the names of the surgeons who were on duty in July 1863, based on their individual service records and other corroborating accounts. For each surgeon, the data collected includes birth and death dates, where and when they studied medicine, as well as any biographical information about their life before, during, and after their Gettysburg experience. Identification of contract surgeons and volunteers proved more difficult without official records and depended on either contemporary accounts or hospital records kept by Dr. Henry Janes, the surgeon left in charge of the hospitals at Gettysburg. The resulting database includes biographical information for approximately

1,200 nineteenth-century medical doctors who served in various capacities during and after the battle of Gettysburg.

How does this approach differ from other recent research on Civil War medicine? William G. Rothstein, author of *American Physicians in the 19th Century* (1985), identified three different ways to approach medical history:

- Development of medical knowledge and technology—what doctors know.

- The health of the populace and impact of medical care on patients—the effectiveness of treatment.

- Behavior of individual physicians as members of a profession—a social history of medicine.

Looking at physicians as members of a profession, Rothstein acknowledged, has been least explored and merited further study. Civil War surgeons and medical history have remained some of the last fields to be fully investigated despite keen interest in Civil War history. This is changing with new scholarship on medical care and the publication and digital accessibility of many more primary sources of military records, letters, and diaries. Other authors have focused on changing medical technology and the impact of medical care on patients. This study focuses on the experiences of individual physicians as members of a profession. Rather than a traditional biography of one famous physician or the account of a single diarist, the study collects as much information as possible about all the surgeons who were at the battle of Gettysburg in order to understand them both personally and professionally as a group. Although Union and Confederate surgeons served in opposing armies, they were members of the same profession. Their experiences were so similar that there was no need to tell separate stories for Confederate and Union surgeons. For the most part, their stories follow similar patterns from education and training to camp life and medical responsibilities. Where there are differences, I have tried to identify and explain them.

The methodology that best fit this approach proved to be *prosopography*, briefly defined as a study that identifies and relates a group of persons or characters within a particular historical or literary context. Distinguished from a biography of one individual or a collective biography of several individuals, prosopography collects and analyzes relevant quantities of biographical data about a well-defined group of individuals with a goal of establishing patterns and relationships that inform social history. The database of surgeons functioned as the first step in the prosopographic process by creating "a set of biographical profiles of each individual in the group under investigation." The second step involved analysis of the data according to the questions that underlie the research.[1]

The questions that emerged during the research process focus on the experiences of the surgeons themselves.

- How well prepared were Civil War surgeons?
- What motivated them to join the army?
- What adjustments did they have to make to military life both personally and professionally?
- Were there significant differences between the experiences of Union and Confederate surgeons?
- How did medical care in the field differ from the work of physicians in military hospitals?
- What work did surgeons perform both during and after the battle of Gettysburg?
- What was the role of the volunteers and contract surgeons who provided assistance after the battle? What was their relationship to the army surgeons?
- As noncombatants, how were surgeons treated when they were left behind with wounded and became prisoners?
- What were the personal and professional issues facing doctors who returned to civilian life after the war?
- How did their wartime experiences influence their contributions to medicine and other fields in later life?

- As professionals who faced death on a daily basis during the Civil War, how did their own lives end?

The profiles of the individual surgeons in this study are based on a wide variety of sources. Some left personal letters and diaries written contemporaneously; others wrote published or unpublished memoirs and accounts afterwards. They appear in official reports and regimental histories. As prominent men in their home communities, some were included in county histories or eulogized in extensive obituaries. Others have left only scant public records of military service, directory listings, school catalogues, or census records to document their lives. Each individual biographical profile tells an interesting but incomplete personal story. Combined, these stories provide a more nuanced and complex narrative than official reports or a single personal memoir could convey. Some surgeons describe a particular aspect of their Civil War experience; others provide different perspectives. Assistant Surgeon Alfred T. Hamilton, 148th Pennsylvania, explained in his contribution to a regimental history that "the story of the soldier, whether of the staff or line, when written on the spot of occurrence has the merit of authenticity *from his standpoint.* It is not possible for each to see everything, nor in the same aspect, nor was it possible for each to be impressed with a fact the same as the other witnesses."[2]

The Gettysburg surgeons named in the text are identified by their rank and regiment at the time of the battle. Whenever possible, I have tried to let them tell their stories in their own words. Considered together in the aggregate, these individual stories reveal patterns, connections, and relationships that offer new insights and provide deeper understanding about the lives and legacy of Civil War surgeons. Far from the unskilled butchers of popular stereotypes, most had received the best training available to them in the United States or abroad and were able to pass qualifying examinations that required advanced clinical knowledge. Some had battlefield experience from the Mexican and Crimean Wars. Younger men brought up-to-date knowledge from prestigious urban schools, while older doctors brought years of practical experience in rural and urban communities. Learning from each other and their shared military experience, they acquired new skills and knowledge that would influence medical practice during and after the war.

INTRODUCTION

JULY 4, 1863

Saturday, July 4, 1863, marked the eighty-seventh anniversary of the Declaration of Independence. Some communities celebrated the day as usual with full festivities. In New York City the Tammany Society event featured patriotic music, orations, a banquet, and patriotic toasts.[1] The *Los Angeles Star* reported a general celebration of picnics, a thirty-four-gun salute, an exhibition of fireworks and a ball, with the day "generally observed as a high holiday."[2] The mood was more restrained in Philadelphia where the day passed without any political demonstrations, "on account of the invasion of the state."[3] In Richmond, Virginia, the capital of the Confederacy, there was no cause for celebration. "This is the Fourth of July. In former days it was saluted with the firing of guns, and was honored by grand parades, orations, dinners, and toasts . . . The day is now changed. We have no holiday. The ruthless enemy who has trampled upon every principle and right commemorated by the day itself, gives no intermission for festive enjoyments."[4] In Washington, President Lincoln delayed his speech until July 7th when he was able to report Union victories in both Vicksburg, Mississippi, and Gettysburg, Pennsylvania.[5]

The previous year, residents of Gettysburg, Pennsylvania, celebrated the Fourth of July as a holiday with family picnics and by "ringing of bells, firing of canons, and stirring martial music."[6] But in 1863, there were no fireworks, military parades, fancy dress balls, or picnics. The cannons and guns that had roared over the town for three days and sent terrified residents to their cellars during the battle were finally silent, except for the sharpshooters' rifles or an occasional artillery shell. Gettysburg residents awoke on July 4th with relief that the Confederates were departing, and horror as they confronted the aftermath of a battle that left thousands of suffering wounded, acres of battlefield strewn with the bodies of slain soldiers, and the rotting carcasses of dead horses and mules. A steady downpour of rain that finally broke the sweltering heat and dust of the previous days of battle could not wash away the lingering smell of blood and gunpowder or the stench of death.

Agnes S. Barr, a young Gettysburg woman, heard the Confederate wagons moving all night long and reported the news of their departure to Surgeon Elias Beck, 3rd Indiana Cavalry, one of the Union surgeons left behind enemy lines at the Presbyterian Church hospital.[7] During the night Confederate troops had indeed vacated the town, and their wagon trains of supplies and wounded were already preparing to move south. Throughout the day skirmishing continued as Confederate sharpshooters, protecting their position along Seminary Ridge, remained a constant threat to citizens and soldiers.

Assistant Surgeon Francis Wafer of the 108th New York Infantry wrote that on July 4th, "The enemy kept a strong skirmishing line in our front, which was very active in firing at every living object within possible range. Our stretcher bearers had removed most of their wounded from our front during the night, but some unfortunates had escaped attention . . . On our men attempting to remove these during the day they were deliberately fired at by the enemy's sharpshooters."[8] He was appalled that Confederate sharpshooters prevented their own wounded from receiving treatment for another day.

Behind the Confederate lines, beginning in the early hours of July 4th, every available wagon was appropriated to transport the Confederate wounded back to Virginia. Surgeons had to make medical decisions about which patients could withstand the grueling trip, knowing that those left behind would become prisoners. At the David Schriver Farm, on Mummasburg Road, Surgeon John Moore Hayes, 26th Alabama, was left with about 760 wounded who could not be moved. William H. Connell, a Union soldier wounded and captured on July 1st, remembered that after the repulse of Pickett's Charge on July 3rd, a surgeon came galloping from the front and ordered Dr. Hayes to send out and gather all the farm wagons he could find, load them with the wounded, and start them toward Cashtown.[9]

Peter Tinsley, chaplain of the 28th Virginia, wrote in his diary for July 4th at Bream's Mill, located west of Gettysburg near the Fairfield-Hagerstown Road:

> I was busily employed in visiting the suffering and attempting to minister bodily and spiritual comfort . . . and in helping to send those who could go, for it has been determined to retreat . . . There is no fighting today except for distant picket firing, yet we are in continual fear that the Hosp. will become a scene of conflict.[10]

Surgeon J. Franklin Dyer, 19th Massachusetts, wrote from a Union field hospital near Gettysburg on July 4, 1863:

> We have a joyful Fourth of July only for the dreadful scenes about us. I am now sitting in a little sheltered tent which one of the men has up while the rain is pouring down in torrents as thousands of wounded men gathered in hospitals about two miles from the front. Our corps and some others have no tents, no houses or barns, all exposed to the rain, and thousands have not yet been brought in. It is impossible to operate fast enough to dress all the wounds in three or four days. I am waiting for the rain to hold up to go to work.[11]

The military battle may have ended with Pickett's Charge on July 3rd, but on July 4, 1863, the work of the surgeons was just beginning. Their work would not end until November 19, 1863, when the last patients left Gettysburg hospitals and Lincoln delivered his now famous address invoking the principles of July 4, 1776, to dedicate a new national cemetery in Gettysburg.

The Surgeons

On July 4th, more than a thousand surgeons and assistant surgeons were on duty at Gettysburg with the Union Army of the Potomac and the Confederate Army of Northern Virginia. By the end of November 1863 when the last hospital closed, more than 1,200 doctors, both military and civilian, had participated in the care of an estimated 30,000 wounded. Rather than the stereotype of ill-prepared and incompetent practitioners, they represent a broad sampling of the medical profession of the 1860s, encompassing diverse backgrounds and experiences. They included surgeons and assistant surgeons commissioned in the regular army as U.S. Volunteers, those commissioned to serve in regiments raised by both Union and Confederate states, acting assistant surgeons serving under government contracts, and civilian volunteers working independently or under the auspices of various relief organizations.

The commissioned military surgeons at Gettysburg during the battle ranged in age from sixty-year-old veterans of the Mexican War to twenty-year-old recent medical school graduates. Despite an overall age span of forty years, a majority of surgeons and assistant surgeons were in their twenties and early thirties with the highest percentage in both armies born between 1830 and 1839. Assistant Surgeon Washington Akin, 125th New York, was typical of these relatively young doctors who served at Gettysburg. Born in 1835, he graduated from Albany Medical College in 1858, practiced medicine in Troy, New York, and was appointed attending physician and surgeon at the Troy hospital before the war. Confederate Hunter Holmes McGuire, medical director of General Richard Ewell's Second Corps, was born in 1835, the son of a prominent Winchester, Virginia, physician. He graduated from Winchester Medical College in 1855 and continued medical studies at the University of Pennsylvania and Jefferson Medical College in 1856 and 1859. He was teaching at the medical college in New Orleans when the war broke out.

One of the oldest, Medical Director Thomas Sim, U.S. Third Corps, was born in Maryland in 1802 and graduated from the University of Maryland Medical School in 1823. Surgeon Lawrence Reynolds, 63rd New York, born in Ireland in 1803, studied medicine in Liverpool, England. An outspoken supporter of the Chartist movement, Reynolds was forced to flee Ireland in 1848 for political reasons. In a history of the Irish Brigade, he was described as "a highly educated and refined gentleman, and very experienced surgeon, a true Irish gentleman and patriot, served with honor as surgeon of the regiment from its first organization;

although advanced in years is still young in vigor."[12] The oldest Confederate surgeon was Assistant Surgeon John Work, 1st Texas, born in 1804, who lived in Breckenridge County, Kentucky, before moving his family to Texas in 1838. Dr. Work had seen previous service as a contract surgeon in the Mexican War for eight months and enlisted in 1862 in a regiment commanded by his son, Philip Alexander Work. His letter of resignation in May 1864 cited his age as sixty years old and "unable to endure fatigues of either field or hospital practice."[13]

At the other end of the age range, Surgeon James Julius Winn, 45th Georgia, was the youngest surgeon serving at the battle of Gettysburg. Born in 1842, he graduated from Atlanta Medical College in 1860, was appointed assistant surgeon in October 1862, and passed the examination for surgeon in April 1863. Several assistant surgeons born in 1843 included William F. Tibbals, 5th Ohio, Albert L. Mitchell, 37th Massachusetts, born in Nova Scotia, and Alexander Comer, 9th New York Cavalry. Mitchell and Comer were among the Canadian students recruited to serve in the Union army. Mitchell graduated with a degree from King's College New Brunswick and an MD from Harvard Medical School in 1863. Comer attended Queens College, Kingston, Ontario.

A comparison of birthdates for Union and Confederate medical staff shows larger percentages of both older and younger surgeons among Union surgeons, while Confederate surgeons were more likely to be born in the 1830–1839 period. This difference may be attributed to the fact that the Union army retained more career military surgeons who were older and more experienced. The Union army also had access to greater numbers of younger recent graduates from Northern medical colleges, while many Southern medical schools closed during the war.

Birthdates of Military Medical Staff on Duty at the Battle of Gettysburg

Birthdate	Union (664)	Confederate (444)
1800–1809	1.6%	0.5%
1810–1819	7.0%	2.0%
1820–1829	29.0%	21.0%

1830–1839	53.0%	70.0%
1840–1843	9.0%	5.0%
Unknown	0.4%	1.5%

The surgeons who came to Gettysburg to assist after the battle included a mix of U.S. Army commissioned surgeons, contracted acting assistant surgeons, and civilian volunteers representing various relief organizations. While the commissioned army personnel dispatched to Gettysburg after the battle were born between 1810 and 1839, the birthdates of acting assistant surgeons and civilian volunteers ranged from 1795 to 1844. The oldest, born in 1795, included Thomas T. Smiley, acting assistant surgeon at Camp Letterman, and George McCook, a civilian volunteer from Pittsburgh. The youngest, born in 1843, were acting assistant surgeons George Mason Ward and John Kelly, who served at Camp Letterman, and Charles Fuller, who served at the Seminary hospital.

Birthdates of Military, Contract, and Volunteer Physicians Who Arrived After the Battle

Birthdate	Union Military (12)	Union Contract (55)	Civilian Volunteers (75)
1790–1799		2%	1%
1800–1809		2%	4%
1810–1819	33.3%	7%	19%
1820–1829	33.3%	31%	44%
1830–1839	33.3%	36%	23%
1840–1844		18%	5%
Unknown		4%	4%

The military surgeons at Gettysburg were all men. While a few women held medical degrees in 1863, they were not eligible to serve as commissioned or contract surgeons, although some volunteered to serve as nurses. One notable exception, Dr. Mary Edwards Walker, persisted in volunteering as an assistant surgeon, eventually received a contract as acting assistant surgeon, and was awarded a controversial medal of honor for her service. She was not the only woman physician at Gettysburg. Among the women who served as nurses, Eliza Wood Burhans Farnham and Susan E. Hall had both studied medicine in New York City, probably at the Hygeio-Therapeutic College. Esther Kersey Painter was an 1860 graduate of the Pennsylvania Women's Medical College in Philadelphia.

Geographically, the surgeons represented every state in both the Union and Confederacy, as residents before, during, or after the war. Pennsylvania and New York regiments together made up nearly 55 percent of the Army of the Potomac's medical staff; Virginia regiments accounted for nearly 27 percent of the Army of Northern Virginia; Georgia and North Carolina each represented about 15 percent. A significant number of immigrants served as surgeons, mainly in the Union's Irish Brigade and German-speaking regiments. The largest number of foreign-born surgeons came from Germany with at least twenty-one German immigrants serving with the Union and at least two in the Confederate army. Fifteen Union surgeons emigrated from Ireland, with some trained in Liverpool or Dublin medical schools; at least two were members of the prestigious Royal College of Surgeons. Twelve Canadians served as surgeons with the Union and one, Surgeon Solomon Secord, 20th Georgia, served as a Confederate.

The surgeons represented diverse socio-economic backgrounds. A medical degree itself did not confer high social or professional status in the nineteenth century. While most Confederate surgeons came from upper class planter and mercantile families, and some Union surgeons came from prestigious and wealthy Northern families, others were the sons of farmers, tradesmen, and mechanics. Surgeon William Riddick Whitehead, 44th Virginia, came from a family whose extensive wealth, from shipping enterprises based in New York City and sugar plantations in Louisiana, supported the best education available and provided an international perspective that connected him to European elites. Assistant Surgeon John Shaw Billings, 7th U.S., on the other hand, came from a modest farm family in Indiana and had to pay for his own education by working in medical school dissecting rooms.

Accounts of surgeons often refer to the strength of their character and their interactions with patients. Their personalities ranged from kind and comforting to stern and domineering. A biographical sketch of Surgeon John Henry Beech, 24th Michigan, noted his deep faith, charity, and membership in the Presbyterian Church. He received a tribute from a member of the regiment describing him as

> a frail, thoughtful man, unobtrusive, patient, and studious. His love for his profession was an enthusiasm. His kindness was womanly. His relation to the regiment caused him to be serious, as one carrying great care with carefulness; yet he was approachable and kind always. As a counselor he was wise in his advice. He was a man careful of detail.[14]

Assistant Surgeon John Blocker, 4th Georgia, was described as "a kind and tender-hearted gentleman who treated the private soldier with consideration."[15] Nurses, hospital stewards, and fellow doctors consistently described other surgeons as overbearing and cold. Multiple reports identify Surgeon Pascal Alfred Quinan, 150th Pennsylvania, as unpopular with both soldiers and colleagues. Although he was well trained at Jefferson Medical College and the University of Maryland, received a perfect score of ten on his Pennsylvania medical examination, and had a decade of regular army experience before the war, his difficult personality was reported by various observers. Assistant Surgeon James Fulton, 150th Pennsylvania, recorded in his diary in June 1863 that when Quinan returned to regimental duty after serving as acting brigade surgeon, "deciding who was able to march and those that are not—his usual morose disposition and harshness toward the privates was only increased by this sudden turn in his position."[16] A visitor at Gettysburg described him as a brute, "smoking and swearing and paying no attention whatever to the frequent appeals made to him."[17] The regimental history tersely commented, "His advent was signalized by an almost immediate reduction of the sick list from 70 to 29 whether wisely or unwisely it would be difficult to say."[18]

The surgeons who cared for the wounded at Gettysburg represented the diversity of the profession. Some were temperance advocates with strong religious convictions, and a few were clergymen; others were alcoholics, adventurers, and freethinkers. They represented a range of religious traditions including Catholics, Quakers, Protestants, and Jews. Their training ranged from apprenticeships and medical colleges in America to advanced university studies abroad. They practiced traditional medicine and adopted ideas from new and competing medical theories. Organizing this diverse group of former civilian physicians into an effective military medical corps proved challenging to both armies.

A COMPETENT MEDICAL DEPARTMENT

On July 4, 1863, the 664 Union and 444 Confederate surgeons who faced enormous challenges and a staggering number of casualties at Gettysburg were better organized and trained for their work than the year before. In the third year of a war that many initially thought would last only a few months, both armies had made significant improvements in the selection process for surgeons and the organizational structures of their medical corps.

At the start of the war in 1861, the Union army had a medical staff of only 114 doctors; twenty-four resigned to join the Confederacy and three were dismissed as disloyal.[19] Staffing newly organized state regiments with qualified medical practitioners presented a major undertaking. Both sides faced the immediate need to recruit, train, and mobilize a medical corps to meet the needs of large wartime fighting forces. The medical staff for each Union regiment theoretically consisted of a commissioned surgeon and two assistant surgeons. Confederate regiments normally had one surgeon and one assistant surgeon, apparently due to objections from the Confederate president and secretary to the Union model.[20] Both sides supplemented their medical staff with contracted acting assistant surgeons, especially for work in the hospitals.

The *American Medical Times* for Saturday June 22, 1861, cited the lack of medical care and supplies for the suffering wounded during the Crimean War in the 1850s and hoped that the United States could learn from those mistakes. As the Civil War began, both federal and state governments on both sides realized they had little experience with organizing and staffing for the medical needs of soldiers in camp and battle.

Even medical professionals expressed concern that unqualified physicians would be selected to provide medical care for newly organized regiments.

> We may estimate by hundreds the numbers of unqualified persons who have received the endorsement of these bodies, as capable Surgeons and Assistant Surgeons to regiments. Indeed, these examinations have in some cases been so conducted as to prove the merest farce. Irregular practitioners, "retired physicians," disabled "political doctors," physicians unable to obtain a livelihood in civil practice from sheer incapacity, have emerged from the "Green Room," full-fledged Army Surgeons.[21]

Regiments, organized and recruited from local communities, initially chose local doctors to serve as their surgeons, often without consideration of medical training, surgical skill, or suitability to military life. By 1863 rigorous examinations of candidates were required for the surgeons and assistant surgeons in both armies. Pennsylvania, for example, began testing for its volunteer surgeons as early as May 1861, and most other states initiated similar examinations. Similarly, the secretary of war of the Confederacy was authorized to appoint army medical boards to examine applicants for appointments as assistant surgeons or for promotion to surgeon. In practice, however, the urgent need to assign medical officers for newly organized regiments often meant that early appointments were made without formal examination.[22] In response to concerns that unqualified medical personnel had received commissions as surgeons, Confederate medical director E. S. Gaillard began sending printed notices to all Confederate surgeons in the fall of 1862 that read: "You are respectfully requested to forward to this office, without delay, the date of your appointment, also to state whether you have appeared before a Medical Examining Board, and if so, with what result."[23] Confederate surgeons like James Hickerson, 37th North Carolina, who declined to take the exam and resigned, gave medical disability as the reason for their resignation in the official record.[24]

The system of examinations provided proof of basic levels of medical knowledge in anatomy, practice of medicine, surgery, and *materia medica*. Doctors who passed the examinations were considered competent to serve. By some estimates four out of five applicants failed to pass the Confederate test and were denied commissions.[25] The Pennsylvania state examination rated applicants on a scale of one to ten, with a score of five to seven required to be commissioned assistant surgeon and at least seven to ten to be commissioned surgeon.[26]

Early battles in the war quickly revealed the weaknesses of the medical organizations of both armies and their inability to respond to the medical needs of the wounded. The battle of First Bull Run, July 1861, by all reports was a medical as well as a military disaster for the Union. William S. King, U.S. medical director of the Army of Northeastern Virginia, had no plan in place to deal with the wounded. William W. Keen, a newly appointed assistant surgeon who was later dispatched to Gettysburg after that battle, remembered his first experiences at Bull Run:

> during the entire engagement, I never received a single order from either colonel or other officer, medical inspector, the surgeon of my regiment or anyone else. It was like the days when there was no king in Israel, and every man did that which was right in his own eyes . . . My experience in this battle is a good illustration of the utter disorganization, or rather want of organization, of our entire army at the beginning of the war.[27]

Louis C. Duncan's history of *The Medical Departments of the United States Army in the Civil War* made clear the lessons of Bull Run:

> it was demonstrated that a number of civil practitioners, however highly qualified and patriotic they may be, do not constitute a competent medical department for an army . . .
>
> As we had no Army we should of course have had no Medical and Hospital Corps. Three years had passed before the Medical Department was in a satisfactory condition.[28]

The problems Duncan described at Bull Run—a lack of ambulances and staff to evacuate wounded, inefficient distribution and deployment of medical supplies, and an inefficient way to organize and staff field hospitals—proved difficult for both armies to solve.

The need for change was apparent to the newly appointed Union and Confederate surgeons general, chosen to replace original appointees who either lacked administrative experience or resisted innovation; but attempts to institute change through legislation met political opposition in both governments. Confederate surgeon general Samuel Preston Moore was appointed in July 1861, replacing David C. DeLeon.[29] Moore tried to pass legislation providing for better organization and supplies from August 1861 to April 1863 without success. Yet by 1864, the Confederate medical department's journal reported:

> Although the organization of the medical department is not as complete as it is believed it could have been, had the ideas and suggestions of its experienced presiding officer met with more favorable consideration, still . . . the objects for which it was instituted have been, if not perfectly, yet to a very great extent, satisfactorily accomplished."[30]

Similar efforts to pass federal legislation with support from the U.S. Sanitary Commission initially stalled in Congress. Legislation proposed by U.S. Surgeon William A. Hammond and Frederick Law Olmsted, secretary of the Sanitary Commission, was introduced in the U.S. Senate by Senator Henry Wilson in December 1861. The bill called for medical inspectors to assume responsibility for sanitary conditions of hospitals and camps; a requirement that hospital construction be based on plans recognized as modern and scientific; a revamped ambulance system; and using merit and scientific accomplishments rather than seniority as criteria for future military medical appointments. Thanks to the lobbying efforts of the Sanitary Commission, the medical reform bill eventually passed in April 1862, but without the provisions for hospital construction or an expanded ambulance corps.[31] U.S. Surgeon General Clement Alexander Finley, a veteran of the "old army" who had been appointed based on his seniority, was described by George Templeton Strong of the Sanitary Commission as "utterly ossified and useless." Finley was forced to retire in April 1862 after a conflict with Secretary of War Edwin Stanton.[32] With the support of the Sanitary Commission,

William Hammond was appointed surgeon general and began to initiate much-needed reforms.

While an army-wide ambulance corps had been left out of the U.S. legislation, Gen. George B. McClellan and his medical director, Jonathan Letterman, moved forward to design a new ambulance system for the Army of the Potomac. Letterman joined McClellan's staff as medical director in July 1862 and immediately set to work to strategize and improve field medical tactics in three main areas: ambulance service for the wounded, more efficient distribution of medical supplies, and a complete restructuring of the field hospital system. The battle of Antietam in September 1862 was the first chance to try out changes, which were then fully implemented at Gettysburg and came to be known as the Letterman system.

The volunteer organizations that provided medical support were also better organized and staffed by 1863. U.S. Christian Commission and Sanitary Commission volunteers were mobilized to respond quickly with supplementary medical supplies and nurses after a battle. At Gettysburg they were among the first to arrive with needed supplies. An official corps of paid women nurses had been formed under the supervision of Dorothea Dix, but women also volunteered as nurses under the auspices of the Christian and Sanitary Commissions, with local groups, or even as individuals. Confederate volunteer organizations were not as comprehensive or structured, but civilian efforts also helped provide medical care. Lafayette Guild, medical director of the Army of Northern Virginia, constantly complained that there were not enough ambulances or horses.[33] After the battle of Gettysburg, the Richmond Ambulance Committee helped feed and transport wounded to hospitals with its own funds and provided care in the Winchester, Virginia, hospitals for three weeks after the battle.[34]

MEDICAL SECTARIANISM

At the time of the Civil War in America, there was no legal definition about who could practice medicine and call themselves a doctor. Care of the sick still mainly took place at home where patients were nursed by family members, usually women, with or without professional medical

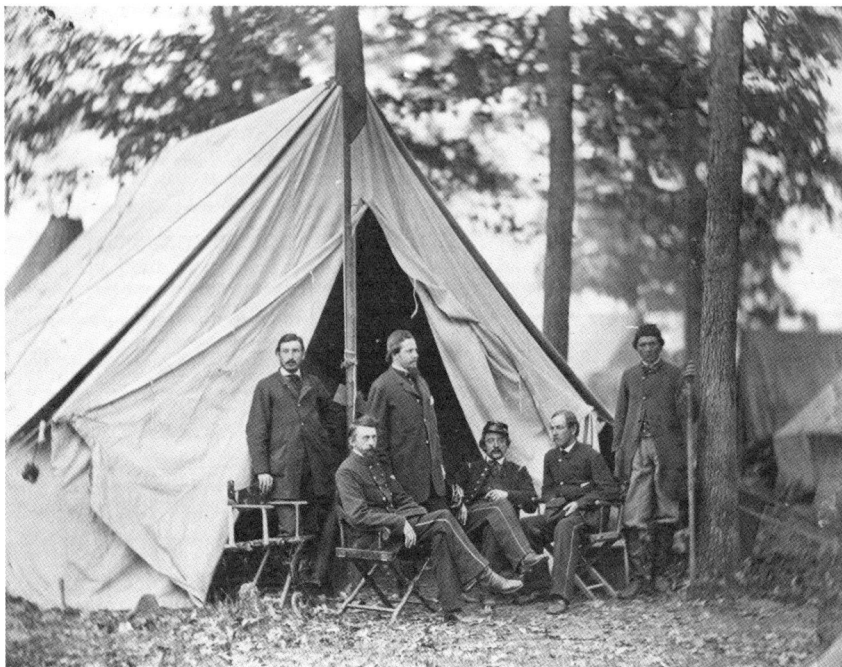

Surgeon Jonathan Letterman, seated left, Medical Director, Army of the Potomac, and assistants, November 1862. Courtesy of U.S. Army Heritage and Education Center, Carlisle, Pennsylvania

intervention. Hospitals were nonexistent except for infirmaries designed mainly for the poor, indigent, and insane in larger cities. Licensing laws that had been in place in the eighteenth century were overturned in most states by the mid nineteenth century, due to the advocacy of new medical systems in competition with the so-called regular doctors. Medical sectarianism took on new importance as a variety of alternative medical theories challenged the exclusive authority of regular physicians and demanded equal recognition.

By the 1860s three medical sects presented challenges to orthodox medicine. Thomsonian medicine, a system patented by Samuel Thomson in 1813, offered to make "Every Man His Own Physician," using botanical medicines that promised a gentler and more effective treatment than the bloodletting and mercury pills favored by regular physicians. After Thomson's death in 1843, plant-based medicines continued to be promoted by botanical and eclectic medical practitioners through the nineteenth century. Samuel Hahnemann, a German physician, announced his new method of treating diseases in 1796 after long study and systematic testing of drugs and dosages. The name homeopathy came from the Greek word for *similar* because patients were treated with diluted doses of drugs that produced the same symptoms as the disease. Hydropathy, widely practiced in Europe and America in the 1830s and 1840s, was based on the notion that water dissolved impurities that could be sweated out and washed away and promoted the additional benefits of hygiene and diet as keys to preventing disease and preserving health.[35] Russell Trall, a graduate of the Albany Medical College, embraced hydropathy in the 1840s and founded the New York Hydropathic and Physiological School in 1853. The school, one of the first in the United States to admit women candidates for the degree of MD, stressed dietary therapies of vegetarianism and Graham flours, sanitation, personal hygiene, and exercise.

Most nineteenth-century physicians adhered to regular or orthodox medicine, based on a theory of disease that focused on correcting imbalances. Inflammation was treated by bleeding and purging; weakened states called for stimulants like opium or alcohol.[36] Because regular physicians used medicines that produced the opposite effect from the disease, regular physicians were dubbed "allopaths" in contrast to their homeopathic competitors, and the term became widely used to designate regular physicians.

Attempts to officially accept homeopathic physicians in the Union medical corps were not successful; the argument for a consistent approach to medical care effectively excluded all but physicians who had attended regular medical schools and identified themselves as allopaths. This was a victory for regular physicians represented by the American Medical Association, which, since its founding in 1847, had deemed it unethical for regular physicians to even consult with homeopaths. The surgeons at Gettysburg were, for the most part, regular physicians who had received an allopathic education available from the most prestigious schools in Philadelphia, New York, Boston, New Orleans, and Virginia, as well as regional schools that proliferated during the decades leading up to the Civil War. But there were exceptions. A few Union surgeons openly practiced homeopathic medicine, and some were graduates of eclectic schools that taught a variety of medical approaches.

CHANGING MEDICAL TREATMENT

Challenges to established practices of early nineteenth century orthodox medicine came not only from competing medical sects but also from younger doctors influenced either directly or indirectly by the Paris model that stressed observation and clinical practice. By 1863, recent graduates of medical school often found their training at odds with older, senior surgeons in the medical corps. Aristedes Monteiro, a Confederate assistant surgeon with the Alexander Artillery Reserves, Virginia, reported that two members of his examining board held opposing views on the proper treatment of gunshot wounds, so he answered that he would use both methods to satisfy them.[37]

Examination question answers make it clear that Civil War surgeons understood current medical knowledge but did not have the benefit of future advances in medical thinking that would dramatically change medical practice. There was general agreement during the Civil War about vaccinating to prevent smallpox, treating malaria with quinine, and performing amputations under anesthesia for compound fractures of extremities. There was less agreement about how to treat hospital infections like gangrene; epidemics like cholera, yellow fever, and typhoid; or chronic conditions of dysentery, rheumatism, and scurvy. Conflicting camps advocated heroic interventions versus nature, contagion versus non-contagion. Although Joseph Lister's findings on germs and antiseptics were not published until after the war in 1867, changes in practice were already underway during the Civil War. U.S. Surgeon General William Hammond fully appreciated the importance of hygiene and had become skeptical of using heroic therapies like purging and bloodletting. In the preface to his *Treatise on Hygiene*, he wrote that "although not doubting the efficacy of proper medication in the treatment of disease, I am sure that . . . [calomel and tartar emetic], the traditional actions of which have been positively disproved by physiological and chemical researches, as well as by the soundest deductions from pathology, are too frequently administered through a strict adherence to the routine which hinders the development of medical science, and cramps the powers of those who labor for its advancement."[38] His Circular No. 6, issued on May 4, 1863, removed calomel and tartar emetic from the medical supply list, eliciting praise from irregular sectarians who were critical of their use and attacks from some allopaths who remained convinced of their efficacy.[39] Although mercury-based drugs continued to be used, medical supply lists of both armies include many herbal medications not dissimilar from those used by botanical medical sects. Quinine, morphine, alcohol, and ether headed the list of *materia medica* for both armies, but they might also include chamomile, peppermint, aconite, and other botanical tinctures. In the Confederacy, shortages of imported conventional medications, due to Union blockades, inspired Confederate surgeon general Samuel Moore to commission Francis Porcher, a botanist and surgeon from South Carolina, to compile a book of medicinal plants found in the Southern states. *Resources of the Southern Fields and Forests*, published in 1863, included folk remedies used by white Southerners as well as those used by enslaved Africans and indigenous peoples.

The *Medical and Surgical History of the War of the Rebellion* contains examples of bloodletting as part of the medical treatment for everything from wounds to pneumonia, but the practice was clearly on the decline among many surgeons. Confederate surgeon Dr. John Julian Chisolm, a graduate of the Medical College of the State of South Carolina in 1850, continued his studies in Paris, returning to Europe in 1859 to observe the treatment of the wounded in the 2nd Italian War of Independence. He was later appointed surgeon in the Confederate army and published the first edition of *A Manual of Military Surgery for the Use of Surgeons in the Confederate States Army*, based on his observations in Europe and his training in Paris. His recommended treatment for wounds argued against blood extraction and for allowing natural healing to take place:

> in our experience the abstraction of blood will occasion a complete prostration of strength, and may be fatal . . . The large success in the treatment of perforating chest wounds in the Confederate hospitals

puts forth, in a strong light, the powers of nature to heal all wounds when least interfered with by meddlesome surgery.[40]

"THE ART AND SCIENCE OF OUR WARFARE"

Writing in the early twentieth century, Capt. Louis C. Duncan, author of *The Medical Department of the United States Army in the Civil War*, complained about the lack of recognition for the work of the Civil War surgeons:

> on the great fields of conflict a thousand shafts tell where batteries stood and battle lines held their ground amid the cannons' thunder . . . The work of the Surgeons alone remains unrecorded, Except for what is embalmed in those cyclopean volumes, the *Medical and Surgical History of the [War of the] Rebellion*, no one has set down the modest story of their unselfish labors.[41]

While Duncan set out to tell an institutional story of Civil War medicine that he hoped would be a useful model for his contemporaries in military medicine, the perspectives of individual Civil War surgeons often have been overlooked as a resource for better understanding their roles—both personal and professional—as they negotiated military regulations, juggled competing responsibilities, and adapted to evolving medical practices. On March 10, 1863, Ellerslie Wallace, professor of obstetrics, delivered his "Charge to the Graduating Class of Jefferson Medical College" in Philadelphia, Pennsylvania.

> on behalf of our profession at large, I would add to congratulation a warm and cheerful welcome into that corps, whose mission is to go out to battle against the great enemy of mankind—to go on "conquering and to conquer" . . . we look confidently forward to improvements which you shall make in the art and science of our warfare—to the honor of our calling, to the pride of your country, to your own undying fame, and to the best interests of humanity.[42]

The metaphor of medicine as a military battle would not have been lost on his audience of graduates, six of whom would serve at Gettysburg.

Assistant Surgeon John Wilson DeWitt, 17th Pennsylvania Cavalry, joined April 10, 1863. William S. Stewart and Jared Free both served as assistant surgeons in the 83rd Pennsylvania Infantry. Assistant Surgeon Daniel W. Richards, 145th Pennsylvania Infantry, joined June 20, 1863. Two other graduates, William L. Hays and George Washington Brougham, served as acting assistant surgeons at Camp Letterman General Hospital at Gettysburg.

The biographical information in this study is based on the surgeons who were at Gettysburg during and after the battle in 1863, following them through their medical training, their transition from civilians to army surgeons, their experiences at Gettysburg, and their careers after the war ended as they returned home or struck out on new adventures. North and South, Union and Confederate, they served as military surgeons for opposing forces fighting for different causes, but they were united, as doctors, facing a common enemy of death and disease.

PART I

BECOMING A SURGEON

CHAPTER 1

Education

MANY PHYSICIANS WHO WERE VETERANS OF GETTYSBURG LOOKED BACK disparagingly on their earlier nineteenth-century education from the perspective of their twentieth-century medical knowledge. Serving in the field during the Civil War, they quickly realized how much they didn't know and how much there was to learn about battlefield medicine. Assistant Surgeon Simon Baruch, 3rd South Carolina Battalion, admitted that he received his medical degree from the Medical College of Virginia on March 6, 1862, "before ever treating a sick person or even having lanced a boil."[1] Only a few months later, as a newly commissioned assistant surgeon, he performed his first operation—an amputation following the technique he had learned from his professor, Charles Bell Gibson—and was commended by the supervising surgeon.[2] The Civil War occurred in the years before new medical and scientific knowledge about germ theory, bacteria, and the use of antiseptics would revolutionize medical practice. Civil War surgeons, even those receiving the best education available, would not know the cause of infections until decades after the war. An 1860 graduate of the Ohio Medical College, Assistant Surgeon John Shaw Billings, 7th U.S., later explained:

> Twenty-eight years ago we had heard nothing of bacteria, antiseptic surgery was unknown, the clinical thermometer and the hypodermic syringe were just new fangled notions that had not come into use and that few of us had even seen. . . . In those days they taught us medicine as you teach boys to swim, by throwing them into the water.[3]

Rise of Medical Schools

The shortcomings of medical education in the United States were widely criticized throughout the nineteenth century by competing faculty members, graduates, students, and the public. In "Practical Essays on Medical Education" published in 1832, Daniel Drake, the founder of the Ohio Medical College, took medical education to task for the shortness of the term of study, the indifference of preceptors, the laxity of the examinations for a degree, the ungraded courses, and the bickering and quarreling among medical educators.[4] Despite these acknowledged deficiencies, formal college instruction was still considered an improvement over the earlier system of training which was limited to a three-year apprenticeship with an individual physician. Apprentices were judged ready to begin a new career as a doctor, armed with a certificate or testimonial from the preceptor or some form of license issued by a medical society. In some rural areas the apprenticeship system continued well into the nineteenth century. A survey by Dr. Frank A. Ramsey in 1850 concluded that 62 percent of practicing physicians in Tennessee had no formal training in a "regular" medical college.[5] Some surgeons at Gettysburg, like Surgeon Nathan Remington Tefft, 122nd New York Infantry, combined apprenticeship with some medical school courses. After completing a common school education Tefft worked as a teacher while he continued his studies at Lansingburgh Academy, near Troy, New York. He studied medicine from 1827 to 1831 under his brother Dr. Lake I. Tefft, in Marcellus, Onondaga County, New York, while he continued to teach during the winter terms to support himself. He then attended one course of lectures at the College of Physicians and Surgeons in New York City during the winter of 1832–33 without completing a degree, and immediately obtained a diploma to practice medicine from the New York State Medical Society at the age of twenty-five.[6]

By midcentury, licensing laws had been abandoned in most states and the primary credential available to a medical practitioner became a degree from a medical college. In Augusta, Georgia, the 1853 announcement advertised, "The Graduates of the Medical College of Georgia are entitled to practice Medicine in this state without licenses from the Medical Board."[7] The number of medical schools in America increased to meet the demand for medical degrees in order to practice medicine. The earliest medical college in the colonies was the Department of Medicine of the University of Pennsylvania in 1765, followed by the Medical Department of Columbia College in New York City in 1767, later affiliated with the College of Physicians and Surgeons (founded 1807). Following the Revolution, Harvard graduated its first medical class in 1783, and the University of North Carolina, Chapel Hill organized a Medical Department in 1796. By 1825 there were twenty-one medical colleges in fifteen states and the District of Columbia and by 1840 that number had doubled and then doubled again in the next decade. Some schools lasted only a few years, others changed names and affiliations or broke away to form new schools. At the outbreak of the Civil War in 1861, there were more than one hundred medical colleges representing various medical sects in twenty-six states and the District of Columbia.

Of the physicians serving at Gettysburg, 96 percent of Union surgeons and 92 percent of Confederate surgeons either received an MD degree or took an equivalent course from a medical college.[8] Those without documented medical college training may have taken courses without graduating, apprenticed to a physician, studied abroad, or attended a college whose records are no longer available. Those with medical school credentials attended at least seventy different medical schools from Boston to New Orleans and from Philadelphia to Keokuk, Iowa. Two Philadelphia schools, University of Pennsylvania and Jefferson Medical College, together account for 436 attendees or about one third of all the Gettysburg surgeons—Union, Confederate, contract, and volunteers. The University of Virginia had seventy-one Confederate attendees and New York University had sixty attendees among both Confederate and Union surgeons. Only six other schools in the South had more than ten students each among the Gettysburg Confederate surgeons. On the Union side, Harvard, Albany Medical College, and Columbia each had more than forty former students and University of Michigan had more than thirty. Seven surgeons studied at homeopathic colleges in Cleveland, Philadelphia, and St. Louis; ten surgeons had studied at eclectic colleges located in New York, Massachusetts, Pennsylvania, and Ohio; and three attended the hydropathic Hygeio-Therapeutic College of New York.[9]

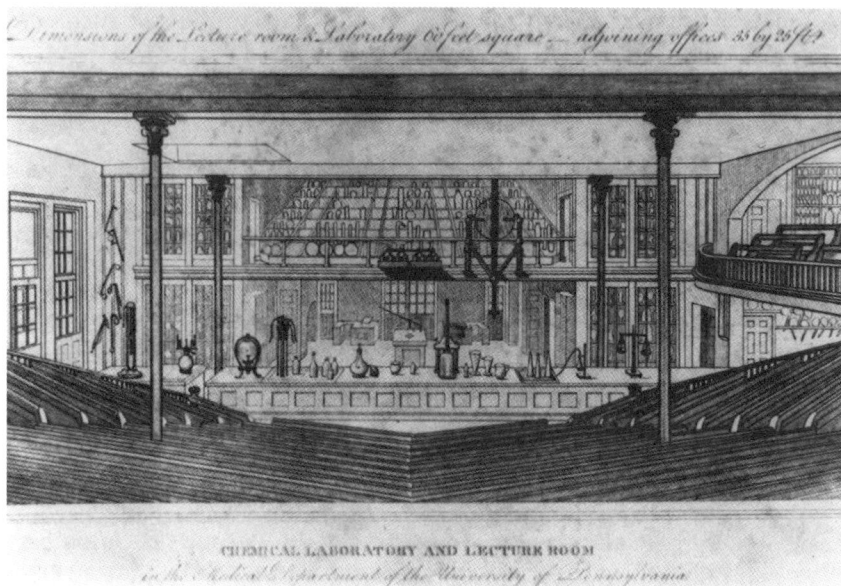

Chemical Laboratory and Lecture Room, Medical Department, University of Pennsylvania. Wood engraving, J. G. Auner, printer 1840–43. Frontispiece of Robert Hare's Compendium of the course of chemical instruction... Courtesy of National Library of Medicine

EDUCATIONAL PREPARATION

How well prepared were the doctors who went from the lecture halls of these medical schools to the field hospitals of the Civil War? Contrary to continued references to untrained or unprepared Civil War surgeons, the individuals who served at Gettysburg represent a remarkably well educated group of doctors. Samuel H. Stout, who served as medical director of hospitals of the Confederate Department and Army of Tennessee, recalled:

> When I attended lectures in Philadelphia more than half a century ago, the number of students in the two schools there (the University, and the Jefferson) was a little more than one thousand, more than half of whom were from the Southern States. Of these latter, a majority were bachelors of arts, or had received a classical education. The Southern States in the slaveholding sections were, therefore, prior to the war well supplied

with educated and chivalrously honorable surgeons and physicians. Such were the men who served at the bedside and in responsible positions in the medical corps of the armies and navy of the Confederacy.[10]

The same could be said for their counterparts in the Union army.

Although there were no specified preliminary requirements to study medicine, students were expected to have "a good English Education."[11] Eli Geddings, a professor at the Medical College of South Carolina, considered "a good working knowledge of English, literature, geography, history (ancient and modern), elementary chemistry and physics, and a reading knowledge of Latin" as indispensable requirements.[12] An analysis of the educational backgrounds of Castleton Medical College students in Maine provides a basis for comparison; of 2,700 students, 128 (4.7 percent) had a previous degree from a college of arts and about 170 (6.2 percent) had one or two years of college.[13] The surgeons at Gettysburg appear to have had a somewhat better educational background than this sampling; 8.7 percent of Confederate and 12.7 percent of Union surgeons were graduates of four-year colleges and an additional 6.8 percent and 4.6 percent had some college training.[14]

A college degree was not required to study medicine. The majority of students, both North and South, who did not attend college, generally prepared for medical school with a college preparatory education provided by one of the many local seminaries, academies, grammar schools, or preparatory programs of English and classical studies offered by four-year colleges. Surgeon Albert Brown Robinson, 10th Massachusetts, for example, attended Monson Academy, Monson, Massachusetts, before graduating from the University of Buffalo School of Medicine in 1859. The Annual Catalogue of Monson Academy for 1854 describes the school's offerings, which were similar to other seminaries and academies at the time. The catalogue lists one hundred boarding students, both gentlemen and ladies, divided between an English Department and a Classical Department in which "studies pursued are those required for admission to college." Subjects taught included Latin, Greek, algebra, and chemistry with an annual tuition of about $21 plus board.[15]

Medical School Curriculum

Graduates of either academies or colleges were able to choose from more than one hundred medical colleges established before the Civil War. While a growing number of homeopathic, eclectic, and botanic schools offered alternative *materia medica* curricula in addition to standard surgery and anatomy, allopathic schools offered a standard set of orthodox courses. Many students from Northern states chose to attend schools within their region. New Englanders typically attended Harvard, Bowdoin, Castleton, and Berkshire Medical Colleges. New Yorkers attended University of Buffalo, Geneva, and Albany Medical Colleges, or New York University and Columbia in New York City. Philadelphia was the exception, attracting almost as many Southern students as those from Pennsylvania and other Northern states. Some medical schools in the South tried to attract students by making the case that a Southern school could better address the particular diseases of the local climate.

Regardless of geographic location, the format and curriculum of allopathic medical colleges in the United States remained largely unchanged throughout the first half of the nineteenth century. Except for minor variations in wording, the annual catalogues of medical schools published almost identical descriptions of course offerings and requirements for graduation: three years of study with a preceptor, two complete courses of lectures, clinical instruction, thesis, and examination. Students who could afford to study abroad in medical schools in Edinburgh, London, Berlin, and Paris often spent a year or more in Europe to supplement their American training. Some Union surgeons earned their medical degrees in Germany and Ireland before emigrating to America. Surgeon Frederick Wolf, 39th New York, graduated from the University of Prague after completing four years of medical study and served in the Austrian army for seven years before emigrating to the United States in 1859.[16]

Correspondence between Surgeon Caspar Coiner Henkel, 37th Virginia, and his friends and family provide personal insights into the life of a medical student at the University of Pennsylvania from 1854 to 1857. Henkel was born in New Market, Virginia, into a family of doctors; his father, Samuel G. Henkel, and uncle, Solon P. C. Henkel, both graduated from the University of Pennsylvania. Finishing his classical education at New Market Academy at nineteen, Caspar began his studies at the Medical School of the University of Pennsylvania in October 1854.

LECTURES

The University of Pennsylvania catalogue for the 1854–55 session outlines the usual course requirements common to other schools: Theory and Practice of Medicine; Anatomy; *Materia Medica* and Pharmacy; Chemistry; Surgery; Obstetrics and Diseases of Women and Children; and Institutes of Medicine. During his first year of lectures, Caspar wrote to Dr. Jacob Neff, another physician in New Market, about his studies:

> I have been tending lectures regularly this winter and a(m) very much pleased with the(m), but it (is) very hard work. I find all a student has to do here is to apply himself . . . to his work and he will be certain [*sic*] . . . he has every chance to improve himself. I have been tending Pa hospital & see there is a great deal of practical knowledge to be gained there from that source . . . I have been tending very closely to dissecting & find there is more to be learned . . . about anatomy that [than] from any others.[17]

The terms of instruction were relatively short in duration as critics pointed out, but they were intense by all accounts. The schedule of classes at Castleton Medical College, for example, included five lectures a day, six days a week for a fourteen-week term totaling 420 lectures. For each lecture, the student purchased a ticket that served as proof of attendance. Students used these tickets to document attendance when attending multiple schools, or to present as evidence of training even without receiving a final degree.[18]

Simon Baruch described the demanding schedule of his first year of medical studies at the Medical College of South Carolina in Charleston in 1860:

> All through the week the hectic routine repeated itself: up early to make a fire and study by candlelight before the boardinghouse breakfast; dash to the first lecture of the day; rush from one lecture room to another; jostle for the position on the stairway to the amphitheater;

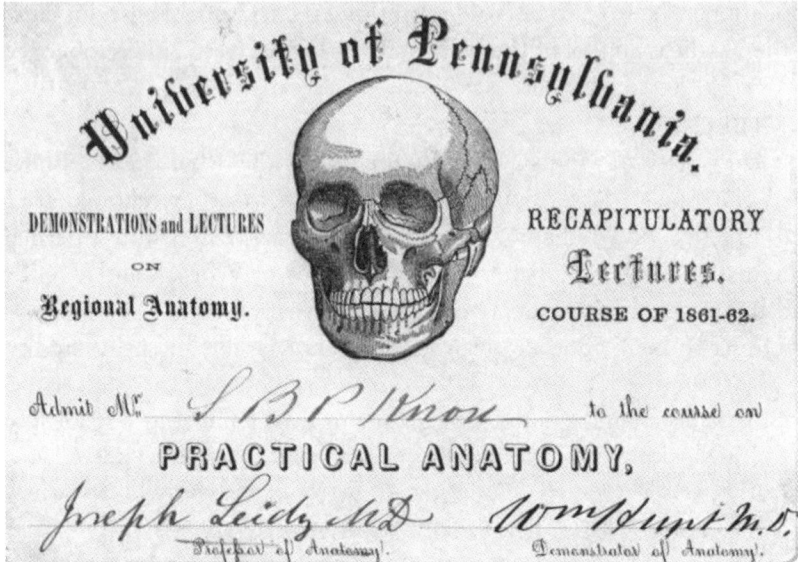

Practical Anatomy Lecture Ticket, University of Pennsylvania 1861-62, signed by Joseph Leidy, Professor of Anatomy. Assistant Surgeon Samuel B. P. Page Knox, 49th Pennsylvania, was mustered into service in January 1863, while attending his second course of lectures at the University of Pennsylvania. He graduated after the war in 1866. Courtesy of Douglas Arbittier, MD, MBA, www.medicalantiques.com

leap forward over the semicircles of seats to the front row, nearest the professor and his revolving table. After supper it was back to the college for dissection. Then long, solitary hours of study, broken only by the watchman's cry—"Past one o'clock and a starlight morning"—"past two o'clock, and a bright moonlight morning"—until it was time even for a student to go to bed.[19]

After completing his first term of courses, Caspar Henkel returned home to study for a year with his father and uncle who served as his preceptors. When he returned to attend lectures as a second-year student, he had more sophisticated opinions and mixed reviews of his professors.

I am very much pleased with lectures. Our lecturers are doing their best, as there is so much opposition in the schools. Dr Leidy, on anatomy, has improved very much in his lectures. Dr Smith is doing his best. He is making every effort to instil the principles of surgery to his class.[20]

I believe I told you in a former letter that I was taking Dr Smith's ticket on "minor surgery." I find it to be a good ticket. We have the opportunity of applying all manner of bandages and dressings to all parts of the body, all splints and the various apparatus used in fractures.[21]

It is not clear what Henkel meant by "opposition," but it may refer to the opposing theories and approaches to treatment that were points of contention among students and faculty of medical schools. Baruch learned from his lectures on theory and practice of medicine with professor Eli Geddings at the Medical College of South Carolina, that, "Whether discussing calomel or cold baths, bloodletting, or surgical procedures, Geddings always noted the current variety of opinion, thus giving his students an excellent picture of American medical thought and practice in 1860."[22] Trained in Europe, Geddings was one of a growing number of American physicians who were advocating for reforms and had adopted the 1835 conclusions of Pierre Louis of the Paris School that bloodletting was ineffective. Some physicians became so disillusioned with all forms of heroic medical treatments that their colleagues accused them of therapeutic nihilism. By the 1850s, when most of the Gettysburg surgeons were in medical school, many of the professors teaching them, like Geddings, had trained in Europe as well as the United States. It was observed that

this group of young fellows brought back from Paris, first, an appreciation of the value of method and accuracy in the study of the phenomena of disease, secondly, a profound, and at the time a much needed, distrust of drugs; and thirdly, a Gallic refinement and culture which stamped them, one and all, as unusual men.[23]

CLINICAL EXPERIENCE

With serious questions about the efficacy of traditional medical theories and increased emphasis on clinical observation, it is not surprising that Henkel and fellow medical students focused on instruction in practical anatomy, surgery demonstrations, and opportunities for dissection. At the beginning of his second year of medical school, Henkel wrote home to his father.

> I have been dissecting about two weeks. I have the head and neck, and have nearly finished it. I have learned more about the brain, from the demonstration Dr Hunt gave me on the brain of my subject; than I could have learnt in a weeks reading. I have also dissected the heart and lungs and think I have a very good knowledge of those parts. There has been a great demand for subjects so far.[24]

On November 19th, Henkel wrote again to his father.

> I finished dissecting my first subject last night. I had the head and neck. I also dissected a good portion of an arm for one of the class. Dr Hunt's lectures on "surgical anatomy" are very good. I have become very well acquainted with him. He always lets me know when he is going to make a demonstration of any part, so that I may be about. There is considerable scarcity of material in the dissecting rooms this winter. I do not think that I can get a subject, suitable for making a preparation, but I will make a strong effort to do so, I will learn all I can about making and injecting a subject.[25]

John Billings underscored the importance of dissection when he later recounted in 1894:

> I graduated in medicine in a two-years' course of five months' lectures each, the lectures being precisely the same for each year . . . In those two years I did not attend the systematic lectures very regularly. I found that by reading the text-books, I could get more in the same time and with very much less trouble. I practically lived in the dissecting-room and in the clinics, and the very first lecture I ever heard was a clinical lecture. The systematic teaching of those times I have had to unlearn for the most part. What has remained is what I got in the dissecting-room and in the clinics.[26]

The importance of the clinics is reflected in the annual announcements of medical schools advertising their advantages over other schools.

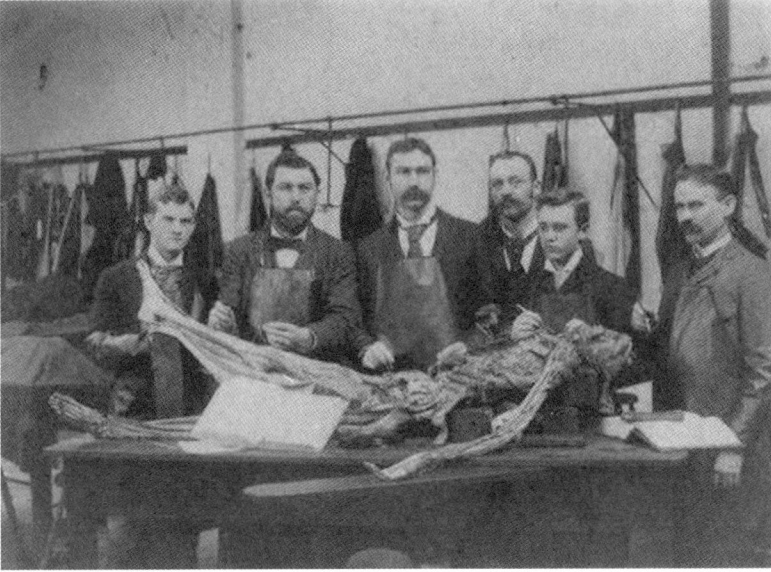

Dissection class, Jefferson Medical College, 1890s. Courtesy of Thomas Jefferson University

The Medical Department of the University of Louisiana took two pages to proudly describe the clinical instruction offered at the Charity Hospital. "There is no great City of the World which can boast of an institution where the Student visits every form of disease so unrestrictedly as in the Charity Hospital—where he can so familiarly look disease in the face." They compared this clinical approach to medical centers of Europe where "the student at a respectful distance, accompanying the Professor in his visits, listens to his speech, looks at the patients in bed, arranged in tableaus . . ." The number of cases reported during the previous year was impressive: 8,050 medical cases; 2,600 surgical cases; and 123 births. Louisiana's reputation for clinical experience at Charity Hospital seems amply justified with about 700 cases at a time in the wards of the hospital.[27] In comparison, Jefferson Medical College reported that, during the year ending March 1, 1855, 1,624 cases were treated and 260 operations performed in the presence of the class. Among them "were major operations as amputation of the thigh, leg, and arms, extirpation of the upper jaw, parotid gland, mamma &c, lithotomy and, lithotripsy."[28]

Caspar Henkel's letters describe his clinical experiences at the Pennsylvania Hospital:

> The clinics at the hospital have been very good so far. We get to see a great many cases of fractures and dislocations, just such practice as we have at home. Dr. Norris is the surgeon on duty now. He is an excellent surgeon and very much of a gentleman. He reminds me very much of Uncle Solon.[29]
>
> Our surgical clinics are excellent this winter, I saw Dr Smith remove a tonsil gland to-day he also operated on two cases of stricture of the lacrymal duct. There was no fistulous opening on the side of the nose. He made an opening into the lacrymal sac with a pointed bistary, just within the lower lid and then introduced a style. He failed to introduce the style into the second case, he will first dilate it with a very small catgut bougie. There are a large number of fractures at the hospital at this time. I see the most simple dressings are used.[30]

Dissection

The medical college announcements of the period were less forthcoming about the sensitive topic of dissection. A single line in the Louisiana Annual Announcement states that "Post Mortem examinations are also made in presence of the Class."[31] Jefferson Medical College announced that "On and after the 1st of October, the dissecting rooms will be open, under the direction of the Professor of Anatomy and the Demonstrator."[32] Hampden-Sydney College reported that "at Richmond, not only is the supply of subjects ample, but the temperature is such as to allow dissection to be continued without interruption from October until March."[33] The usual winter term of lectures coincided with the coldest months to facilitate dissections in an era before refrigeration or embalming and when alcohol was the only method available to preserve subjects.

Although physicians agreed that it was critical for students to dissect a human body before entering medical practice, cadavers remained difficult and often illegal to obtain throughout most of the nineteenth century. Archaeology projects on the campuses of the Medical College of Georgia at Augusta (1989) and the Medical College of Virginia in

Richmond (1994) revealed evidence of the dissecting rooms and the disposal of human remains at those medical colleges in the nineteenth century. Central to the story at Augusta was Grandison Harris, who was purchased in Charleston, South Carolina, by the faculty of the Georgia Medical College in 1852, and served as the porter, janitor, and teaching assistant, first as a slave and then as an employee until 1904. In addition to his other duties, one of his tasks was to obtain bodies for dissection as a so-called "resurrection man." It is well documented that he robbed graves or purchased bodies of poor and unclaimed dead—mostly from the Black community. In the archaeological investigation of the site more than 10,000 bones were collected and determined to be 77 percent male and mostly African-American.[34] College janitors, faculty, and students all participated in the constant search for cadavers, but there were also grave robbers who were willing to work with medical colleges to obtain bodies for a price. Southern schools had access to a greater number of bodies from the population of enslaved African Americans, as clearly evidenced by a Catalogue of the Medical College of Virginia for 1859: "from the peculiarity of our institutions, Materials for dissection can be obtained in abundance, and we believe are not surpassed if equaled by any city in our country."[35] Henkel's letters refer to the scarcity of subjects at the University of Pennsylvania in his second year. Northern schools had to engage in both legal and illegal methods of obtaining bodies for their dissecting rooms that included unclaimed bodies from the almshouses and prisons as well as grave robbing. While most of the illicit activities involving faculty and students went undetected or unreported, occasional run-ins with the law occurred. In November 1830, a grave that had been marked so that disturbance could be detected was found empty in the town of Hubbardton, Maine, 7 miles away from Castleton Medical College. Three hundred men of the town and the sheriff marched to Castleton and demanded the body. The decapitated body, hastily concealed beneath floorboards, was soon discovered, while a student left the building with a bundle under his overcoat and deposited the head in the haymow of a nearby barn. Eventually, the bundle and head were returned to the sheriff, but only after guarantees that there would be no arrests.[36]

Student Rowdyism

Accounts of grave-robbing among medical students did little to allay public fears or improve the reputation of medical students as being wild and dissipated. Caspar Henkel's letter to his father in February 1857 alludes to both student rowdyism and public concerns about medical school cadavers.

> There has not been any rowdyism shown by the students this session. The professors have been complimenting the present class very highly. The city authorities have been making considerable noise about the subjects from the alms-house being used for dissecting. I suppose that is the reason that subjects have been so scarce this winter.[37]

Student rowdyism was sometimes directed against professors as in the case of Dr. John Redman Coxe, professor of *Materia Medica* at the University of Pennsylvania, who was forced to resign.

> The medical school appears to be now in a state of perfect anarchy and confusion, students having taken the government into their own hands and compelled the distinguished professor of Materia Medica to discontinue his lectures . . . After hissing and hooting outside the room, finding that no noise which they could make without could not . . . stop the lecture . . . a band of about twenty rushed into the theater and with clubs and other instruments began to beat on the benches in such a manner as to compel the lecturer to be silent.[38]

A friend from New Market Academy, George R. Calvert, wrote to Caspar Henkel about his observations of dissipated behavior among medical students in Richmond, Virginia.

> There is—as you no doubt know—a Medical College in this city—I do not know its reputation or the qualifications of its professors, but I do know that a great number of the boys do not study. There are about 8 of them boarding at "Broad Street Hotel" about a mile from us. I went up to see one of them and thus became acquainted with the greater number of them. I received knowledge to this effect from one of them: "We

go to the theatre 5 nights out of the seven and on returning home sometimes play at cards until 2 or 3 o'clock in the morning—sometimes we go to a house of ill-fame—the home of the 'fille de joie,'—and we generally get to lectures about 9 o'clock."[39]

COST OF MEDICAL EDUCATION

A nineteenth-century medical education represented a considerable investment. Henkel's letters to and from his father discuss his need for funds.

> You will please send me some money as soon as convenient. My expenses have amounted to $300, since I left home, that is tickets, board, thesis & all, I shall spend as little money as possible. I can make out with the clothing I have till Spring.[40]

Henkel's father regularly sent him money through the mail, cutting $50 bills in half and sending them separately to prevent theft. Other families established accounts with business associates to provide funds for students who were away from home. A medical school education could cost between $750 and $1,000 depending on the school and the location. Country or rural schools like Castleton Medical College in Vermont, or Berkshire Medical College in Massachusetts, were able to offer lower fees for tuition and board. While the faculty of these schools might be comparable to those in larger cities, the rural schools lacked the clinical opportunities of urban hospitals. Many students divided their training among two or more schools to take advantage of lower fees, study with different professors, and obtain more clinical experience.

The cost of two terms at Castleton Medical College for 1847–1848 would have included:

- Fees for two terms of lectures   100
- Matriculation fees for 2 years   10
- Dissection   3
  (Cost of $15 for cadaver divided among 6 students)
- Graduation fee   16

- Room and Board for 32 weeks   64
- Text books   35
- 3 years for cost of Preceptor   300
- Bd and Rm with preceptor   248
- Total   776[41]

Costs at urban schools like the University of Pennsylvania and Jefferson Medical College were considerably higher.

- Fees for two terms of lectures   210
- Matriculation fee one year   5
- Hospital Fees   20
- Practical Anatomy   20
- Graduation fee   30
- Room and Board (32 weeks)   96
- Preceptor   300
- Bd and Room with preceptor   248
- Total   929[42]

For the most affluent students costs were not a major factor. Surgeon William Riddick Whitehead, 44th Virginia, left an account of his education that exemplifies the unlimited opportunities open to the sons of wealthy Southern planters and merchants who considered themselves not just Southern elites but members of a national and international aristocratic community.[43] Born in 1831, Whitehead attended boarding school in New Jersey, graduated from Virginia Military Institute, and studied medicine at the University of Virginia from 1851 to 1852. In the spring of 1853, he "graduated at the Medical Dept of the U of Pennsylvania, with a view to establish myself in that city for the practice of my profession, but decided otherwise and during the following summer sailed for France . . ."[44] During the winter of 1853–54, he attended the surgical wards of the Charity Hospital in Paris and studied operative surgery at the Ecole Pratique. In August he left Paris on a grand tour to Strasbourg, down the Danube to Linz, and admitted to visiting the hospitals in Vienna only occasionally. In December 1854, he offered his services to the Russian embassy in Vienna and enlisted as a surgeon in the Crimean War, studying under Nicolay Pirogoff, a famous Russian surgeon. Whitehead decided to return to Paris in 1855 and continue his studies:

> It began to dawn upon my intellect that, possibly, able surgeons are <u>always</u> students; really I wished to become a medical student again, and had an earnest desire to seek more knowledge of my profession by a renewed and diligent study of medicine . . . My eyes had been opened to the advantages of a more careful practical study of Anatomy and also of surgery . . .[45]

His vivid descriptions of the hospital wards, the examinations, and distinguished faculty at Paris provide a detailed picture of what study in Paris entailed. Student life for Whitehead was one of comfortable privilege. He lived in "an unfurnished apartment of three small rooms with a little kitchen. . . . furnished this apartment to my taste, took breakfast at my rooms, and dined at restaurants."[46] In August 1860, he received the degree of Doctor of Medicine from the Academy of Paris and left two weeks later to become instructor at New York Medical College as professor of clinical medicine.

Surgeon John Curtis Jones, 4th Texas, received his MD from Edinburgh University and studied with Joseph Lister, who authored a publication on germ theory and antisepsis in 1867 that would change medicine. Surgeon Nathan Hayward, 20th Massachusetts, graduated from Harvard in 1850 and planned to enter Harvard Medical School, but went instead to Germany where he studied at Berlin and Göttingen until the spring of 1854. He returned home to receive his MD from Harvard's Tremont Medical School in 1855. A talented sketch artist, his drawings of college life at Harvard, published in 1850, depict the pranks and hazing as well as more serious aspects of upper-class college life.

Not all students had equal access to the unlimited educational opportunities of the wealthy. Those of limited means made sacrifices to study medicine, often taking years to complete their studies, while working as teachers, druggists, clerks, and other occupations to support themselves and pay for their education. Simon Baruch emigrated to America from Germany in 1855 and worked for several years in the general store of the Baum family of Camden, South Carolina, before beginning his medical studies at the Medical College of South Carolina at Charleston. When the school closed in 1861 after the outbreak of war, he transferred to the Medical College of Virginia, graduating in 1862. John Billings, while living with his family in Indiana, convinced his father to help him through college despite their limited means. Billings graduated from Miami University in Oxford, Ohio, "living on bread, milk, potatoes, eggs, ham, etc. such things as I could cook myself." He then paid his own way through medical school by living at the hospital and taking care of the dissecting rooms. His friend S. Weir Mitchell remembered that "of these years of privation . . . he never recovered from the effect of one winter in which he lived on seventy-five cents a week."[47]

GRADUATION

Caspar Henkel was a serious student anxious to complete his degree and begin a career as a physician. He paid particular attention to the final requirement for the thesis and examination, choosing the topic of "Herneas."

> They require us to hand in the thesis by the first of February. I am going to hand it in tomorrow. Some of the boys are getting very uneasy about the examination. There is no use in getting into a figit yet. The examinations do not commence till the middle of March.[48]

On March 5, 1857, his father offered advice:

> As you are approaching the time of your examination, do not get into a pucker. Take things easy and leasurely, and when you call on the Professors for examination, recollect that they are only men, and do not feel backward in giving your views in every question propounded. Do not answer until you fairly understand the question . . . With the fund of information you have you need not be uneasy.[49]

March 23, Henkel reported to his father:

> I got through with my examinations last Saturday at 3 O'clock. The professors balloted to-day at 12 O'clock. I have just returned from the University with my notice to appear at the commencement to be held at the Musical Fund Hall next Saturday. I feel now as if I had a mountain off my shoulders—although in reality the work has just now commenced. I got through very well with all the professors. I did not miss any questions before four of the professors.[50]

Armed with an MD degree, new graduates had to make choices about how best to pursue a career in medicine. Caspar Henkel was anxious to begin practicing medicine with his father and uncle in New Market, Virginia, despite concerns that there were too many doctors and too few patients; "I have been theorizing long enough. I want to see how it will bear in practice. I think there is business enough for us all if we just hunt it up."[51] He remained in practice there until the Civil War. Some graduates returned home to practice with their preceptors; others moved west to new communities where they hoped there would be less competition and more opportunities. Billings and Whitehead both secured teaching positions in medical schools. With the outbreak of war in 1861, many recent graduates saw military service as a continuation of their medical training and an opportunity to acquire professional credentials in surgery. Simon Baruch was among those who took the examination for assistant surgeon immediately after graduating to join the Confederate medical corps. But whether they were recent graduates of a medical school or had been in private practice for several years, few newly recruited surgeons and assistant surgeons were prepared for the battlefield wounds, chronic diseases, and unsanitary conditions they would encounter in wartime medicine.

CHAPTER 2

Joining

ON APRIL 13, 1861, ONE DAY AFTER CONFEDERATE GUNS FIRED ON Fort Sumter, John Nicholas K. Monmonier wrote from his home in Baltimore, Maryland, to the Honorable Jefferson Davis:

> Dear Sir,
> Being Desirous of joining the Army of the Confederate States, I hereby offer you my services. My education was one in which Military Tactics formed an important part and I have always been anxious to lead a military life. At present Sir, I am a Second Lieutenant of one of the companies of the best drilled Infantry Corps (Independent Grays) and perhaps equal to any in the States. Within the past three years, sir, I graduated in medicine from our School the University of Md. Last though not least, I like many others in our good old state sympathize with you but are kept down by that Masterly Inactivity (policy) of our quasi Governor. I should also say, sir that I offer you my services as an assistant surgeon.
> Yours respectfully sir, Jno. N.K. Monmonier, MD
> 225 E Balt. Sy., Balt Md.[1]

Monmonier followed up with letters on June 3, to both Surgeon General Dr. DeLeon, and Secretary of War LeRoy Pope Walker, reiterating his desire to join the Confederate army: "Being forced from (Baltimore, Md.) my home by the oppression exercised there; viz, suppression of free speech, I am determined to serve the Confederate States in some manner."[2] If unable to secure a commission as assistant surgeon, he was willing to serve in any capacity. Twenty-six years old and single, he was appointed assistant surgeon November 6, 1861, and assigned to duty as Assistant Surgeon, 8th Louisiana Infantry.

In New York State, William W. Potter of Cowlesville, New York, also responded to the outbreak of war.

> On the 15th day of April 1861, three days after the fall of Fort Sumter, the President called for 75,000 men and, in apportioning the number for each state, New York's quota under this call and a subsequent one made May 3rd, was fixed at 38 regiments of infantry. To raise, arm and equip, officer, and get this force ready for the field became the duty of the Governor [Edwin D. Morgan] and his military staff. His surgeon-general, Dr. S. Oakley Vanderpoel, at once issued a notice to medical men throughout the state who might desire to serve as sur-geons and assistant-surgeons, to assemble in Albany on the 25th and 26th days of April 1861, for examination as to their fitness for these positions in the volunteer forces then raising.[3]

Potter went on to explain that at first he despaired of obtaining an appointment, despite a successful examination, because at the beginning of the war regimental colonels followed a longstanding practice of nominating their own medical staff: "Most of these early appointments were obtained by men of influence with the several colonels, men much older and more experienced in affairs than I."[4] Dr. Potter was eventually commissioned Assistant Surgeon, 49th New York, on September 16, 1861 at the insistence of the local Union Defense Committee.[5] He was twenty-three years old, recently married, and had graduated from the University of Buffalo Medical Department two years earlier.

The first call for enlistments in the spring of 1861 assumed that the war would be of short duration. As the three-month Union regiments mustered out, new calls came for additional Federal troops. In July 1861, Surgeon J. Franklin Dyer, 15th Massachusetts, began his Civil War journal:

> The three months' regiments had been sent forward, but it was soon discovered that they were insufficient, and a call was made for three

years' troops. One or more regiments were to be raised in Essex County. I considered this a just and righteous war on our part, and I should not be doing my duty if I did not take part in it.[6]

Assistant Surgeon John Tullar Brown, 94th New York, continued to practice medicine in Fairport, near Rochester, New York, "until the month of August 1862 when he could no longer stay at home with the call of 600,000 more . . . was examined before the State Board of Military Surgeons and commissioned on the 17th of Sept. as Assistant Surgeon to the 105th NYSV."[7]

A Sense of Duty

The majority of surgeons—both Union and Confederate—volunteered out of a sense of duty. No one states that more clearly than Theodore Dimon of Auburn, New York. In his diary for April 16, 1861, he references the president's initial call for 30,000 militia from New York State, "Taking a strong interest in these movements, after several conversations with our leading physicians here as to the Surgency of this regiment, and finding none of them disposed to take that position, I concluded it to be my duty to offer myself for it."[8] In his unpublished account he later made clear his political position on the war.

> It became then with me not only a peculiar Republican incentive to sustain the right and propriety of my vote, but a clear duty as an ordinary citizen to maintain the government and laws of the country, to be ready to do anything I could in its support. Consequently, I offered to be Surgeon, as I was professionally fit for that Service, of a Regiment raised in Cayuga County New York, to enter the U.S. service in maintenance of the Government against this rebellion, which had become so formidable as to require the service of all loyal citizens to put it down. Accordingly, I was mustered as surgeon of the 19th N.Y. . . . for 3 months on the 22nd of May 1861.[9]

With battle lines drawn, military surgeons throughout the country had to make decisions about which side they would support. As an assistant surgeon in the U.S. Army, Lafayette Guild was directing the federal military hospital at the Presidio of San Francisco in April 1861 when the war began. A March 13th letter written on his behalf to Confederate secretary of war L. P. Walker states that Guild had already "signified his intention to his family to resign his present position so soon as he would learn that Alabama had seceded. I therefore [hope] that in making your appointments you will reserve a position for him as he will doubtless [come] home soon."[10] Guild resigned from Federal service, returned home to Tuscaloosa, Alabama, and accepted a Confederate surgeon's commission in July 1861, eventually becoming medical director of the Army of Northern Virginia. Edwin F. DeGraffenried, serving at U.S. Forts Leavenworth and Garland, and David C. Jones, serving on the Texas frontier, also resigned their commissions to serve in the Confederate army as assistant surgeons in the 4th Alabama and 5th Texas. They were among the twenty-four surgeons who resigned from Federal service to join the Confederacy. John Meck Cuyler, born in Savannah in 1810 and an 1829 graduate of the Medical College of Georgia, made a different decision. He had spent his entire career in the U.S. Army since 1834. When the war came, he chose to remain and served as medical inspector with the Army of the Potomac.

The "duty" that motivated surgeons to join the war effort and volunteer their services took various forms. Some clearly held strong convictions about their respective causes. Charles S. Bigelow was born and grew up in Virginia, but, when war came in 1861, he was so eager to eradicate any connection to his Northern family that he legally changed his name from Bigelow, his father's Vermont family name, and took his mother's Virginia family name of Morton. As Charles S. Morton he served as Surgeon, 57th North Carolina.[11] Assistant Surgeon Abner Embry McGarity, 21st Georgia, wrote to his wife in April 1863 that "Nothing but the defence of the rights of my country and its people could induce me to stay from you. But I am perfectly willing to endure present privation for the procurement of future liberty and independence."[12] A number of Union surgeons had strong abolition ties. Zabdiel Boylston Adams Jr. was an ardent abolitionist for whom the war to end slavery was a "high and worthy and holy" goal. The same day Bostonians learned of the Southern attack on Fort Sumter, Adams left his medical practice to volunteer, serving as Surgeon, 32nd Massachusetts.[13] Assistant Surgeon Francis Julian LeMoyne, 9th Pennsylvania, was the son of noted abolitionist, Dr. F. Julius LeMoyne, who served as president of the Washington (Pennsylvania) Anti-Slavery Society and was a regional agent for the American Anti-Slavery Society.[14]

Even those with more moderate views had to make decisions about how to fulfill their duty to country. After graduating from Cleveland Medical College in 1855, Smith Buttermore of Connellsville, Pennsylvania, practiced medicine for five years in California before returning east and settling in Harrison County, Virginia. "When the war broke out, all business on the border especially was thrown into confusion and he being unable therefore to prosecute his profession in the old way accepted a commission in the Confederate Army . . ."[15] Buttermore served as Assistant Surgeon, 31st Virginia. Sylvester Farmer shared the anti-secession sentiments of his neighbor and friend, Alexander H. Stephens, who nonetheless served as vice president of the Confederacy. Likewise, "when it became evident that fighting had to be done, and troops were called for to do it, Dr. Farmer offered himself to the Confederate cause" and served as Surgeon, 16th Georgia.[16] Thomas Sim of Frederick, Maryland, was a slaveholder, but volunteered to serve in the Union army and became medical director of the U.S. Third Corps.

While many who committed to the Confederate cause belonged to long established planter families or mercantile families whose wealth depended on maintaining the slave economy, others were more recent arrivals to the South. Daniel Parker, Assistant Surgeon, 8th Alabama Infantry, was born in Northfield, Vermont, in 1835, but left in 1856 to teach school in Marion, Alabama, earning enough money to graduate from the University of Louisiana medical school in 1860. Parker remained in Alabama, practicing medicine in Marion in 1861, until he enlisted as a corporal and then was appointed Assistant Surgeon, 8th Alabama, July 3, 1861.[17] Solomon Secord, a physician from Kincardine, Ontario, was living in Georgia, possibly for health reasons, when the war began. Although he was reported to have abolitionist sentiments, he remained in Georgia and served as Surgeon, 20th Georgia, from 1862 until he resigned in 1864 and returned to Ontario.

Duty to home and family sometimes conflicted with duty to country. Assistant Surgeon William Child, 5th New Hampshire, reveals multiple reasons for enlisting in his letters home to his wife. He wrote frequently about family finances, worries he will not receive a bounty of $200 for enlisting, but admits he is caught up in the excitement of war and army life. "My duty is perfectly plain to me—and at this time every man has a responsibility—has a duty which he can not avoid if he would"; he also questioned, "am I doing right to leave my family alone?"[18] Assistant Surgeon John S. Richards, 34th North Carolina, resigned in November 1863, to return home to Albemarle and Green Counties. A letter to Secretary of War Seddon complained that several thousand inhabitants of Albemarle and Greene Counties had been left without a physician and enclosed a petition from residents asking for approval of Dr. Richards's resignation.[19] Assistant Surgeon George T. Dougherty, 59th New York, enlisted May 23, 1863, but had difficulty in collecting his pay because his predecessor was still officially in the position. Dougherty resigned August 5, 1863, because "My family is depending upon me for support, and if there is no possibility of receiving compensation for my services, and my expenses and outfit &c. I shall be compelled for the sake of my family, if for no other reason, to return to Brooklyn and resume my practice."[20]

Financial Gain

The U.S. Army pay of $165 a month for a surgeon or $110 a month for an assistant surgeon was an incentive for some physicians to seek commissions. Confederate pay for surgeons similarly ranged from $165 to $200, and $110 to $150 for assistant surgeons.[21] The earnings of a mid-nineteenth-century physician could vary considerably. Those from upper class families often had independent wealth apart from their medical practice; doctors in larger cities with teaching and hospital opportunities could attract enough students and wealthy patients to make a comfortable living. On the other hand, recent graduates practicing in small towns and rural communities often struggled to make a living, supplementing limited medical income with farming or an appointment as local postmaster. Assistant Surgeon James D. Benton, 111th New York, wrote home to his father on October 4, 1862, that "It is not patriotism that has made me take this course but I wanted to make money for my family. If it had been patriotism I should have been sick of it long since but as it is not my plunk [pluck] is good."[22] William Child wrote to his wife in 1863 wondering if he should stay in the army or resign: "What had I best do? I am earning as much or more than I could at home. I like the business much, only that it takes one away from home."[23] Assistant Surgeon Benjamin Barr, 10th Pennsylvania, sought a higher paid commission as surgeon of colored troops. "I am a married man with a wife and four children; have had ten years practice, the last three in the army; am 35 years of age—can I have a position in the colored troops in my Regiment going out of service . . . the pay of Asst. Surgeon is hardly sufficient to maintain my family. I am a poor man & have labored hard to obtain what I have & certainly think I deserve as much again."[24]

EDUCATION

Medical students, recent graduates, and young doctors found many opportunities to further their medical education by serving in the Union and Confederate armies. Assistant Surgeon Charles Richards, 28th Virginia, had completed one year of medical classes at the University of Virginia when he enlisted in May 1861 as a private. Writing to the medical director in Manassas, he turned down an offer to be detailed as a hospital nurse and reiterated his desire to procure a situation in a hospital, "in order that I might gain a more perfect knowledge of the Practical part of medicine to the study of which I have devoted the last two years."[25] After being hospitalized in Richmond, Virginia, with intermittent fever he was detailed as hospital steward. From October 1862 to March 1863, he was able to complete a second course of lectures at the Medical College of Virginia, receive an MD degree, and pass the examination to be commissioned assistant surgeon.[26] Assistant Surgeon Charles Fanning Wood, 3rd North Carolina, was unable to afford medical school before the war due to reversals in his family's financial position, but his interest in pursuing medicine continued. At 18 he earned $100 teaching in a country school for three months, using part of his salary to purchase medical books. He next worked in Wilmington, North Carolina, as a clerk in a lawyer's office for $25 a month and spent his free time in the office of

Dr. James F. McRee, who served as his preceptor and provided access to his extensive medical library. In 1860, Dr. McRee helped Wood secure a position in the drug store of Louis B. Erambert, a staunch secessionist. In September 1861 Wood joined the Wilmington Rifle Guards but became ill after the Seven Days Battles and was sent to recover at Moore Hospital in Richmond. The surgeon in charge, Dr. Manson, arranged for Wood to be detailed for duty at the hospital with the privilege of attending classes at the Medical College of Virginia.

> I was given night charge of the ward only, and sleeping in the Dispensary with its partition reaching not half to the wall, I could hear the slightest sound and so kept the nurses at their duty. I matriculated at the College in October, took out my tickets with $115 sent from home by my father. I had been a medical student since 1856, but this was my first opportunity to attend lectures.[27]

Wood passed the examination for assistant surgeon in February 1863, even before the courses ended, and was assigned Assistant Surgeon of the 3rd North Carolina.

Even those who had completed medical training looked for opportunities to enhance their training, Surgeon James Langstaff Dunn, 109th Pennsylvania, was a graduate of the Western Reserve Medical College in 1850, but while his regiment was stationed in Philadelphia in the winter of 1861–62, he attended medical classes in addition to his assigned duties examining recruits. He was able to attend lectures free of charge, and he paid $10 for a "subject" and $15 to Dr. Agnew of Blakely Hospital for private instructions.

> We go through all the different surgical operations on the "subject," such as ligating arteries, dressing wounds, applying bandages, and in fact everything an Army Surgeon would be likely to be in need to know . . . I have learned more since I came here than I did in two winters in Cleveland . . .[28]

Dunn particularly appreciated the opportunity to interact with medical colleagues.

I am thrown into the society of six or eight surgeons of the different Reg'nts who are from all parts of the state. I find them first rate fellows. We meet every night in the college and guide each other on the different operations in surgery. Some of the professors meet with us. I stand all right here among the Jeffersons in the College. I have joined the acquaintance of some of the first medical men of America and have their esteem and friendship. This must be advantage to me in my future career as a surgeon or medical man.[29]

Surgeons in the field often continued this kind of study group, meeting in the evenings to read and discuss medical texts. Older or more experienced surgeons acted as preceptors for the younger recent graduates.

For some, hospital experience seemed to offer broader educational opportunities than service in the field. Surgeon John Wilson, 11th North Carolina, an 1850 graduate of Jefferson Medical College, wrote to Medical Director William A. Carrington in Richmond on May 15, 1863, requesting transfer to a hospital position to gain more medical experience than possible in the field:

> If it is not incompatible with the public interest, I respectfully ask for a transfer from field to hospital services. It has been now thirteen years since I commenced the practice of medicine and my present expectation is to make it my business for life. Under these circumstances I desire to avail myself of the best opportunities that public service can offer of studying diseases and of comparing the results of private with those of hospital practice. An experience in the field of rather more than a year enables me to see that no great deal is to be gained in that quarter. In so far as the change would bring increased pay it would be highly acceptable as my present salary has proved utterly insufficient for myself and family.[30]

More than a dozen Canadians served as medical staff in the Union army at Gettysburg. Assistant Surgeon Francis Moses Wafer, 108th New York, was born in Canada and studied at the Medical School of Queens College, Kingston, Canada West. In March 1863, following the close of the winter session, Wafer was recruited to serve in the Union army as an assistant surgeon, intending to serve for six months between medical school sessions. He reported, "Many students of Canadian schools availed themselves of this privilege, in order to profit by the new & extensive field thrown open for the study of *Practical Surgery*."[31] He returned home in July 1865, having paid the high price of impaired health in exchange for his medical experience during the war.

FOREIGN-BORN

Canada was not the only country that supplied surgeons. The large number of German and Irish immigrants in the 1840s and 1850s were represented among the surgeons. Confederate assistant surgeons Simon Baruch, 3rd South Carolina Battalion, and Carl H. A. Kleinschmidt, 3rd Arkansas, both came to the United States in their teens and subsequently completed their medical education. Kleinschmidt studied medicine at Georgetown University Medical School, declined a commission in the U.S. Army, and chose Confederate service because his sympathies were with the South.[32] Union surgeons at Gettysburg included at least twenty-four German-born and twenty Irish-born doctors in addition to other nationalities. Some came as children with emigrating families; others came as adults, escaping the political upheavals and uprisings that occurred throughout Europe in support of democracy. Political activists who emigrated remained committed to the cause of freedom and many saw the American Civil War as a continuation of the political struggles in their homelands. Surgeon Lawrence Reynolds, 63rd New York, for example, was born in Ireland in 1803 and described as

> a native of Waterford, a highly educated and refined gentleman, and very experienced surgeon, a true Irish gentleman and patriot, served with honor as surgeon of the regiment from its first organization; although advanced in years is still young in vigor. . . . He was a distinguished Chartist in England and was also amongst those of his countrymen who had to fly from Ireland in '48, his only crime being that he loved his country dearly.[33]

Surgeon Francis Huebschmann, 26th Wisconsin, was born in Weimar, Germany, and graduated from the University of Jena in 1841 before emigrating and settling in Milwaukee, Wisconsin. He remained active throughout his life in politics as a school commissioner and an advocate for suffrage and equal rights for the foreign born. Immigrants from Europe came from diverse backgrounds, sometimes representing competing sides of conflicts in their home countries. Two Union surgeons, Samuel Brilliantowski and Frederick Wolf, emigrated from the Austrian empire under different circumstances. Brilliantowski, 41st New York, emigrated with his family at the age of ten, one of several hundred Polish exiles deported from Austria for their role in the uprisings against Austrian rule in 1831. He arrived in New York City in 1834, studied medicine, and was active as a member of the educated Polish community in New York that continued to advocate for Polish freedom.[34] Wolf, 39th New York, grew up in a wealthy family in Prague but interrupted his academic studies in natural history after his father's failed business left the family without adequate resources. To better support himself, he decided to study medicine at the University of Prague, served as an assistant surgeon in the Austrian army during the 1848 insurrections in Lombardy, and then served for another four years in Slovenia and Poland. Rather than reenlist, he decided to emigrate to America in 1859, only to be caught up again, "with his avocation as a field surgeon, entering the US A[rmy]. in September 1861 as Medical Volunteer Officer in the so-called German division of the Union his commission as a surgeon of the 39th Regt. NY Volunteers 21st Dec. 1861."[35]

A few German physicians came to the United States specifically to volunteer for the Union cause. Two young doctors aged twenty-eight and twenty-nine, Assistant Surgeon Gustav Jacobi, 52nd New York, and Assistant Surgeon George Rebay, 45th New York, departed from Hamburg, Germany, on September 6, 1862, on the *Borussia*, arrived in New York on September 24, and promptly enlisted October 10th in Albany, New York. Assistant Surgeon Carl Uterhart, 119th New York, also came to fight in the Civil War. Born in 1835, he studied medicine at the University of Jena and Friedrich Wilhelm University in Berlin. In 1862 he left his medical practice and sailed to America to join the Union army at Stafford Court House, Virginia, on March 4, 1863. On November 3, 1864, he was promoted to surgeon of the 9th U.S. Colored Troops Heavy Artillery Regiment and served until May 1865.

ADVENTURERS

For some, the Civil War offered adventure. Uterhart was among the surgeons who clearly relished travel and had a taste for adventure both before and after their Civil War experiences. After returning to Germany, Uterhart served as medical officer of the 1st Grand Ducal Mecklenburg Dragoon Regiment No. 17. He then may have moved to South America before going to Australia on an emigrant ship and served as surgeon superintendent of Queensland. In 1878 he returned to Germany and practiced medicine until his death in 1895 at the age of sixty.[36] Surgeon Andrew Jackson Ward, 2nd Wisconsin, enlisted August 5, 1861, in Madison, Wisconsin, at thirty-seven years of age. He had already left his home in Milford, Pennsylvania, to serve in the Mexican War and the gold fields of California. According to his own account in a biographic sketch in his government file,

> When twenty two graduated at the Pennsylvania University—the same year joined Stevenson's Regt. of vols & went to California. Acting first as Hospt. Steward & subsequently as assist. Surgeon during the war with Mexico. I remained one year after the regiment was disbanded, practicing medicine at Sutters Fort where I had before been stationed. On my return to the States in 1850, sought a new home in Madison Wisconsin . . .[37]

Surgeon Thaddeus Hildreth, 3rd Maine, interrupted his medical studies at Bowdoin College to go to the gold fields with family and friends, arriving in California on November 27, 1849, aboard the steamship *Oregon*. The following March, Thaddeus and his brother George were among the first miners to claim a rich strike called Hildreth Diggins, which grew into a town of 6,000 miners that they named Columbia. While his brother remained in California, eventually owning a saloon and serving as city marshal, Thaddeus returned home to Gardner, Maine, and graduated with a medical degree from Dartmouth College.[38] Surgeon James William Claiborne, 12th Virginia, after receiving his medical degree in 1848 from the University of Pennsylvania, went to California with his brother Gilbert in 1849, sailing by way of Cape Horn. He practiced medicine at Jamestown, California, for nine years and served as a justice of the peace before he returned to Petersburg, Virginia, in 1858. The hardships of isolated and overcrowded mining communities in California provided a training ground for their Civil War experiences. Theodore Dimon recognized that his regiment was suffering from scurvy dysentery caused by lack of fresh vegetables based on his earlier experiences in California.[39]

Some Civil War surgeons already had firsthand battle experience from their participation in the Crimean War. While Americans officially remained neutral in the war between Russia and Turkey, aided by its allies, France and Britain, American public opinion leaned in favor of Russia. Anti-British sentiment, particularly in the South, reflected British antislavery policies and opposition to American expansion in Central and South America. Russian agents in Paris successfully persuaded a number of young American surgeons studying abroad to join the Russian army, hoping their participation would strengthen pro-Russia feelings in the United States. The American students were offered high pay and speedy promotions, in addition to the opportunity to practice surgery.[40] Surgeon William Reddick Whitehead, 44th Virginia, an 1853 graduate of the University of Pennsylvania, was pursuing advanced medical studies in Paris and Vienna. On December 18, 1854, he went to the Russian Embassy in Vienna and offered the "services of an American Physician." In his unpublished memoir he recounts serving with Pirogoff, a great Russian surgeon, and treating patients with Asiatic cholera until December 1855, when he received orders releasing him from service and he returned to Paris to complete his studies. In his account, he mentions his "friend Dr. Reid of Norristown PA."[41] After graduating from the University of Pennsylvania in 1849, Division Surgeon Louis Wernwag Read, U.S. 3rd Division, Fifth Corps, was also studying in Europe when he entered the Russian service in 1855, participating as a surgeon in the siege of Sebastopol. At the conclusion of the conflict Read spent six months in the hospitals of Paris before he returned to Norristown to begin his practice in 1857.[42] Surgeon Erwin James Eldridge, Cobb's Georgia Legion, was another medical student studying in Vienna after he graduated from Jefferson Medical College in 1854. He volunteered to serve as a surgeon for Russia in the Crimean War and was decorated for his service.[43] On the British side, Surgeon Francis Reynolds, 88th New York, a native of County Kilkenny, Ireland, and a Fellow in the Royal College of Surgeons, Ireland, served on the British medical staff during the Crimean War before emigrating to the United States.[44]

THE EXAMINATION

For those who decided to serve, the path from civilian physician to military surgeon could be a daunting and confusing process. For most, the first step was the dreaded examination. Although early assignments were often local or state appointments, both armies soon adopted consistent examinations, written and oral, administered by examining boards. Surgeon James Langstaff Dunn, 109th Pennsylvania, visited Harrisburg in June 1861, to meet with Governor Curtin and wrote home that he "saw the exams for Surgeons; some of them will hardly pass as the examinations are very strict and severe. Only such men as are good surgeons will pass muster. How important it is that these men should understand their business, for when sick we look to them for help, and when wounded we need the skillful and steady hand."[45] Francis Wafer provided a detailed description of his military entrance examination. As a Canadian student, he was still required to hold a diploma from an American school of medicine or medical society. He was directed to the New York Medical Society in Albany, and after examination by several "Censors" in a range of medical subjects, he received certificates of proficiency, which he submitted in exchange for a parchment diploma written in classical Latin after payment of a graduation fee of $16. The same day, he went to the Surgeon General's Office to take the examination and "was presented with writing materials, a sufficiency of foolscap & sixteen printed questions, including all the principal branches of Medicine . . . after writing seven hours, answering some fully and attempting them all, I handed in my paper."[46] Thomas Fanning Wood had not yet completed his first session of medical lectures at the Virginia Medical College in Richmond in 1863 when,

> The great day in February came and I was to appear before the Board. It was very cold— . . . We had not long been seated in the cold room— no fire at all—before a boy brought in a blank sheet of fools-cap with the name of the subject written on the first line . . . my subject was "Typhoid Fever". . . . I was fortunate because I had charge of fever cases for months and had kept records of my cases. In addition I was saturated with the writings of Louis and Huss. The French school being in great favor I made use of all the quotations I could from the great masters, and I thought I did very well.[47]

He was next called to appear before a board of three physicians for oral examination on diseases of the chest, physical and general anatomy of the arteries, and surgery for fractures. "I left the room with a feeling that I had succeeded, although there was no intimation of it from any members of the Board."[48] Wood was ordered to report immediately to the surgeon general for assignment, but others had to wait weeks and months for commissions and orders.

In July 1861, J. Franklin Dyer was appointed acting surgeon of the 19th Massachusetts after passing his examination. "A few days after . . . I commenced examination of the men in camp, rejecting such as were found unfit . . . my home was thenceforth 'in the field.'"[49] John H. Brinton of Philadelphia decided to take the Federal examination for "brigade surgeon," in the regular army, later known as "surgeon of volunteers," rather than join a Pennsylvania regiment. On July 3, 1861, he traveled to Washington to take the examination, "chiefly a written one was not very rigid, and at its conclusion I was informed that the result was satisfactory, and that I might return home and await my commission."[50]

Getting Outfitted

Brinton had to wait until September 4, 1861, before he received orders assigning him to duty in the Department of the West. During July and August, he purchased supplies to outfit himself for military service. "My uniform I purchased at Hughes and Muller, tailors in Chestnut Street.

A

SURGERY.

1.—What are the symptoms of a wound of the Lung—and how would you check Pulmonary Hemorrhage?

2.—How would you Trephine the Skull—and what fills up the opening made by the Trephine?

3.—What is a Hydrocele—what an Hæmatocele, and what is Varicocele?

4.—Describe the circular operation for Amputation of the Thigh.

5.—Describe the dressing usually applied to a Fracture of the Femur.

6.—Describe the method of reducing a Luxation of the Head of the Femur on the Dorsum Ilii.

7.—In how many ways may Hemorrhage be arrested?

8.—Name the best styptics for the arrest of Venous Oozing.

9.—Why are Gunshot Wounds tedious in healing, and what are their chief dangers?

10.—How would you treat a Gunshot Fracture of the Humerus?

Surgery Questions for Pennsylvania Surgeons Examination. Courtesy of Pennsylvania State Archives, RG 19

. . . My saddle and horse equipments, I bought of Lacey & Phillips, the leading harness makers of the city."[51] William Child wrote home that "I have one suit of military clothes consisting of a blue flannel blouse with bright brass buttons—vest same and pants. I have shoulder straps with a bar in each end—the mark of First Lieut. I wear a black hat with the letters MS of silver within a gold wreath. This signifies medical staff. I have purchased a complete suit of India Rubber. Have bought also a pocket ink stand and pocket pen holder."[52] Most newly commissioned surgeons did not have the opportunity or resources to shop in the best stores. A new uniform purchased in Philadelphia cost James Langston Dunn about $50, including overcoat.[53] James Benton wrote home to his father on August 14, 1862, from Auburn, New York, where his regiment was waiting to be mustered into service.

> The officers and staff and the medical staff met last night and ordered their accoutrements from New York. The medical officers all send for the same articles . . .
> Sword 12.00
> Sash 7.00
> Sword Knot 1.50
> Belt 2.75
> Shoulder Straps 6.50 and 2.50
> Spurs 1.50
> Saddle & Trappings 35.00
> The Colonel has taken great pains to get these articles as cheap as they can be purchased, They cost about 33 1/3 percent less than the 75th Regiment had to pay.[54]

The total amounted to nearly $70 and even with the discount Benton had to ask his family to lend him money to cover these expenses, Surgeon William W. Potter, 57th New York, was able to pay off about $130 in expenses and articles needed by an officer from his first pay of $196.24 in November 1861.[55] On September 12, 1862, William Watson of Bedford, Pennsylvania, recently assigned as surgeon to the 105th Pennsylvania, wrote home, on his way from Harrisburg to Washington, that he has not had a photograph taken to send home because he had not succeeded in getting a uniform. "You have no idea of the exorbitant prices that are charged for everything pertaining to Military. I will not have sufficient money so I intend asking Gideon to lend me fifty dollars . . . It will be impossible for me to do without a horse."[56] As officers, surgeons and assistant surgeons were required to purchase their own horses and received an allowance for forage. Horses were particularly important to surgeons who had to carry not only their own personal possessions but were also responsible for medicines and surgical kits. After many pleas to his family to help him find a horse, Watson eventually acquired a captured Confederate horse for $35 that he described as thin and run down but "gets over ground pretty well."

JOINING THE REGIMENT

Surgeon George Stevens, 77th New York, left Saratoga Springs with the Bemis Heights Battalion on Thanksgiving Day, November 21, 1861. "As the long train of cars bore us from the station at Saratoga Springs, the thousands who had gathered to witness our departure united in cheer after cheer until all the groves and vales of that charming resort rang with the echoes of the tumultuous shouting."[57] Ten days after leaving

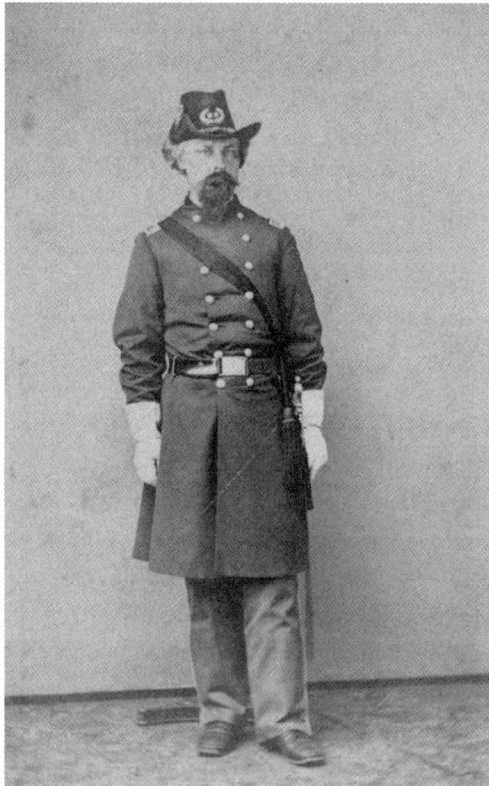

Union surgeon Charles J. Nordquist, 83rd New York, Hallett & Brother, New York.
Courtesy of Library of Congress Prints and Photographs Division

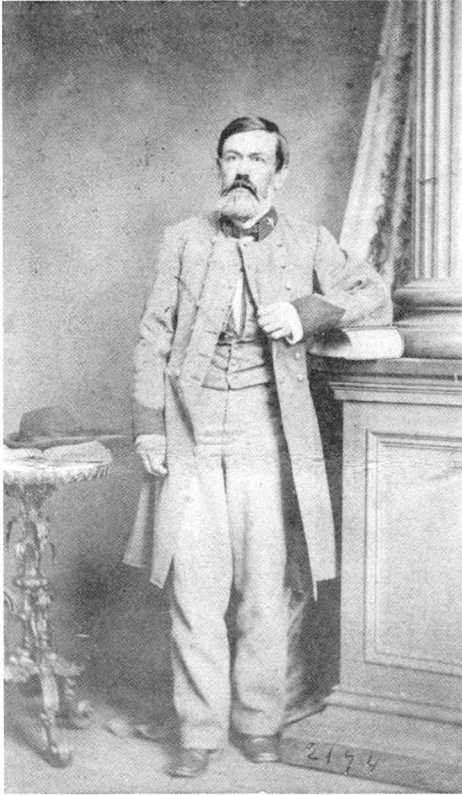

Confederate assistant surgeon Robert H. Worthington, 7th Virginia, Charles Rees, Richmond, Virginia. Courtesy of Peck Medical Antiquities

Concord, New Hampshire, to join his regiment William Child wrote to his wife from Newport News, Virginia.

> You can not imagine what a change from quiet, sleepy dull Bath the exciting scenes here in Virginia. It is now 9 o'clock P.M. imagine to yourself a level field perhaps fifty acres. On one side a forest of oak and pine—on the other the James River. On this field are encamped perhaps twenty thousand men. Our Reg. is on the North side of the encampment—and our hospital tent is the outside tent of all. I am now writing and shall sleep in a good covered hospital wagon. To the South of me as far as I can see right and left are the camp fires. Away off to

the East is the Brigade Band discoursing music—and all over the field are sounding the Regimental trumpets and drums. In the intervals of music and trumpet blasts may be heard the braying of mules and neighing of horses. Oh, I wish you were here this moment. I could go into battle I know.[58]

After the pomp and circumstance of parades, martial bands, and cheering crowds, surgeons in their newly purchased uniforms and equipment were about to face the hardships of army life and the realities of war.

CHAPTER 3

In the Field

ASSISTANT SURGEON ABNER EMBRY McGARITY, 21ST GEORGIA, echoed the experience of many Civil War surgeons when he wrote home on March 14, 1863, "If I had known, before I left home, what I now know, I should have brought fewer fine shirts and more syrup and honey and blankets."[1] Regimental surgeons sent into the field had to adapt quickly to the realities and rigors of camp life. Assistant Surgeon Thomas Fanning Wood, 3rd North Carolina, later wrote that "The difference between a home—a fixed abiding place in a hospital, a comfortable bed, good fare, congenial companions about me, and the hardships of the battle field were very great."[2] Assistant Surgeon Cyrus Bacon, 2nd U.S., joined the Army of the Potomac in November 1862 after several months of hospital duty in Frederick, Maryland. "My first nights I took cold easily . . ." he wrote in January 1863, "But now I am quite a soldier. do not take cold so easily, and dwell in comfort. I think, could I but have books, I would like this camp as well as a Post."[3] Surgeon William Watson, 105th Pennsylvania, wrote home to his father on September 20, 1862:

> This is my second night in camp. Last night I slept upon the ground in a tent without sides. Had as comfortable a night's rest as if I had been in my own bed at Home. Think I will like Camp life well—although it is a very hard life . . . I will send my trunk home by Express as no officer is permitted to carry more than a Carpet sack.[4]

Camp

Surgeons accompanied their regiments in hastily assembled camps for short stays, and more comfortably fitted quarters for longer periods between marches and battles. They shared the hardships of long marches without tents and with only the personal and medical supplies that they could carry on a pack horse. A typical camp consisted of a parade ground where the regiment drilled, surrounded by guard tents at the front and a color line delineating the beginning of the encampment. Behind the color line were rows of tents for enlisted men organized by company; then the kitchens, noncommissioned staff, sutler, and police guard; and a row of company officers. Tents for the Field and Staff officers at the rear of the camp included quarters for the surgeon, assistant surgeons, and a hospital tent. Sinks for enlisted men and officers were placed to the sides and rear of the camp to avoid contamination. Behind the officers' tents were the wagons, stores, and tents for teamsters and servants; horses and other livestock were placed at the very rear of the camp. Assistant Surgeon Daniel Holt, 121st New York, wrote that "To see ten or fifteen thousand men encamped at night with their camp fires and hear their music and singing, is no small affair, yet one soon becomes used to it and thinks little about it." He goes on to say he "should rather enjoy this sort of Gipsey [*sic*] life. To be sure you often go to bed hungry and cold, and rise in the morning worse than a foundered horse, yet there is a sort of fascination about it, that compels a man on despite the hardships."[5]

Surgeon's Mess

As officers, surgeons did not receive regular army rations and were responsible for purchasing their own food. Descriptions of eating arrangements appear frequently in their diaries and letters. Supplies could be purchased from commissary stores, sutlers, or by buying or foraging food from the surrounding community. Assistant Surgeon John Billings, 7th U.S., wrote home to his wife from camp: "It will cost me about sixty or seventy dollars a month to live here, for everything is exactly double what it is anywhere else . . . The Commissary supplies us with fresh bread four times a week and there is very good butter at the sutler's, so that we are faring sumptuously."[6] Daniel Holt was less enthusiastic when he wrote home

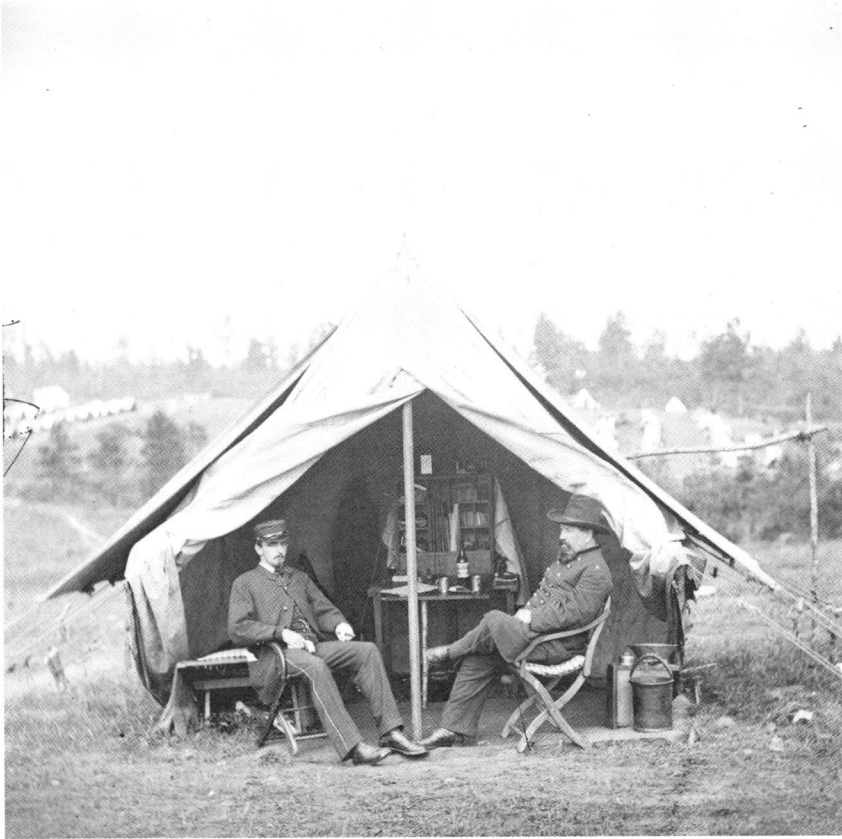

Dr. Charles K. Irwin, 72nd New York Infantry, in camp at Culpepper, Virginia, September 1863. Born in Ontario, Irwin studied medicine in Toronto and graduated from the Albany Medical College before settling in Dunkirk, New York. Courtesy of Library of Congress, Prints and Photographs

in September 1862 that "I am sometimes almost famished for want of something to eat . . . I have stood and looked on and been ashamed that I with shoulder straps should fare so much worse than any of our men, for they are regularly served with government rations and good ones too, while I have to purchase the best I can and have no means of cooking it after it is purchased."[7] Two weeks later he reported that the situation had improved: "Five of us, consisting of us three surgeons, Lieut. Keith of Company 'B' and the Hospital Steward form a mess. We have a black cook, and while in camp have three regular meals daily; but on the march everything is changed.—Uncertainty attends every step."[8] Most surgeons messed with other doctors or officers to help offset the costs. Surgeon William W. Potter, 57th New York, explained how they established an officers' mess with "each paying a pro rata share that was determined by a committee, as in an ordinary club. Were thus enabled to have a greater variety of food at much less expense, than if we had broken up into several smaller messes."[9] Between October and November 1862, William Watson had to live frugally, "having nothing but Bacon, bread without butter, and Coffee."[10] With only $2 to spend on food, he was happy that his assistant surgeon, "Dr Wenger, being rather flush, has sustained the entire expense of our Mess ever since his arrival and I only hope he may still have enough to stave off starvation till the Paymaster comes."[11] In January he was still without money for food and "if it were not for 'old Pap,' my cook, I would be compelled to beg my rations or starve. Old Pap has a little money which he expends . . . for me in the purchase of Crackers, Coffee, and Sugar."[12]

SERVANTS

Separated from wives and families, Union and Confederate surgeons, like other officers, relied on servants to perform the daily domestic chores of feeding their horses, maintaining their quarters, and cooking their meals. Letters and diaries provide glimpses of the important but often underreported role that these servants played in camp life. While only some are specifically identified as "colored," the prevalence of Black servants in both armies suggests that most were African American. As might be expected, Confederate officers, including surgeons, brought their enslaved body servants to accompany them into war. Assistant Surgeon Spencer Glasgow Welch, 13th South Carolina, mentions frequent changes in servants in his letters home. On the march to Pennsylvania in June 1863, he remarks, "My servant, Wilson, says he 'don't like Pennsylvania at all,' because he 'sees no black folks.'" But after the battle, Welch reports that "My servant got lost in Maryland. I do not think it was his intention to leave, but he was negligent about keeping up and got in rear of the army and found it too late to cross the river."[13] On September 1, 1863, he

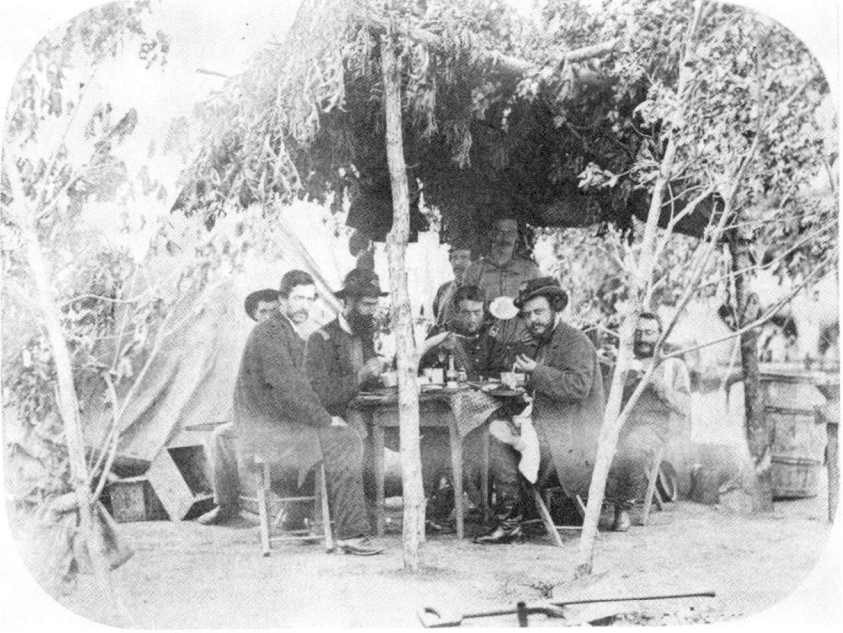

Second Wisconsin Officers' Mess. Surgeon Alexander Jackson Ward seated on the left. Courtesy of Wisconsin Historical Society

writes that "My new servant Gabriel arrived yesterday from South Carolina," but by mid-January, he writes that "I had to give Gabriel a little thrashing this morning for 'jawing' me. I hate very much to raise a violent hand against a person as old as Gabriel, although he is black and a slave. He is too slow for me and I intend to send him back by Billie when he goes home on furlough. I must close as Gabriel is bringing in my dinner." By May he had another servant named Alick who was making extra money washing soldiers' clothes.[14]

Confederate surgeons relied on enslaved Black servants to forage, cook, and serve meals. Division Surgeon Samuel Brown Morrison, Confederate Second Corps, wrote home in August 1863 that Sam "is a very good cook & suits me well. Seems to delight in getting me something good to eat—is very successful in his trips to the country in way of getting things to eat. We have been abundantly supplied with chicken, potatoes, some tomatoes, cabbage . . ."[15] Since they were not military personnel, personal servants were not restricted to camp and had freedom of movement to go back and forth on errands between home and camp. On one occasion, Morrison sent Sam home to Rockbridge, Virginia, to exchange one horse for another.[16] Assistant Surgeon Clayton Glanville Coleman, 24th Virginia, addressed a letter to his wife in Louisa County, Virginia, as "Sent by Servant George," writing on August 26, 1863 that "As I purpose sending George over home tomorrow, I will Write you this note by him."[17] Not every Confederate surgeon owned slaves and some hired servants. Surgeon Harvey Black, 4th Virginia, wrote to his wife from camp in Martinsburg on September 26, 1862 about his need for a servant:

> I don't know what I will do for a servant. I get along tolerably well in warm weather, but in the winter when we have tents to pitch and wood to get and horses to feed, it will be more difficult. Say to John Black that if he should come across a boy that would only suit me tolerably well, to hire him and send to me. I have been trying wherever I have been but can not find one; indeed, nearly all the Negroes have been taken from this country.[18]

Union surgeons also had servants, many of whom were drawn from the growing numbers of newly freed slaves commonly called "contraband." The roles of these servants and their relationships to Union surgeons did not significantly differ from the enslaved servants who served Confederate masters. William Watson was in camp with his regiment for only about ten days when he wrote home to his father in September 1862, "I am going to Alexandria tomorrow to have the Medical Purveyor fill a requisition for Hospital Supplies. I will see if I can't pick up a good Colored boy to do my cooking. I have one of the Hospital Attendants performing this work for me at present."[19] There is no indication that he succeeded in finding a servant on this trip, but in January 1863 he wrote home describing his observations of prejudice against African Americans among soldiers:

> You have no idea how greatly the common soldiers are prejudiced against the Negro. An officer can scarcely retain a colored servant. I

have seen with pity and indignation [a] poor, unfortunate and inoffensive contraband kicked, cuffed and maltreated without cause. The soldiers do this because they think the Negro considers himself their equal and that before long he will be made so by Congress and the administration.[20]

Daniel Holt was antislavery in his political views, often citing the curse of slavery, but he acknowledged that there were limits to racial equality. Writing home to his wife on December 18, 1862, from camp in Belle Plain Landing, Virginia, he provided a detailed description of his daily living arrangements with his Black servant:

The mess consists of two—Josh and myself. He (Josh) is maid of all work. On him devolves the duty of rising in the morning, making fires, sweeping out the tent, making up bed, and feeding Fannie [his horse]. That done, he proceeds to get breakfast; and here carries in our kit and stock in trade, which consists in all told of two dishes made of a canteen which I found upon the ground after the boys left.

Despite the fact that they were sharing a tent and eating the same food, Holt goes on to explain,

It would not answer, you know, to have a Nigger eat at the same table with you, so to keep up the distinction which man has created. Josh has to keep back until his master is helped. I can sometimes hear him swearing with the men back of the tent, about the cold victuals he has to eat after I am through. Well, if he does not like it he will have to leave, for with all my love for a black skin I never yet saw one with whom I would be willing to be on perfect equality . . . not because I feel that by nature I am better than they, but education—early as life itself is against it. It is engrafted in me—I cannot help it.[21]

Two months later, Holt sent Josh away because he had "become insolent and saucy, and demanded an increase of pay, so I thought he had better go. I can get another as good and cheaper."[22] While contraband early in the war may have traded their services for the protection of the Union army, African-American servants eventually felt emboldened to demand regular wages. Dr. Child wrote home in April 1864 about increased expenses because "During the first year we had a servant for nothing—this year we must pay seventeen dollars each for two months."[23]

Some servants were young children who became attached to regiments and officers in less formal ways. William Potter noted on June 27, 1862, that after the Seven Days Battle, he was taken prisoner with wounded at Savage Station, where "a sergeant of the regular army transferred a colored boy, a servant of his captain, to my custody, who passed as my servant thereafter." When Dr. Potter was exchanged July 17, 1862, "The little colored boy, who became separated from me on my arrival at Libby, now came running up with tears in his eyes, begging to go along too."[24] Presumably, he remained with Dr. Potter through the war. On the march after Gettysburg, Surgeon James Langstaff Dunn, 109th Pennsylvania, wrote home that

> I picked up a nice smart little contraband as black as jet on the march near White Plains, Va. He is smart as can be, can cook and do almost everything. His master was hunting him to send him South but he hid in the woods until evening came along, then came out of his hole and I picked him up. He is about 12 years old, says if I will learn him to read and write he will go home with me and work for me all his life.[25]

Some servants formed enduring relationships with surgeons that lasted beyond the war years. Assistant Surgeon Edgar Parker, 13th Massachusetts, appears in the 1865 census for Framingham, Massachusetts, with fourteen-year-old Wilson Baylies, a Black servant born in Virginia, who later became a barber. Lucy Johnson and her husband served as cook and groom for Acting Assistant Surgeon John Nice Jacobs; he later provided employment for Lucy and her family after the war in Kulpsville, Pennsylvania, and took care of her until her death in 1905.[26] Surgeon Theodore T. Tate, 3rd Pennsylvania Cavalry, a Gettysburg resident, recounted, "in the winter of 1862, I picked up Nelson Royer some place in Virginia and hired him as a servant. He proved to be a good man and I kept him from that time until the Reg. was mustered out in August 1864."[27] Nelson Royer who was with Tate at Gettysburg, subsequently enlisted in the 25th U.S. Colored Troops as Nelson Roy, 44, born in Goochland, Virginia, was discharged in December 1865, and eventually made Gettysburg his home.

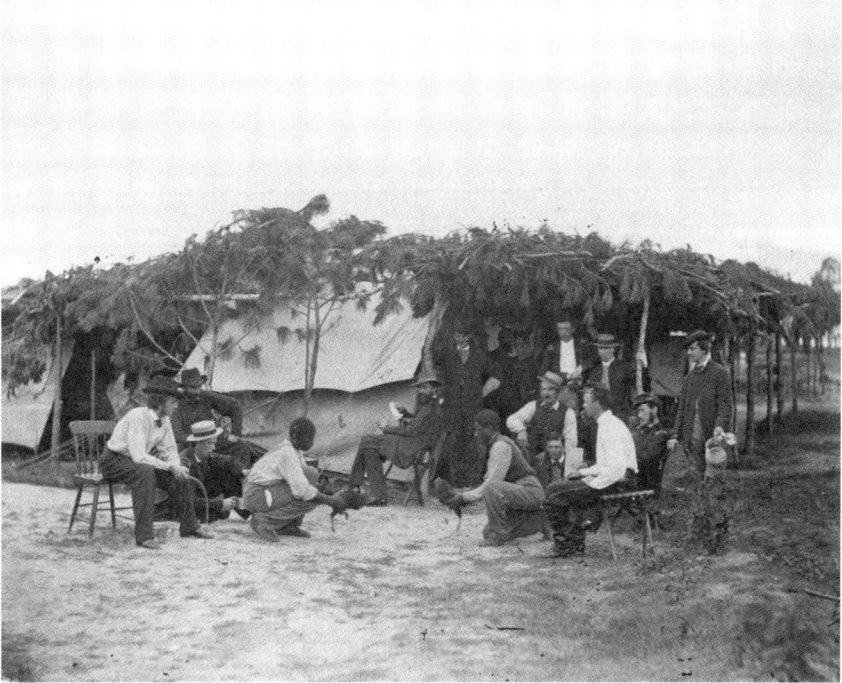

Headquarters of Brig. Gen. O. B. Wilcox in front of Petersburg, August 1864. Surgeon Patrick A. O'Connell seated second from right in uniform. "George" and "John" probably refer to the cocks being held by two unnamed young Black servants. O'Connell served with the 28th Massachusetts at Gettysburg but later received a commission as U.S. Volunteer. Courtesy of U.S. Army Heritage and Education Center, Carlisle, Pennsylvania

Daily Routine

Daily life in camp for surgeons followed a set military schedule. Daniel Holt wrote to his wife early in October 1862, from a camp in the field near Bakersville, Maryland:

At early dawn, we rise, wash and prepare to eat breakfast; that over, Surgeon's Call is sounded and from one hundred and fifty to two hundred patients present themselves for treatment. The time required to attend all this consumes two or three hours and then the hospital has to be visited and those in sick quarters—that means those who are too unwell to come up to call, but who are not sick enough to go into the barn which we have taken possession of for a hospital. We have to make from twenty-five to thirty of these calls daily, seeing that the medicines prescribed are faithfully given and that the condition of the men is comfortable, &c.—the diet of the sick in bed is also to be looked to—Sanitary condition of camp must be attended to, and a general supervision of the health of the men made and reported, You may think we have hardly time for all this, and indeed you think correctly, but it has to be done daily, and sometimes we have to see a patient several times a day.[28]

Assistant Surgeon Cyrus Bacon, 2nd U.S., described the repetitive nature of the work: "I get up at reveille, or as soon as my fire is warm. [I] have had sick call soon after [arising] but shall have it later hereafter. Sick call does not number more than 30 men and my work is done before breakfast. The papers are a little wearisome, but all in all the work is not hard."[29] Assistant Surgeon William H. Taylor, 19th Virginia, remembered:

When our medical duties were over for the day, we governed ourselves according to circumstances. If the troops were moving we went with them and partook of their adventures, whatever they might be. If we were in camp it was always, to me at least, a problem to know what to do to enliven the usually tedious hours. I preferred to read, if there was anything to read which was only occasionally the case . . . other devices for passing the time were playing cards or chess, chatting with one another and strolling idly about.[30]

Inactivity in winter quarters prompted younger surgeons to engage in snowballing and "kicking at football on the parade." Others like William Child used the time to study medical books with fellow doctors or medical students. In February 1863, William Potter wrote, "The times are very dull in camp these days as the roads are so bad that riding is not agreeable, so we are committed to the dull routine of eating, reading, and sleeping in the daytime. In the evening we have quite jolly times. Some of the officers are very good singers . . ."[31]

Surgeon's Call

The surgeon's workday—winter and summer, in camp and on the march—began with the bugle announcing sick call. In response, "some who were whole and needed not a physician, as well as those who were sick, reported at the surgeon's tent for prescriptions. Much used to be said by the soldiers in regard to the competency or incompetency of army surgeons."[32] William Watson reported that "Quinine" or 'Old Quin,'" as the surgeons were often called, "gets many a deep though not loud cursing—especially from the lazy vagabonds who try their very best to play sick and so get off duty."[33] When his assistant surgeon, Dr. Wenger, refused to excuse a fellow who was in the habit of "playing off," Watson was amused that the soldier "went off muttering and growling that he would go to the 'old man.'" Although only twenty-six years old, Watson, as surgeon, was often referred to as the "old Doctor."[34] Daily interaction with the men was an important function of the regimental surgeon's responsibility to monitor the health of the troops. A surgeon's medical decisions could mean life or death to soldiers in the field. A history of the 63rd Pennsylvania regiment explains the mixed reviews that surgeons received from the men in their care.

> While there were some noble, humane and self-sacrificing physicians in the army, who were an ornament to the class and a God-send to the poor, broken down, fever-stricken or wounded soldiers, unfortunately they formed a minority to the unskilled quacks whose ignorance and brutality made them objects of detestation to the soldier . . . We had a number of other doctors, some good, some middling, and some worthless.[35]

Surgeon Castanus Blake Park Jr., 16th Vermont, was so highly regarded by his regiment that when he left in October 1863, the enlisted men presented him with a silver tea set, noting:

> You won our confidence by manifesting a skill in the art of healing which few possess; then by untiring diligence and continued watchfulness, you almost robbed disease of its terrors and death of its victims. But this is not all. Your whole intercourse with us was characterized by gentlemanly deportment and kindly consideration. Neither the annoyances of dealing with unpleasant subjects, nor the necessary inconveniences of camp life, induced neglect or sourness.[36]

Regimental histories that praised the work of their surgeons suggest that most surgeons took their medical responsibilities seriously, and many recognized the importance of trust and attentiveness in the doctor-patient relationship between surgeons and soldiers. Thomas Wood described his first surgeon's call where he encountered a case of shingles that was not familiar to him. After providing a lotion, he went back to his tent to consult his copy of *Watson's Practice*, and afterwards "made it a duty to study my cases, even though I considered myself familiar with them."[37] Daniel Holt's letters home describe his devotion to his patients and his hard work on their behalf.

> I am at this time sitting upon a cannister of black tea, with a surgical case upon my lap for a table, writing this amid almost momentary interruption. Someone comes for an excuse from duty—another for relief from guard—another does not feel well enough to attend battalion drill—still another prays for excuse from dress parade, and others still want their discharge papers made out and they sent home. This is all competent for the Surgeon, and these calls are as frequent as every few moments a day. The men soon learn where to go. Dr. Valentine swears at them and sends them away. I do not so.—Although I hate the annoyance as much as he does, yet I cannot say to a sick man, or even to one who is not violently indisposed, "return to your quarters, and do your duty or go into the guard house" when I know that he is willing to do all that is reasonably required of him.[38]

Holt's workload was particularly heavy because his fellow assistant surgeon, Stephen Valentine, was often "sick," a polite term for his drunkenness. Valentine was dismissed for incompetence before the battle of Gettysburg, but Holt thought "that if the whisky bottle had not been quite so near the head of his bed he would have been well to-day."[39]

Reports of drunkenness occasionally appear in the diaries and letters of fellow physicians, but formal complaints of drunkenness were probably underreported. Complaints leading to court-martial or dismissal that cited incompetence or neglect of duty were probably linked to chronic alcohol and drug abuses. Based on the records compiled for the Gettysburg Surgeons Database, 2 percent of the surgeons of both armies clearly struggled with alcohol problems of varying degree. This percentage represents nine Confederate and fourteen Union doctors. For example, Assistant Surgeon Alexander D. Hamilton, 5th Alabama Battalion, was tried for both drunkenness and neglect of duty but acquitted on both counts.[40] The military records of Assistant Surgeon Thomas Harold Wilson Upshur, 2nd North Carolina, describe chronic alcoholism; he was court-martialed in 1862 for drunkenness, reprimanded, and given a month suspension. In September 1863 he was in a Richmond hospital for chronic hepatitis and gastric disorders and a February 25, 1864, letter from Surgeon General Moore made clear that "a continuation of his dissipated habits will not be permitted and if he offends again charges will be brought against him."[41] Union surgeons were more likely to be dismissed for drunkenness, perhaps reflecting the greater supply of Northern physicians available to replace them. Among the Gettysburg cohort, Assistant Surgeon Edward Gardner Marshall, 124th New York, was dismissed "on account of habitual intoxication" on August 7, 1863, and Surgeon George W. Jackson, 53rd Pennsylvania, was removed for drunkenness in December 1864.[42] Not all alcoholics were charged with drunkenness. Cyrus Bacon, Assistant Surgeon, 2nd U.S., recorded his impressions of Charles Colton in October 1862, soon after Colton joined their brigade as Assistant Surgeon, 17th U.S.

Poor fellow he has already had attacks of Delirium Tremens and it is with difficulty he is now able to steer clear. Yet [he] is never [visibly] drunk. If he reforms he will make one of the most brilliant men of the army.[43]

On February 18, 1863, he wrote that Dr. Colton "is slightly affected with delirium tremens and most excessively irritable," and on May 25th wrote, "Colton was sick again yesterday."[44] Although Colton was accused of failing to attend to a patient who died, there was no mention of alcohol abuse, and he was acquitted.[45]

MEDICAL PRACTICE

Letters, diaries, and accounts of Civil War surgeons can seem limited because they provide so little personal insight into clinical practice in the field. The picture that emerges from a few surviving accounts suggests that regimental surgeons in the field had to make do with minimal tools and limited medications compared with their counterparts working in hospitals. William Taylor later described his personal experiences as a regimental surgeon, acknowledging that surgeons in the field did their best with limited resources:

> Early in the morning we had sick-call, when those who claimed to be ill or disabled came to be passed upon. Diagnosis was rapidly made, usually by intuition, and treatment was with such drugs as we chanced to have in the knap-sack and were handiest to obtain. In serious cases we made an honest effort to bring to bear all the skill and knowledge we possessed, but our science could rarely display itself to the best advantage on account of the paucity of our resources.[46]

Taylor admitted that serving in the field, "afforded only the most limited and meagre opportunities for acquiring comprehensive and actual knowledge of the methods of medical and surgical service."[47] Surgeon Caspar Henkel, 37th Virginia, wrote home to his father on February 23, 1863, complaining that "Surgeons are leaving the field whenever they can. I fear I shall have to remain in the field all the time, as I generally am left to bear the blunts. One consolation, field service is considered the most honorable position, if its duties are more onerous, and the opportunity of seeing operative surgery is far superior."[48]

Some surgeons, however, expressed their preference for regimental service because it afforded them a greater degree of independence and the opportunity to establish a more personal rapport with their patients. Recent studies on contemporary doctor-patient relationships have identified four main elements in those relationships: knowledge, trust, loyalty, and regard.[49] When Daniel Holt wrote home about his role as a regimental surgeon, he clearly recognized the importance of these relationships in his ability to provide medical care:

> My heart is with the boys and the regiment; and they appear to be suited to the "old doctor" as they good naturedly call me . . . I have cured many a man who was really unwell by simply making him believe that his sickness was all in his mind.[50]

Regimental doctors had plenty of practical experience but little time to consult books or other colleagues. Julian Chisolm pointed out in his *Manual of Military Surgery* that "Those killed in battle are but a handful when compared to the victims of disease."[51] He stressed that keeping an army in health was even more important than curing wounds from the battlefields, but a regimental surgeon had to be skilled in both departments. William Taylor's assessment of regimental medical care accurately depicted the more mundane treatment of everyday chronic complaints rather than the dramatic heroics of battlefield surgery:

> The prevailing diseases were intestinal disorders, though we had a share of almost every malady. Occasionally we suffered seriously from measles. Smallpox was effectively kept in check by vaccination. Intermittent and other malarial fevers at times incapacitated regiments to an extent which was really portentous. Our management of these various diseases presented, as far as I know, nothing unusual or novel. None of the well-developed cases remained long under my care, for they were sent from the camp to the hospital to be treated by the surgeon . . . A modicum of surgical practice was furnished by the accidents that occurred.[52]

Seriously ill cases were usually transferred to general hospitals where they could receive long-term care. Assistant Surgeon James Benton,

111th New York, explained that "as soon as a man is taken sick he is immediately sent away unless it be with some slight disorder from which he will recover in a few days . . . it would not do to have the ambulances filled up with sick and be compelled to leave the wounded on the field."[53]

The diseases and chronic complaints of camp proved difficult to combat; surgeons often had to make decisions based on their own observations, or through trial and error. Limited by the medical supplies available to them, and without fully understanding the causes of many diseases, surgeons in the field struggled with treatment for the most common complaints. Chronic diarrhea, for example, resulted in more deaths in the Union army than any other disease and almost as many deaths as from gunshot wounds. Some cases of diarrhea were caused by water-borne diseases spread through contaminated water, and surgeons were increasingly aware of the need for pure drinking water. Assistant Surgeon Alfred T. Hamilton, 148th Pennsylvania, an 1858 graduate of the Hygeio-Therapeutic College of New York who also attended regular medical courses at Bellevue and the College of Physicians and Surgeons in New York, promoted sanitary conditions and the importance of clean water as part of his duties. In the regimental history he described the large amount of sickness in the camp from December 1861 to April 1863, "Notwithstanding a well policed camp ground and comfortable quarters, we labored under the great disadvantage of having drinking water polluted more or less by surface drainage into the springs."[54] Looking back, he thought "it would have been economical had we been supplied, while in camp, with distilled water for drinking purposes."[55]

Other causes of dysentery were attributed to unripe fruit, spoiled or uncooked meat, and other dietary causes. Surgeons suffered from dysentery along with troops. Daniel Holt wrote about eating undercooked meat resulting in "cramps in my stomach and bowels to such an extent that I verily thought my last day had come. Opium nor ether had the least effect."[56] Cyrus Bacon wrote in his diary describing self-treatment of his own diarrhea.

> Was so unwell today, I did but little, took a dose of Rhein (rhubarb) as bowels had for a few days been almost inactive. Had much headache.

With the action of the Rhubarb began a dysentery. To check this I use Morphine. (The secondary effects of opii, upon me are very unpleasant. Always when taken in quantity making me very sick.) And my dysentery was so severe I was obliged to use large quantities. Therefore I was kept with nausea and vomiting and very sick 'til June 27th.[57]

This regimen of a cathartic like rhubarb to move the bowels, followed by opium to slow the bowels, corresponds with the recommendations outlined in Joseph Woodward's 1863 U.S. Army publication on camp diseases.[58]

Some regimental surgeons identified another cause of camp diarrhea as "scurvy dysentery," resulting from an army diet lacking fresh fruits and vegetables. Theodore Dimon, while serving as a regimental surgeon in July 1861, was taken to task for supplying his men with fresh vegetables against the orders of Charles Stuart Tripler, then medical director of the Army of the Potomac.

I was summoned by an orderly to report myself to Dr. Tripler's quarters forthwith. I found the doctor very indignant and angry at what he called insubordination in regard to the fresh fruit question. I said to him, "Sir, this with me is not at all a question of military orders or orders on service, or of respect and obedience to my superior officers in this respect, but simply a question of professional practice and personal responsibility. It is to me the same as if an order should be issued to me either not to cut off any limb shattered by a ball or to cut off all limbs that were at all injured. I am not a hospital steward. You can dismiss me from this service or relieve me from the responsibility in any other legitimate way, but as long as the professional responsibility remains with me, nobody but God Almighty can, without my consent, interpose between me and my patients, whether in or out of U.S. service."[59]

Tripler dismissed him, grumbling about "these volunteer surgeons," but the regiment was allowed to obtain cucumbers, green corn, melons, and apples from the sutlers. In his next monthly report, Dimon's regiment had only six off duty for sickness compared to other regiments with 150 to 200 sick with dysentery. Tripler came to inspect the regiment himself and asked Dimon, "on what professional ground I placed my curing my men of dysentery with green corn and cucumbers. I told him that I considered the dysentery we had now to be scurvy dysentery such as I had met with in California . . . [60] Dimon's interchange with Tripler illustrates the conflicts that sometimes developed between the new volunteers recruited from civilian practice and old-school regular army doctors. Despite the evidence of "scurvy dysentery" that Dimon provided him, Tripler made few adjustments, believing that dried vegetables boiled in soup provided adequate nutrition. Surgeon Franklin Dyer, 19th Massachusetts, was still complaining a year later in June 1862 about "sickness due to lack of fresh vegetables" and the unwillingness to admit that troops suffered from scurvy. On June 14, 1862, he recorded in his journal: "We have had potatoes issued but once since we came on the Peninsula, and even vinegar but seldom. We reported cases of scurvy sometime since, but its existence was denied at headquarters of the army. 'The troops should not have scurvy. Their rations are plentiful and good.'"[61] Tripler refused to recognize the problem and it was not until Jonathan Letterman replaced him as medical director of the Army of the Potomac in June 1862 that increased rations of fresh fruits and vegetables significantly improved the health of Union soldiers.

Confederate documents indicate that fresh vegetables were distributed to troops in the summer of 1862, and as late as March 1863, Confederate Surgeon General Moore issued an official circular on the incidence of scurvy, noting, "The only certain method of preventing scurvy is by issuing with the soldiers rations at suitable proportions of vegetables & vegetable acids." Attached was one list of plants to be collected in camps: "wild mustard; wild garlic and onions; water cress; shoots of polk [poke] stalk; sassafras; sorrel; lambs quarters; artichokes" and a second list of items to be obtained through the Commissary, "vinegar, pickles, bottled cold slaugh, sour crout. [sic] dried and canned fruits, horse radish, peas, potatoes & beans, molasses, cabbage sprout, turnip greens, lettuce, radishes, hominy course [sic] and fine, garden vegetables of every description."[62]

Some camp diseases were best prevented by sanitation and personal hygiene. Surgeon Harvey Black, 4th Virginia, shared his treatment for scabies with his wife, who was also experiencing an infestation. "The remedy which I think cut it short for him was Fowler's solution, though he used the Sulphur ointment for about one week . . . This is becoming a favorite remedy in the army . . . Another suggestion [is] in regard to washing your clothes."[63] Chisolm's *Manual of Military Surgery* advised surgeons that "cleanliness of the encampment and of the tent, with frequent ablutions of the body and clothing of soldiers, should never be absent from his thoughts."[64] Soap was listed on the schedule of medical supplies for good reason. While Civil War surgeons did not understand germ theory and the need for antiseptics, they "had correct ideas as to ordinary cleanliness and decency and we policed the camp in accordance with them, but there was no excessive care, nor anything approaching the refinement of present-day sanitary science . . ."[65]

Policing the sanitary conditions of the camp was the responsibility of the surgeons. Camps were regularly moved to new locations to prevent contamination from latrines and garbage. Tents were routinely struck to dry out the ground beneath. Cyrus Bacon wrote on March 10, 1863:

> The camp is broken up, leveled, policed and reset by general order. The 3rd 4th and 12th were censured for filth. Dr. Craig makes an inspection of my Hospitals. [He] compliments me on their neatness. Dr. Ramsey too, gives the police of the camp a compliment. Has been snowing this morning so we set the tents rapidly, intending the first dry day to air and cleanse the ground within them.[66]

Inspections of camp were carried out regularly. J. Franklin Dyer wrote in February 1862, "Day by day we go through the same routine, I rise at surgeon's call which is at seven-thirty o'clock. This I always attend. Sunday morning inspection at eight o'clock, first of men and arms in line, and then inspection of quarters, which occupies us nearly all the forenoon. This inspection I make and report the condition of quarters to the colonel."[67]

Reports

Medical reports allowed both armies to assess their troop strength as well as to document and improve medical care, but they were one of the more onerous and bureaucratic aspects of the job. Surgeons were expected to make daily, weekly, monthly, and quarterly reports to their commanding officer and to the supervising medical staff. Requisitions for paper attest to the volume of reporting that was required. In addition to reports on patients and diseases, they were also responsible for accounts of medical supplies and hospital expenses. William Watson wrote home that "I have constantly employed the last few days in moving camp and preparing my monthly reports. Dr. Sims [Medical Director Thomas Sim] is so particular about the Reports that it requires a great deal of time and labor to get them up neatly and correctly. My last report was both difficult and tedious to make out. I was compelled to report in detail the seat and character of all wounds—the different operations performed and their result."[68] W. W. Potter wrote on December 31, 1861: "I was busy, during all [of my] spare time, with the quarterly return of medical and hospital property, and stores. The return was a complicated and perplexing one to make up at first, but I finally mastered it . . ." In May 1862 he wrote that he "was occupied with my monthly report, which must always be sent in promptly, lest there be complaints from headquarters."[69]

While these reports document health and diseases in both armies and provide statistical and other evidence for historians, they served an immediate need for the military command. Medical staff wanted to know about diseases, numbers of patients, etc.; military commanders wanted to know how many men they had available and able to fight. Medical decisions excusing men who were legitimately too sick to drill and march could conflict with a colonel's need to have sufficient forces. If surgeons were too permissive, the ranks could be depleted of active soldiers; if they were too strict and denied furloughs or discharges, it could be a fatal decision. A bound volume found in the mess kit of Surgeon Isaac Scott Tanner, 21st North Carolina, includes handwritten copies of monthly and quarterly reports for sick and wounded. Listed are the number of cases of each disease, and the names of soldiers who were killed or died. Each report tallies the number of sick brought forward from last quarter;

new cases taken sick and whether they have been sent to a general hospital, returned to duty, on furlough, discharged, deserted, or died; and how many remained sick or convalescent.[70]

The number that was of interest to the military command was how many were fit for duty. This was particularly true in anticipation of a major battle. In May 1863, after the battle of Chancellorsville resulted in Union defeat and withdrawal back across the Rappahannock River, both armies remained in place for the rest of the month. By June both armies began preparing for another campaign. Charles Fanning Wood wrote,

> The Spring campaign was about to commence, the rest was broken after a while by an order to examine all the men in camp and send to the hospital all not able to march. After I had completed the examination, the Surgeon, Dr. Washington, noticing how large the list was, went over my examinations and struck some of my excused men from the list.[71]

Newly commissioned, Surgeon Walker Washington, 3rd North Carolina, had only recently passed the examination for surgeon in April 1863, and was less experienced than Wood. At least one of the men whose medical excuse was countermanded died on the march. Wood attributed Washington's misjudgment to his desire to be conscientious, distrust of opinions of others, lack of experience in the field, and not being acquainted with the individual officers and men.[72]

On June 4, John Billings wrote about the Union army's preparations to march:

> I packed up all my goods—also the hospital stores and medicine—struck the tents—packed my two wagons, got a hot breakfast, got food for two days packed in my haversack, secured an ambulance all to myself by a little diplomacy, and when the assembly sounded I was seated on Dick [his horse] smoking a cigar and placidly contemplating the universal rush and confusion around me.[73]

On June 12th Billings was still waiting to leave when "orders came to pack up—the sick were sent off—all surplus baggage was sent to the rear . . . We may move in an hour, to-day, to-morrow, or next week."[74] For James Fulton, Assistant Surgeon, 150th Pennsylvania,

> In the morning of June 11th we were all up in time to get the men Break-fast before starting for the Hospital the ambulances coming we got the men aboard and started them and soon our Brigade was in motion taking the direction toward Falmouth.[75]

By mid-June both armies were marching north toward Pennsylvania.

PART II
GETTYSBURG

CHAPTER 4

Gettysburg Battle, July 1

By mid-June 1863 both armies were on the move, abandoning their camps in Virginia and heading north toward Maryland and Pennsylvania. "No one who has not seen the train of an army in motion can form any just conception of its magnitude," George T. Stevens, USA Surgeon 77th New York, wrote, estimating that if placed in a single line the wagons would extend over 70 miles.[1] The *Valley Spirit,* Chambersburg, Pennsylvania, described the march of the Confederates as they arrived in Chambersburg:

> First came an immense body of cavalry, steadily and quietly, every man with his hand on his carbine, and his eye glancing suspiciously at each open window and door . . . First came a brigade, then an artillery, then its ambulances, and then its baggage train. . . . fully fifty thousand men, two hundred and ten cannon, twelve, twenty-four and thirty-two pounders, and over two thousand wagons.[2]

Assistant Surgeon Spencer Welch, 13th South Carolina, wrote to his wife from Franklin County, Pennsylvania, on June 28, 1863, that "We are taking everything we need—horses, cattle, sheep, flour, groceries and goods of all kinds, and making as clean a sweep as possible."[3]

While the Confederate army was amassing supplies of food, livestock, and medicines seized from the communities along its route, the Union army was making efforts to streamline its baggage trains. Jonathan Letterman, medical director of the U.S. Army of the Potomac, complained in his memoir that military commanders too often favored food and ammunition as more essential than medical supplies, to the dismay of medical personnel. The normal allowance of medical transportation that Letterman had established in the fall of 1862 was further reduced by order of Commanding General Joseph Hooker on June 19th, despite Letterman's objections. "Notwithstanding my verbal and written opinion against such reduction, which compelled this department to send away a large portion of its hospital tents, mess-chests, and other articles necessary upon the battle-field, and proved, as I foresaw it would, a source of embarrassment and suffering, which might have been avoided."[4]

Assistant Surgeon John Shaw Billings, 6th U.S., wrote in his official report, "On this march, all the ambulances were collected into a train which followed immediately behind the Division, and was superintended by a medical officer detailed for the purpose. Transportation was allowed in the proportion of one wagon for the medical supplies of two regiments, and this train of wagons followed close behind the ambulances."[5] On June 21st, when the Fifth Corps received the order to further reduce baggage, Billings was obliged to discard even his own mess furniture.[6] Union troops and officers marched long days and nights, sleeping on the ground, often without tents, and with little opportunity for food preparation beyond coffee and hardtack.

Marches could be as dangerous and deadly as actual battle. John Stuckenberg, Chaplain, 145th Pennsylvania, wrote, "It was such a march which men say they dread more than a battle."[7] Thomas Fanning Wood, Assistant Surgeon 3rd North Carolina, described that on marches "The Assistant Surgeon's place was behind the Regiment, now stopping to write a rear pass for some poor fellow overcome by fatigue, carry a canteen of water to one fellow by the wayside . . ."[8] The summer heat took a heavy toll on the marching troops of both armies. Stevens described men of the U.S. Sixth Corps falling from exhaustion and heat stroke, "with faces burning with a glow of crimson, and panting for breath." In one stretch of four days, they marched 100 miles in their haste to reach the battlefield and on July 1st, they marched 38 miles in a single day.[9] Surgeon J. Franklin Dyer, 9th Massachusetts, wrote on June 28, 1863, that "My position during this march has been no sinecure. The superintendence of

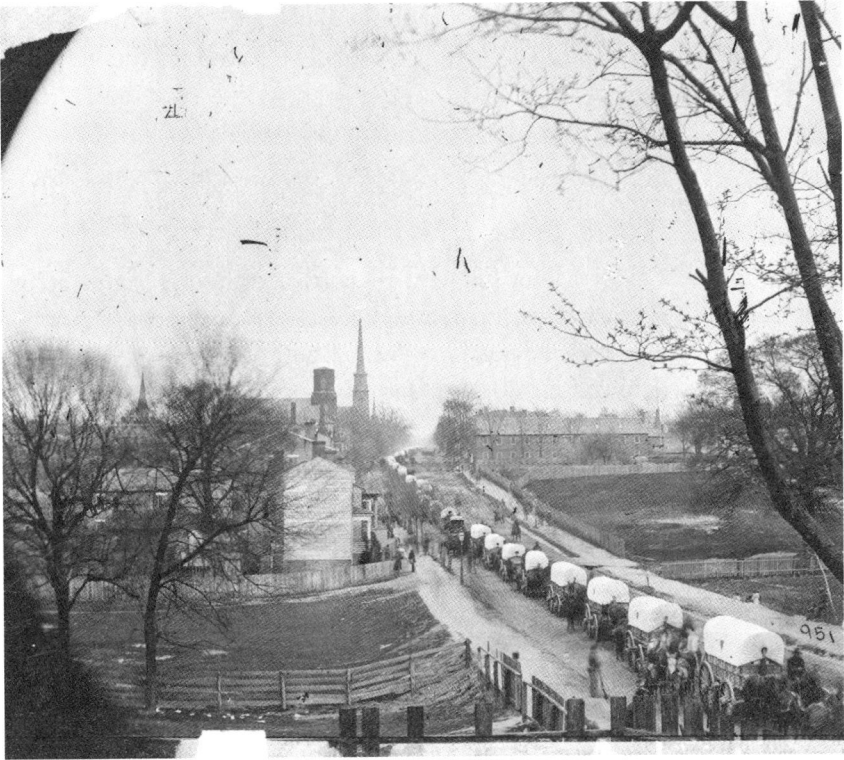

A *New York Times* article of April 8, 1865, estimated that Gen. William Sherman's army had a wagon and ambulance train of 4,500 vehicles that stretched over 45 miles with 100 wagons per mile. During the retreat from Gettysburg, the trains of General Ewell's Corps reportedly extended nearly 20 miles. Courtesy of Library of Congress, Prints and Photographs Division

the medical department of the division requires much labor, and besides General Gibbon requires everyone on his staff to use his utmost endeavor to prevent straggling."[10] The two armies heading northward occasionally skirmished in cavalry battles along their routes, but it was understood that a major battle would take place at some point. Eventually their paths crossed at the small town of Gettysburg, Pennsylvania, not far from the Maryland border. Assistant Surgeon Alfred Hamilton, 148th Pennsylvania, observed, "The march was severe on the men, many fell out to be picked up by ambulances, many died . . . the condition of our men from long marches, loss of sleep, lack of rations . . . will give the civilian an idea of how far spent the physical man was when we went into the fight and kept it up for three days."[11]

July 1st

On the morning of July 1st, Assistant Surgeon John Dewitt, 17th Pennsylvania Cavalry, reported that he "was on the line in attendance upon the wounded of [U.S. Major General Richard] Anderson's troops before 7 o'clock am," and that the firing commenced two hours before he reached the front.[12] Dewitt was part of Gen. John Buford's cavalry division that had spent the night of June 30th in Gettysburg anticipating the approach of nearby Confederate forces. The Confederate Third Corps commanded by Gen. A. P. Hill was already nearby and moving toward Gettysburg. Spencer Welch, part of Pender's Division in Hill's Third Corps, described that, on the morning of July 1st, "about five o'clock we began moving. We had not gone more than a mile and a half before our suspicions of the evening previous were fully verified and our expectations realized by the booming of cannons ahead of us in the direction of Gettysburg . . . It was Heth's Division ahead of ours fighting . . ."[13]

Buford's cavalry was able to hold their position against Hill's Third Corps until Gen. John Reynolds arrived with the Union First Corps. Assistant Surgeon James Fulton, 143rd Pennsylvania, recorded in his diary for July 1st that his regiment broke camp early and began marching to Gettysburg, a distance of 4 to 8 miles. When they reached the Theological Seminary, the men threw down their knapsacks and went into the field. As assistant surgeon, Fulton's role was to follow the men to the front and provide immediate care at a dressing station, but he soon realized that neither his steward nor the hospital orderly carrying the hospital knapsack with supplies had followed him. He was on his way back to look for them when Assistant Surgeon Whiteside Hunter, 149th Pennsylvania, ordered him to the division hospital for special duty. Returning to the Seminary, Fulton learned that Surgeon George New, 7th Indiana, had already designated the Seminary building for the First Division hospital.[14] New later recalled that he "opened the first hospital for the wounded, the Lutheran Theological Seminary. [Later] I went back into town with other Medical Officers who took possession of several large rooms, halls, hotels, etc., being first also to open hospitals in the town for the wounded."[15]

The wounded carried from the battlefield north of town began to fill every available space in Gettysburg. Despite the chaotic nature of the battle scenes and the seemingly random placement of wounded seeking shelter, Union hospital sites were selected according to a prescribed plan for establishing division field hospitals for each corps at a safe distance

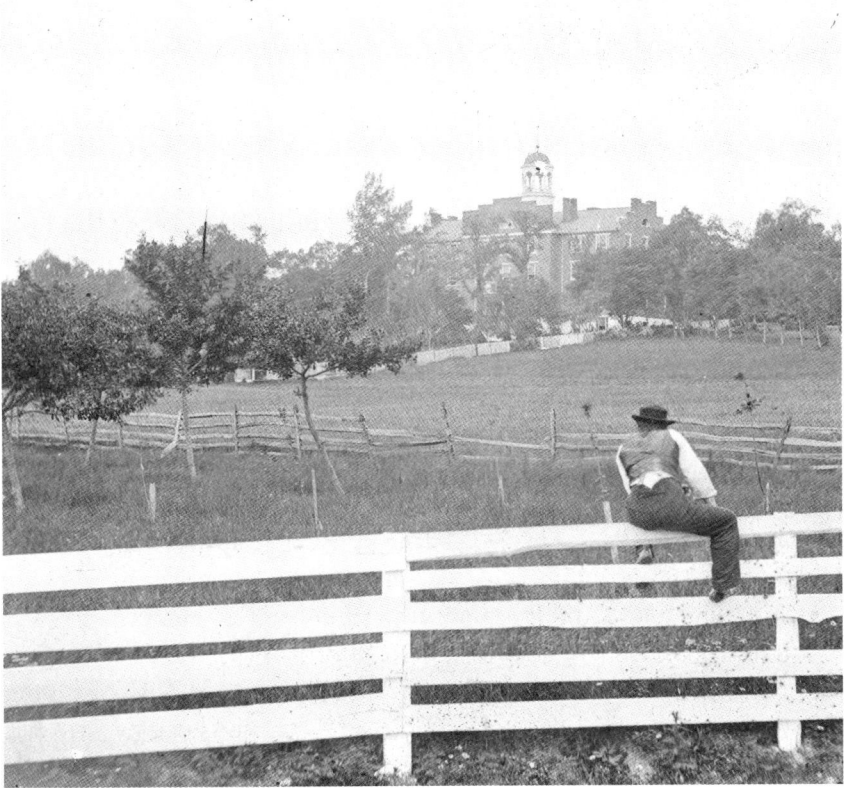

Seminary Building, July 15, 1863. The 1832 Seminary building was designated as a hospital for the Union First Corps on July 1st and later controlled by Confederate forces during the battle. The building was still being used as a hospital when this photograph was taken. Photograph by Mathew Brady. Courtesy of Library of Congress, Prints and Photographs Division

behind the line of battle. Just as military commanders studied the field to gain the most advantageous battle positions, the medical staff had to anticipate the course of military engagements to situate dressing stations and field hospitals in locations that were near enough to the fighting to be effective but shielded from direct fire for the safety of patients and doctors. The changing battle lines throughout the day on July 1st necessitated relocating Union hospital sites to safer ground, while the most seriously wounded and surgeons to care for them had to be left behind.

Union Cavalry Hospitals

The first casualties of the cavalry divisions fighting along McPherson's Ridge northwest of town were treated at dressing stations near the battlefield or found shelter in nearby barns, houses, and the Lutheran Seminary. Seriously wounded were transported by ambulances to the rear. Among the first medical staff on the scene, Surgeon Abner Hard, 8th Illinois Cavalry, as division surgeon, had originally selected the Railroad Depot in town as his hospital site on June 30th, but he described how on July 1st,

> We removed our wounded to the Presbyterian church near the center of town and were engaged in amputating the arm of a rebel soldier, when a messenger announced a dispatch from General Buford that we must fall back. Hastily arranging for the care of the wounded, by leaving Surgeons Beck, Rulison and Vosburg to attend them, we left the church to find the street crowded by the retreating Eleventh corps . . .[16]

In her account of the hospital in the Presbyterian church on Baltimore Street, Gettysburg resident Agnes Barr named Assistant Surgeon Simon Sanger, 6th New York Cavalry, in addition to William Rulison, Hiram Vosburgh, and Elias Beck, as the surgeons who boarded with her family during the battle.[17]

Union First Corps Hospitals

Arriving in Gettysburg on the morning of July 1st, Thomas Hewson Bache, Medical Inspector, and John Theodore Heard, Medical Director, served as senior medical officers on General Reynolds's First Corps staff. Bache later recounted how his first responsibility was to select locations for field hospitals: "It was not at the moment my place to attend to anything but the selection of field hospitals in the town, and I must repress my desire to follow up the slope to the left of it with the division with which I was marching. I took my way straight into the little town . . . My duty as staff surgeon gave a free foot after my duties were performed in town, to go directly to Seminary Ridge." At some point that morning, he was identified as attending to the wounded at Professor Charles Krauth's house on the Seminary grounds. Bache participated in discussions among the surgeons as to whether they would be able to hold the Seminary position. "That difference of opinion, however, made none in what we had to do and did, in the line of our duty in caring for the wounded and seeing to their transportation to the hospitals in town. This filled the full measure of the time of all of us, until after 3 o'clock in the afternoon, at which period the battle was still raging as fiercely as ever." He described how he then rode toward the front to observe the battle and assisted in treating the wounded until the tide of battle turned and Confederate forces took Seminary Ridge. He then walked back to town, having given his horse to a wounded officer. "The town was in full possession of the enemy and we surgeons and assistants, prisoners of war at large within our narrow bounds . . . This and the next two days in Gettysburg were to me and all the other surgeons a time of unremitting exertion and care . . ."[18] Both Bache and Heard remained with the First Corps hospitals in town, boarding at the home of Catherine Foster on Washington Street until July 5th.

At about 11 o'clock James Fulton recorded in his diary, after reporting to his division surgeon, William Humphrey, 149th Pennsylvania:

> I found that the Catholic and Presbyterian churches on High Street had been selected as hospitals for the third Division. . . . Jo [Hospital Steward Josiah Lewis] and I took what tea we had with the Sugar—we had not been in Town long until the wounded Began to come in Jo and Myself Began to look around for a place in which we might make tea and Soup.[19]

As Fulton was setting up the 3rd Division hospital site at the Catholic church, General Reynolds was already being carried off the field, one of the early casualties of July 1st. Fulton was kept busy providing the wounded in his hospital with soup and bread assisted by the Myers family and other nearby residents. Among the surgeons operating at the 3rd Division hospital at St. Francis Xavier Roman Catholic Church and the nearby United Presbyterian and Associated Reform Church were Surgeons Pascal Quinan, 150th Pennsylvania; Francis Reamer, 143rd Pennsylvania; Robert Loughran, 80th New York; and Assistant Surgeon Howard Gates, 80th New York. Assistant Surgeon Whiteside Hunter, 149th Pennsylvania, taken prisoner on July 1st, may have been with them as well as Division Surgeon William Humphrey.

Around noon, a pause in the fighting allowed some of the residents of Seminary Ridge to vacate their homes and seek safer quarters. The First Corps had been able to hold their lines against the Confederate forces. Fighting resumed in the afternoon as Confederate general Richard Ewell's Second Corps and the U.S. Eleventh Corps arrived on the field. By four o'clock on July 1st, the Union forces, unable to hold their defensive line, began to retreat south through the town of Gettysburg toward Cemetery Hill. As the Seminary building was overwhelmed by Confederate soldiers, the Union wounded and the surgeons who remained became prisoners. Although originally designated as a 1st Division hospital, most of the surgeons left behind at the Lutheran Seminary were from the 3rd Division of the First Corps: Surgeon Amos Blakeslee, 151st Pennsylvania and his assistant surgeons, Jonas Kauffman and Warren Underwood, and Assistant Surgeon Charles E. Humphrey, 142nd Pennsylvania. Assistant Surgeon Abram Haines, 19th Indiana, remained with the wounded of the 1st Division.

The retreating First and Eleventh Corps troops continued fighting through the town of Gettysburg as they withdrew toward the high ground of Cemetery Hill where reserve Union forces had already arrived. Jacob Ebersole, USA Surgeon 19th Indiana First Corps, later recounted:

> About 4 o'clock, I was ordered to go into Gettysburg to take possession of the railroad depot and establish our hospital therin. This depot was

at the north edge of the town. In the afternoon, the Eleventh Army Corps, under Howard, met the rebels to the north and were fiercely driven back through the city past my hospital. Here my hospital steward, a worthy and faithful man, came hastily to me in great alarm and perturbation, and said "Shall I go to the front or stay with you" He being an enlisted man greatly feared being taken prisoner . . . I replied to him, "Do as you think best, but whatever you do, act quickly." He snatched up his hat or coat and hastened below to the street . . . This was just before sunset. Looking from the upper windows of the hospital, I could see our lines being repulsed, and falling back in utter confusion. . . . I remained here a fortnight, working day and night, till again ordered to join our army, which was in pursuit of Lee.[20]

The First Corps 1st Division hospital also occupied the nearby Adams Express Office staffed by surgeons from the Iron Brigade: Surgeon John Beech, 28th Michigan; Assistant Surgeon John Hall and Surgeon Abram Preston, 6th Wisconsin; Assistant Surgeon Alexander Collar, 24th Michigan; and Assistant Surgeon Peter Arndt, 2nd Wisconsin. From the north window of the building, Dr. Hall had a "perfect view" of the retreat of the Eleventh Corps. In his journal of July 2, 1863, he wrote, "Away went guns and knapsacks and they fled for dear life, forming a funnel shaped tail, extending to the town. The rebels cooly and deliberately shot them down like sheep. I did not see an officer attempt to rally or check them in their headlong retreat. On came the rebels and occupied the town, winning at that point a cheap victory."[21]

At a hotel across from the Railroad Station, probably the Washington House Hotel on Carlisle Street, wounded of the First Corps 1st Division were being cared for by Surgeon James L. Farley, 84th New York, and Surgeon Algernon Sidney Coe, 147th New York. While Coe was tending to an officer in another building, some Brooklyn men began shooting from the upper floor of the hotel as the Confederates entered the town. In an 1885 letter to the *National Tribune*, Coe described the chaotic scene he encountered on returning to the hotel.

The surgeon of the regiment [Coe] with the surgeon of the Fourteenth Brooklyn Regiment [Farley] occupied a large hotel in the lower part of the town, which was very much exposed to the shells of the enemy during the first day, and from the shells of the Union army during the next two days of the battle. In the morning of the first day's battle, the hospital was soon filled with the wounded of these two regiments many of them were wounded slightly. In the confusion, the slightly wounded had the freedom of the hotel. They ransacked the building and found a quantity of liquor of all descriptions; they soon got somewhat intoxicated.[22]

After some of the wounded fired at the enemy, Coe managed to diffuse the situation by disarming the inebriated men and convincing the Confederates not to shoot them. No mention is made of Farley, though his fondness for drinking suggests he may have been among those imbibing. Coe recounted how Confederate and Union soldiers were soon sitting together on the steps joking and exchanging stories about past battles.

The First Corps 2nd Division hospital was located at Christ Lutheran Church on Chambersburg Street. Melvin H. Walker of the 13th Massachusetts described how "An operating table was placed in an anteroom opening off the Main hall and here our surgeon worked with knife and saw without rest or sleep, almost without food, for 36 hours before the first round had been made . . ."[23] Among the surgeons identified there, Assistant Surgeon Edgar Parker, 13th Massachusetts, and Surgeon Charles Alexander, 16th Maine, were wounded on July 1st on the steps of the church during the Union retreat through town.[24] Surgeon Charles Nordquist, 83rd New York, remained as one of the operating surgeons.[25] Other surgeons at Christ Lutheran Church included Assistant Surgeon William F. Osborn, 11th Pennsylvania, who boarded at the Smith McCreary House with the chaplain and another surgeon of his regiment, probably Surgeon James W. Anawalt, 11th Pennsylvania.[26] Other 2nd Division surgeons who remained with their wounded at various locations also became prisoners on July 1st. Assistant Surgeon George P. Tracy, 90th Pennsylvania, reportedly taken prisoner on July 1st and "paroled on the spot," was probably captured at one of the battlefield dressing stations.[27] Surgeon John Windsor Rawlins, 88th Pennsylvania, and his hospital steward, Frank Murphy, stayed behind at the Elias Sheads House on Oak Ridge to care for wounded there.[28] Caroline Sheads reported nursing seventy-two wounded soldiers during the battle, and a Confederate officer allowed her to keep five Union prisoners as attendants to help care for them.[29] One of those prisoners, Asa Sleath Hardman, 3rd Indiana Cavalry, recounted how he

> was one of the seven selected, and remained on the field in that immediate vicinity during the remainder of the battle. After the Rebel lines had swept past, the wounded in our immediate vicinity claimed our undivided attention, and as fast as possible we carried into the house, a large two-story building with full basement, 72 of the worst wounded that lay in the yard. All the night we worked, doing the best we could for the wounded who lay on the field; the most we could do was to provide temporary shelter, remove their bloody garments, bathe their wounds, and see that they had plenty of water. If they had any desire to eat and their own haversacks were empty, we supplied their wants from the full haversack of the nearest dead soldier.[30]

The 2nd Division of the First Corps suffered heavy losses on July 1st. Most of the 16th Maine were either killed or taken prisoner as they withstood the Confederate assault and allowed other regiments to retreat. All three of their medical officers, Surgeon Charles Alexander, Assistant Surgeon William Winslow Eaton, and Assistant Surgeon Joseph Benjamin Baxter became prisoners; both Alexander and Eaton were wounded.[31]

The retreating First Corps established new division hospitals behind the Union lines on Cemetery Hill with Surgeon Alexander Jackson Ward, 2nd Wisconsin, serving as the medical officer in charge, while senior members of the First Corps medical staff, John Theodore Heard and Thomas Hewson Bache, and many of the surgeons, remained with the wounded in town. The 1st Division hospital was located near White Church on the Baltimore Pike with Surgeon George W. New, 7th Indiana, in charge; the 2nd Division located near Conover Farm with Surgeon Enos Chase, 104th New York, in charge; and the 3rd Division at Jonathan Young Farm with Surgeon Adrian Theodore Woodward, 14th Vermont, in charge. Assistant Surgeon John Tullar Brown, 94th New

York, described how he performed "several important surgical operations at 2nd div hospital, in the absence of senior medical officers through the 2nd, 3rd and 4th days until they were released. . . . as the 1st surgeons were all captured with the hospitals in the village and retained through the battle."[32]

Union Eleventh Corps Hospitals

After a short lull, the fighting continued in the afternoon of July 1st with the arrival of two divisions of General Ewell's Confederate Second Corps, marching south from the direction of Carlisle and two divisions of the U.S. Eleventh Corps marching north from Emmitsburg. Daniel Garrison Brinton, 2nd Division Surgeon of the U.S. Eleventh Corps, observed the fighting underway from Cemetery Hill where his division remained in reserve.

> During the day the medical officers were busily engaged in choosing and arranging a hospital. Its location was altered twice owing to the approaching fire of the enemy, but finally it was definitely established in a large barn 1 mile back from the cemetery. The wounded soon began to pour in, giving us such sufficient occupation that from July 1st till the afternoon of the fifth I was not absent from the hospital more than once and then but for an hour or two . . . Four operating tables were going night and day.[33]

The main field hospital of the Eleventh Corps was established at the Spangler farm under the direction of Surgeon James A. Armstrong, 75th Pennsylvania, as officer in charge. The 2nd Division surgeons who remained on Cemetery Hill in reserve throughout the first day of fighting were joined by Eleventh Corps surgeons of the 1st and 3rd Divisions who were able to evade capture and retreat to Cemetery Hill. Surgeon Robert Hubbard, 17th Connecticut, was on the field on July 1st near the Alms House earlier in the day but was able to make it safely to Cemetery Hill where he remained at the Corps hospital until July 14th.[34]

The 1st and 3rd Divisions of the Eleventh Corps had had little time to establish division hospitals in town before they were swept into the battle. Some wounded from the fighting on Barlow's Knoll were taken to the Adams County Almshouse located north of town. As the Eleventh Corps retreated south through town toward Cemetery Hill, Trinity German Reformed Church and the schoolhouse on High Street became refuges for their wounded. Assistant Surgeon Abraham Stout, 153rd Pennsylvania, later provided an account of his experiences on July 1st for the regimental history:

> I was captured between the Poor House and the town. Colonel D.B. Penn [7th Louisiana Infantry] saw me and dismounted. He walked by my side. . . . told me I was his prisoner, (and) taking me to the German Reformed Church, said to me: "You ought to take this church for a Hospital" . . . In less than an hour, it was filled with wounded, mostly Union men. I was in attendance there three days . . . after that we removed the wounded to the public school building.[35]

Ruben Ruch, a wounded soldier of the 153rd Pennsylvania, described ten or twelve amputation tables in one room of the German Reformed Church and doctors with sleeves rolled up to their shoulders at work there.[36] The first day of fighting took a heavy toll on surgeons of the Eleventh Corps: Assistant Surgeon Jacob Laubly, 68th New York, was wounded; Assistant Surgeon Daniel Bishop Wren, 75th Ohio, was captured and held prisoner until November 1863. Surgeon Francis Huebschmann, 26th Wisconsin, nine of his assistants, and 500 wounded were caught between the firing lines and remained prisoners for three days at the German Reformed Church. According to one account by J. H. Blakeman of the 17th Connecticut, one of the wounded on Barlow's Knoll on July 1st, some Union wounded were transported by wagon and ambulance to the schoolhouse and church on the edge of town on July 2nd, "under fire of our artillery, hoping we would be killed by our own guns."[37] This matches a description of Surgeon Huebschmann who "became annoyed by the senseless bombardment and sniping of the southern troops at the hospital. He boldly lay down his instruments after an operation and walked out into the open fields . . . He implored in a booming voice to the troops to stop firing at the wounded."[38] Lt. Col. Rufus Dawes of the

6th Wisconsin succinctly described the Eleventh Corps situation at the end of the day on July 1st. "Our dead lay unburied and beyond our sight or reach. Our wounded were in the hands of the enemy."[39]

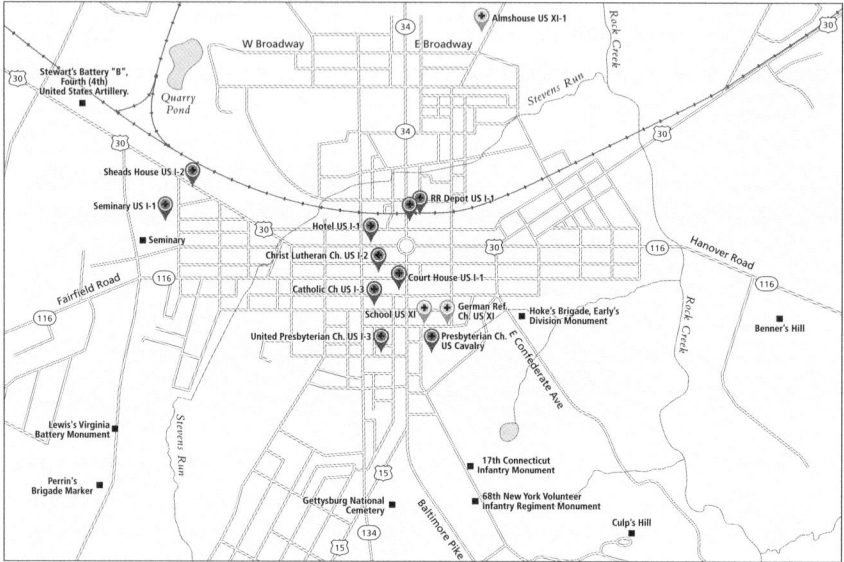

Union Hospitals in and near the town of Gettysburg July 1, 1863.

CONFEDERATE HOSPITALS

By the end of the day on July 1st, Confederates held the town of Gettysburg and positions north and west of town, but they too had suffered severe losses. Some Confederate wounded remained in homes and buildings in town; others were treated in dressing stations or transported to a field hospital. The Confederate hospitals were located behind the various troop positions surrounding the town of Gettysburg.

Hill's First Corps, the first to arrive from the west, established its hospitals in the area west of town between Chambersburg Pike and Fairfield Road. Based on the surgeons associated with various sites, Heth's division hospital was located at the Samuel Lohr Farm along Chambersburg Pike with additional hospitals further in the rear at Cashtown and Fairfield. Senior medical staff included Dr. Henry H. Hubbard, chief surgeon, and William Alexander Spence, division surgeon, 47th Virginia.

Pender's division hospital was established nearby at the Andrew Heintzelman tavern and farm under Pleasant Allen Holt, division surgeon. Assistant Spencer Glasgow Welch, 13th South Carolina, on duty at the Pender division hospital, wrote,

> Most of the casualties of our brigade [Perrin] occurred this day [July 1] . . . When I arrived at the hospital my ears were greeted as usual at such time with the moans and cries of the wounded. I went to work and did not pretend to rest until next morning after daylight. I found that Longstreet had come and that McLaws's Division of his corps was encamped near our hospital. Kershaw's Brigade was almost in the hospital grounds.[40]

Arriving that night, a member of Kershaw's Brigade described the Pender division hospital, located near the Samuel Lohr Farm:

> About three o'clock at night . . . we saw in the plain before us a great sea of white tents, silent and still, with here and there a groan, or a surgeon passing from one tent to another relieving the pain of some poor mortal who had fallen in battle on the morning of the day before. We had come upon the field hospital of Hill where he had his wounded.[41]

General Robert Rodes's division of Ewell's Second Corps arrived midday from the north and established field hospitals north of Gettysburg under the supervision of Hunter Holmes McGuire, medical director, and Harvey Black, senior surgeon. The hospital at the Samuel Cobean Farm along the Carlisle Road may have functioned as a corps hospital staffed by surgeons of various divisions. Rodes's division hospitals were located along the Mummasburg Road and included the farms of David Schriver and Jacob Hankey. Late in the day on July 1st, General Jubal Early's division arrived from the east. Early's division hospitals were located mainly along the Harrisburg Road at the Elizabeth Weible farm, Christian Benner farm, Ross house, and Kime house.

The Union retreat to Cemetery Hill established the battle lines for the next two days of fighting, with the Union occupying the high ground in the so-called fishhook configuration of the high ground, and the

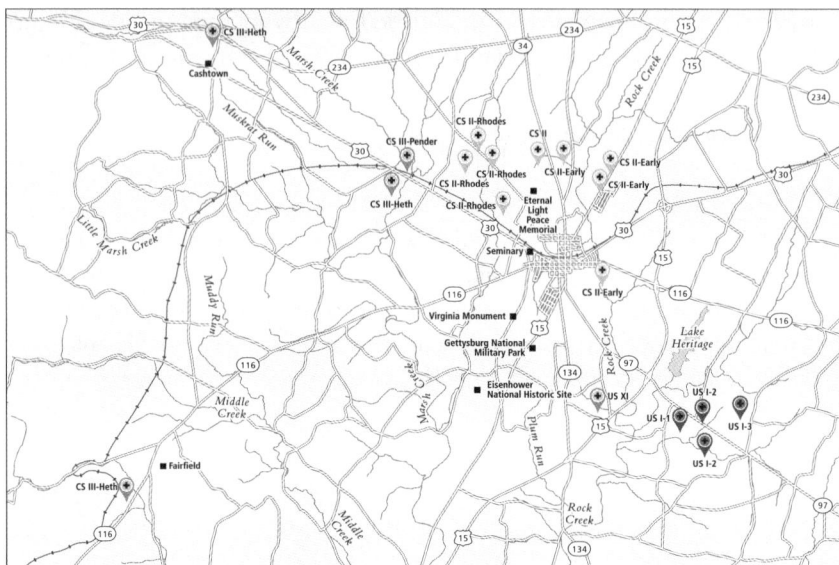

Union and Confederate Hospitals July 1, 1863.

Confederate forces spread out in a long line centered along Seminary Ridge and extending to the west, north, and east. The medical staff of the Union First and Eleventh Corps was now divided between those at the hospitals established on Cemetery Hill and those held as prisoners with the wounded left in town.

In both Union and Confederate hospitals, the work of caring for the wounded of July 1st continued. Surgeon Francis Patterson, 2nd North Carolina Battery, and chief surgeon of Daniel's Brigade was hard at work in the hospitals of Rodes's Second Corps division: "Already the ground was covered by the wounded and mangled, while three of the Medical Staff, including Dr. Frank Patterson, the brigade chief of that department, were hard at work, their coats off and sleeves rolled up, to stem the torrent of death, having a couple of impromptu tables for operating purposes."[42] Assistant Surgeon William W. Gaither, 26th North Carolina, in Pettigrew's Third Corps Brigade, spent all night of July 1st bringing wounded from the field and worked with them all the next day and night.[43] Although it is difficult to separate the impact of the first day of fighting at Gettysburg from the battle as a whole, one estimate of casualties (killed, wounded, and captured) suggests that Union troops totaling 18,000 men suffered 9,000 casualties while the 30,000 Confederate troops may have suffered 7,000 casualties.[44] The next two days would triple the number of casualties and stretch the limits of the medical staff of both armies.

CHAPTER 5

Gettysburg Battle, July 2–3

THE MORNING OF JULY 2ND BEGAN QUIETLY WITH ONLY SCATTERED skirmishing. Harriet Bayly's farm north of Gettysburg on the Carlisle Road was within the area now controlled by Confederates, but nevertheless she ventured out to do what she could for Union wounded left on the field. A member of a local Gettysburg relief society, she had prepared a "market basket full of bread and butter and wine, old linen and bandages and pins."

> There was no fighting that morning. Getting down into the valley I found our wounded lying in the broiling sun, where they had lain for 24 hours with no food and no water . . . The very worst needed a surgeon's care, but while my niece and I gave food to the hungry and wine to the faint I looked after their wounds . . . While busy at work, a German Surgeon came along, saying he had been directed to look after the Union wounded. As he could not speak English, nor I German, I was content to hear his expressions of "goot" "goot" when he examined the work I had done. He was as gentle as a woman in his touch, and it did me good to see how tenderly he handled those wounded men.[1]

The German doctor was probably one of the Eleventh Corps surgeons taken prisoner on July 1st who remained with wounded prisoners at the Alms House.[2] Other Gettysburg women also provided assistance to the Union surgeons caring for wounded in their homes, churches, and other buildings in town.

Many Union wounded from July 1st, like those that Harriet Bayly encountered, remained on the field behind enemy lines without medical treatment, shelter, or water for several days. Treatment of enemy wounded was uneven. Surgeons of both sides gave their own wounded priority, and while there are many accounts of enemy wounded receiving prompt care as prisoners, others received little or delayed medical attention. For example, the instruments and supplies of the First Corps surgeons at the Lutheran Seminary were confiscated when the Confederates took possession of the building. Lt. Col. George McFarland of the 151st Pennsylvania, wounded on the afternoon of July 1st, described how "As soon as the rebels took possession of the hospital, they seized and carried off all the instruments, chloroform, and appliances and thus deprived Surgeon Blakeslee and his assistants . . . the means of amputating shattered limbs or dressing painful wounds . . ."[3] Union wounded at the Seminary had to wait until July 3rd for their surgeons to perform the first amputations with smuggled instruments.

Union surgeons at the hospitals in town had a different experience and were allowed to continue to perform operations after the Confederates took control. At Christ Lutheran Church, Melvin Walker of the 13th Massachusetts described one surgeon operating for thirty-six hours, noting that "A Confederate guard was placed over the hospital, but otherwise we were left to ourselves."[4] Assistant Surgeon James Fulton, 143rd Pennsylvania, noted on July 3rd, "By this time the wounded that had been brought in from the first day had all been operated upon that required an operation most of them being pretty comfortable or as much so as they could be made under the circumstances . . ."[5]

Thomas Hewson Bache, medical inspector of the U.S. First Corps, remained with the wounded, and may deserve credit for persuading General Ewell's staff to let the surgeons in town retain their medical supplies and instruments. An Alumni Register of the University of Pennsylvania describes Bache's work at Gettysburg and notes that he resisted an order of General Early to surrender his medical stores and was complimented by Union and Confederate officers for his work.[6] In addition to his military position, Bache was also a great-great-grandson of Benjamin Franklin and came from a distinguished Philadelphia family with medical, scientific, and military credentials. A fellow surgeon described him as "tall and thin in exact uniform," displaying a military rigidity "only found in that family."[7] He would have been in a position to negotiate with General Early and his chief surgeon, Samuel Morrison, and may have known Ewell's medical director, Hunter Holmes McGuire, from their time together in Philadelphia. Bache, an 1850 graduate of Jefferson Medical College, became attending physician at Children's Hospital in Philadelphia and was an active member of the medical profession there. McGuire, an 1855 graduate of Winchester Medical College, later attended classes at Jefferson and taught private quiz classes in operative surgery in Philadelphia until he organized an exodus of Southern medical students from Philadelphia in 1859 after John Brown's raid of Harpers Ferry. McGuire had already exhibited his support for treating surgeons as noncombatants. In 1862, he helped establish the so-called "Winchester Accord," an agreement between the two armies that confirmed the status of surgeons as noncombatants. Even after the war, he remained an advocate for proper and respectful treatment of military surgeons both nationally and internationally.

UNION HOSPITALS

On Cemetery Hill additional Union troops continued to arrive in Gettysburg during the morning lull in the fighting and throughout the early afternoon of July 2nd, as the remnants of the First and Eleventh Corps were gradually joined by the rest of the Army of the Potomac: The Twelfth Corps arrived on the afternoon of July 1st; the Third Corps divisions on the afternoon of July 1st and early morning of July 2nd; the Second Corps on the morning of July 2nd; and the Fifth Corps divisions on the morning and afternoon of July 2nd. Assistant Surgeon John Billings, 7th U.S. of the Fifth Corps, reported how "about six A.M., July 2d, the Division marched into position and formed line of battle on the right of the somewhat horse-shoe shaped line in which our Army was drawn up. . . ."[8] Also described as a fishhook, following the high ground of Cemetery Hill, the Union position afforded a compact line of defense. The Sixth Corps was the last to arrive on July 2nd.

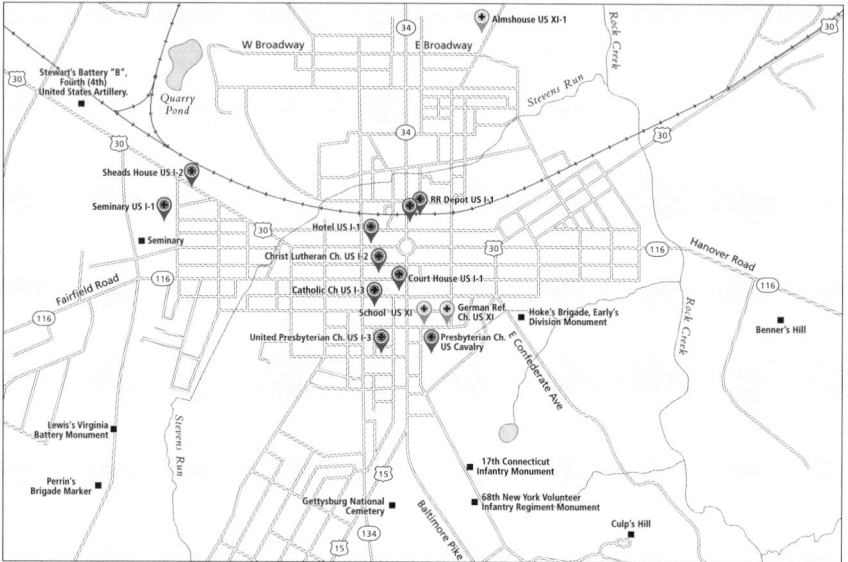

Union Hospitals in and near the town of Gettysburg, July 3, 1863.

Arriving in the afternoon of July 1st, the Twelfth Corps first established its field hospital behind Power's Hill but later moved to a safer location at the George Bushman Farm. The medical director, John McNulty, had apparently ignored the order of July 1st from General Meade to leave all baggage trains except ammunition and ambulances in the rear at Union and Westminster, Maryland. While the other Union hospitals found themselves without hospital tents and cooking equipment, McNulty's Twelfth Corps was fully equipped throughout the battle. Surgeon H. Ernest Goodman, 28th Pennsylvania, was the medical officer in charge.

Field hospital sites were chosen to be as close as safely possible to the front to minimize transportation of seriously wounded, but some Union hospitals set up directly behind the lines along Taneytown Road had to move farther to the rear during the battle. The heavy shelling on July 2nd and July 3rd forced several division hospitals to relocate. On July 2nd, the Second Corps established hospitals near the Granite Schoolhouse but moved to a site along Rock Creek on July 3rd. They would move again after the battle due to flooding. Third Corps hospitals under

Surgeon Thaddeus Hildreth, 3rd Maine, were first located in houses and barns along the Taneytown Road, then moved farther back to the Jacob Schwartz farm along White Run. The Fifth Corps first set up their hospitals at the Jacob Weikert farm and other nearby houses with Surgeon Augustus M. Clark, 4th U.S., in charge, but they later moved across Rock Creek to locations nearer Two Taverns at the farms of Michael Fiscel, Jane Clapsaddle, and Jesse Worley. Last to arrive on the afternoon of July 2nd, the Sixth Corps hospitals were established near the John Trostle house with Surgeon Cyrus Nathaniel Chamberlain as the medical officer in charge.

Union corps hospitals were organized at the division level according to the more centralized system that Jonathan Letterman had established for the Army of the Potomac, beginning in May 1862. During engagements, the divisions established their hospitals under a designated surgeon-in-charge, with three appointed operating teams each made up of a chief surgeon assisted by three additional surgeons. Operators were specifically chosen based on their skill rather than seniority or rank. One surgeon was detailed to provide food and shelter and another to keep the records. These operating teams administered chloroform or ether, performed surgery, and dressed wounds. Hospital stewards, cooks, and nurses were assigned to assist the hospital surgeons.

Assistant Surgeon William F. Breakey, 16th Michigan, described the work of the surgeons at the Fifth Corps 1st Division hospital following the structure outlined by Letterman.

> Two or three operating tables were kept occupied all the afternoon, each with its staff detailed by the division surgeon in charge, the duties of each determined by detail, or by the same professional courtesy which would govern a like case in civil practice. The various positions on the staff being frequently interchanged. I kept records, administered chloroform, made operations and dressed wounds in turn . . .[9]

Breakey also explained the decision-making process for amputations and the importance of keeping accurate records, even on the battlefield.

No grave or capital operation was undertaken without a full consultation and concurrence of the most prominent surgeon present. The assent of the patient was always asked, when the patient was conscious enough to be consulted, and I do not remember that it was ever refused. The name, rank, command, home and address of friends, together with inventory of effects and character of injury and operation, if any, were entered in official record by a member of the staff detailed for that duty.[10]

At the division hospitals of the Second Corps, established on the morning of July 2nd in the area of the Granite Schoolhouse, Surgeon Justin Dwinelle, 106th Pennsylvania, reported, "The Hospital of the Second Division was located before the battle commenced at the stone barn and orchard of Miss Sally Patterson on the Taneytown Road immediately in the rear of the Second Corps which occupied the left centre of the line of battle."[11] The 1st and 3rd Division hospitals were located nearby in a barn and at the edge of woods near the schoolhouse. Surgeon William W. Potter, 57th New York, had arrived in Gettysburg with the 1st Division of the Second Corps a little after daylight on July 2nd.

Just after our regiment had assumed its appointed position, I received an order to report to the division hospital as assistant to Dr. Charles S. Wood, one of the chief operating surgeons of the [1st] division. The place selected for the hospital was in an oak opening east of the Taneytown Road . . . After breakfast, I laid down and slept for several hours, as all was quiet.[12]

He awoke at noon, had dinner, and, since there was still no fighting, rode to Cemetery Hill where he had an excellent view of the field, watching as the U.S. Third Corps moved toward Emmitsburg Pike and the Confederate batteries opened fire. He returned to the hospital, found that his division hospital had been moved due to heavy shelling, and eventually found his way to the new location.

Union Hospitals, July 3, 1863.

CONFEDERATE HOSPITALS

Unlike the Union system initiated by Jonathan Letterman, which placed responsibility for hospitals and ambulances with medical staff, Confederate quartermasters continued to oversee hospital and ambulance logistics, sharing the responsibility for choosing hospital sites with the division surgeon in charge of medical care. As additional Confederate divisions arrived at Gettysburg, hospital locations were chosen relative to troop positions on the field. Hill's Third Corps hospitals, established on July 1, were already located northwest of Gettysburg along the Chambersburg Pike with Heth's division hospital near the Samuel Lohr farm and Pender's division hospital nearby at the Andrew Heintzelman tavern and farm. Anderson's Division arrived late in the day on July 1st and established a hospital farther south at the Adam Butt farm and school. Ewell's Second Corps hospitals on July 1st were located north and east of Gettysburg with Rodes's division hospitals along the Mummasburg Road north of Gettysburg and Early's division hospitals along the Harrisburg Road to the east. Johnson's Division arrived late on July 1st and established hospital sites east of town along the Hunterstown Road, including the W. Henry Montfort, Martin Shealer, Henry Picking, and Christian Benner farms. During the night of July 1st and over the next two days, Longstreet's First Corps arrived and established hospitals to the rear of positions southwest of Gettysburg along the Fairfield Road. McLaws's Division arrived during the night of July 1st and established hospitals at Francis Bream's Black Horse Tavern and at the farms of John Crawford, John Cunningham, and Samuel Johns. Hood's Division arrived at noon July 2nd and established a hospital at the John Edward Plank farm. Pickett's Division arrived last on the morning of July 3rd and set up hospitals at Francis Bream's Mill, the William Myers house, and the John Currens farm.

Confederate Hospitals, July 3, 1863.

While the Union medical corps consistently organized its field hospitals at the corps and division level, Confederates organized their hospitals at the brigade level. Confederate surgeons frequently reference the important role of their brigade surgeon. Regimental surgeons who took on the additional responsibilities of brigade surgeons had a second assistant surgeon assigned to their regiment to help fulfill both roles. The responsibilities of brigade surgeons are illustrated by Surgeon Thomas Salmond, 2nd South Carolina, serving as Kershaw's brigade surgeon on July 2nd when he "came on the field and directed in person the movements of his assistants in their work of gathering up the wounded."[13] Brigade surgeons were also likely to serve as operators in the hospitals based on their rank. In Longstreet's First Corps, for example, McLaws's Division, headed by Division Surgeon Francis Patterson, occupied four locations corresponding to the four brigades, each headed by the brigade surgeon: John Gilmore, 13th Mississippi, of Barksdale's Brigade at John Crawford Farm; Thomas Salmond of Kershaw's Brigade at Francis Bream's Black Horse Tavern; George Todd, 10th Georgia, of Semmes's Brigade at Samuel Johns Farm; and Erwin Eldridge, Cobb's Georgia Legion of Wofford's Brigade, at the Cunningham Farm.

JULY 2ND AFTERNOON

The lull in the fighting ended on the afternoon of July 2nd. The Confederate attack on the Union position began with an exchange of artillery bombardment followed by the Confederate assault on the Union right flank with heavy fighting on Little Round Top, the Peach Orchard, and Wheatfield. As the surgeons in the U.S. Fifth Corps were called into action with their regiments to resist the Confederate attacks, John Shaw Billings of the 2nd Division reported that "About half past three o'clock P.M., the Division was brought into action . . . I accompanied my regiment until they were under fire, and was then ordered to repair to a large stone house and barn near the base of Round Top, and there establish a field hospital . . ."[14] The Weikert house and other local homes were often chosen for hospital sites because they offered shelter, water supply, and supplemental supplies of food and material for bandages. Billings explained,

> On entering the house, I found it unoccupied and bearing evident traces of the hasty desertion of the inmates. A good fire was blazing in the kitchen stove, a large quantity of dough was mixed up, the bake-pans were greased; in short everything was ready for use. I immediately set

my attendants at work baking bread and heating large boilers of water. In five minutes I was joined by the other medical officers detailed for the hospital.[15]

Billings's account also makes clear that the ambulance trains assigned to each division provided adequate medical supplies. Each ambulance carried basic medical supplies, and Autenrieth medical wagons, stocked with additional medical supplies and equipment, accompanied the ambulance trains as part of Jonathan Letterman's medical corps reforms.

> The ambulance train reported to me fifteen minutes later, having with it three Autenrieth wagons, and by the time the operating tables were set up, and materials for dressings arranged, the wounded began to pour in. I performed a large number of operations of various kinds, received and fed 750 wounded, and worked all that night without cessation. An agent of the Sanitary Commission visited me in the evening, and furnished me with a barrel of crackers, a few lemons, etc. Of stimulants, chloroform, morphine and materials for dressing, the Autenrieth wagons furnished an ample supply.[16]

Sanitary Commission wagons also delivered additional food and medical supplies to the Second Corps and other Union hospitals on the evening of July 2nd.[17]

Assistant Surgeon Cyrus Bacon, 2nd U.S., worked with Billings and echoed the experience of the 2nd Division surgeons at the Weikert house.

> At about 5 pm the regiment goes into action. Soon the wounded begin to pour in upon us and now all are very busy . . . The men found some dough prepared for bread which was, some of it, seized and baked by them. I had a lunch off it. It is nearly midnight before retiring. When with Dr. [Edward T.] Whittingham. I go and lie under an apple tree [to] get a little sleep."[18]

William Breakey, working at the 1st Division hospital of the U.S. Fifth Corps at the Lewis Bushman farm, described the system of triage used by the surgeons to sort the wounded and treat the most urgent cases first.

> The wounded came back from the front thick and fast. The operating tables were put up and the work of caring for the wounded went on til far into the night. Actual heaps of amputated limbs accumulated at these tables. The wounded brought to these tables were of the gravest character and that needed the promptest care. Many of the slight wounds were dressed at the front, and of those coming to the Field Hospital the less severe had to wait till the graver and more urgent cases had been attended.[19]

REGIMENTAL SURGEONS

Not all surgeons served in hospitals during a battle. While Union and Confederate surgical teams were assigned to the specific hospitals of their corps, regimental surgeons remained close behind their troops to administer immediate aid at improvised dressing stations. Surgeons and assistant surgeons not assigned to hospitals followed their regiments onto the field of battle equipped with supplies from the regimental hospital knapsacks, setting up aid stations in buildings or sheltered areas. Different terms are used to describe these temporary locations near the front where the wounded first received aid before being sent to a division hospital in the rear. Nathaniel Bierly, a musician in the 148th Pennsylvania, was describing a regimental aid or dressing station when he recounted that on July 2nd at 4 P.M., Colonel McKeen "told us to go to a certain rock that afforded some shelter, to assist Dr. Hamilton in dressing the wounds of those who were wounded on the field."[20] Assistant Surgeon Thomas Fanning Wood, 3rd North Carolina, later described:

> In company with Dr. Coke of the 1st, I established a field dressing station at the foot of the hill in an abandoned farm house. There was a large spring at the door of the house, and everything adapted to our purpose, and especially we were secure from the fire from the front lines. . . . Coke and I were kept busy with the wounded day and night, until we were exhausted, and when our lines were withdrawn we went to the rear to the Division Hospital . . .[21]

The work of regimental surgeons near the line of battle placed them in considerable danger. A number of surgeons and assistant surgeons were wounded during the fighting on July 2nd. Surgeon John Brennan, U.S. 1st Sharpshooters, wounded on July 2nd, had been praised with other surgeons for "coolness displayed in going wherever the discharge of their duties, which often called them to the extreme front, demanded their presence."[22] When the 1st U.S. Sharpshooters were dispatched on the afternoon of July 2nd to determine the position of Confederates, Brennan probably was wounded during heavy fighting with the 10th and 11th Alabama regiments of Wilcox's Brigade. Assistant Surgeon Joseph Stewart, 71st New York, also wounded on July 2nd, was part of Sickles's Third Corps, engaged in the heavy fighting in the Wheatfield later in the evening. Surgeon John Stevenson, U.S. 3rd Maryland, was wounded when Twelfth Corps regiments were moved from Culp's Hill to reinforce

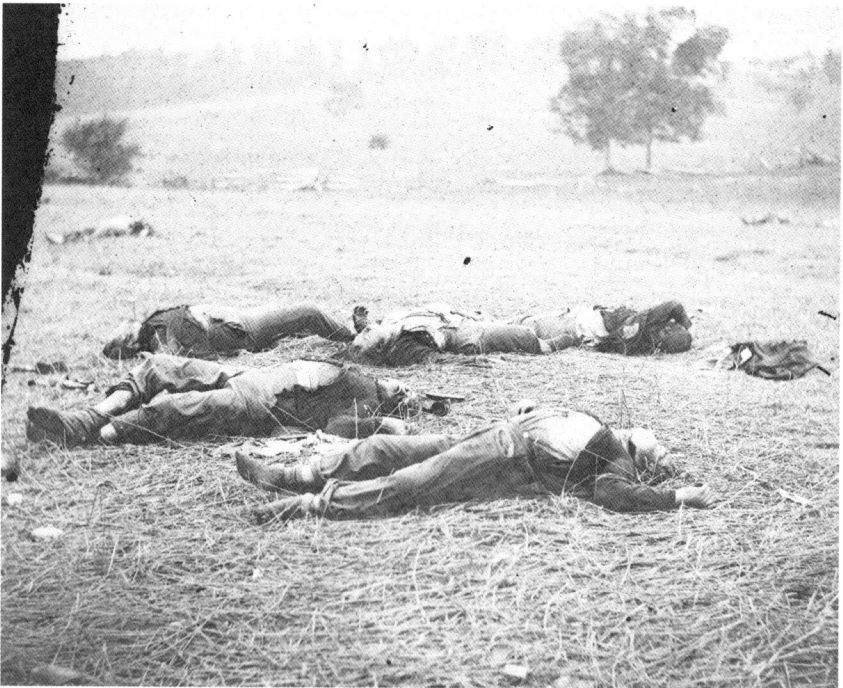

Union dead, of U.S. Third Corps near Rose Farm, Timothy H. O'Sullivan, July 5-6, 1863. Courtesy of Library of Congress, Prints and Photographs Division

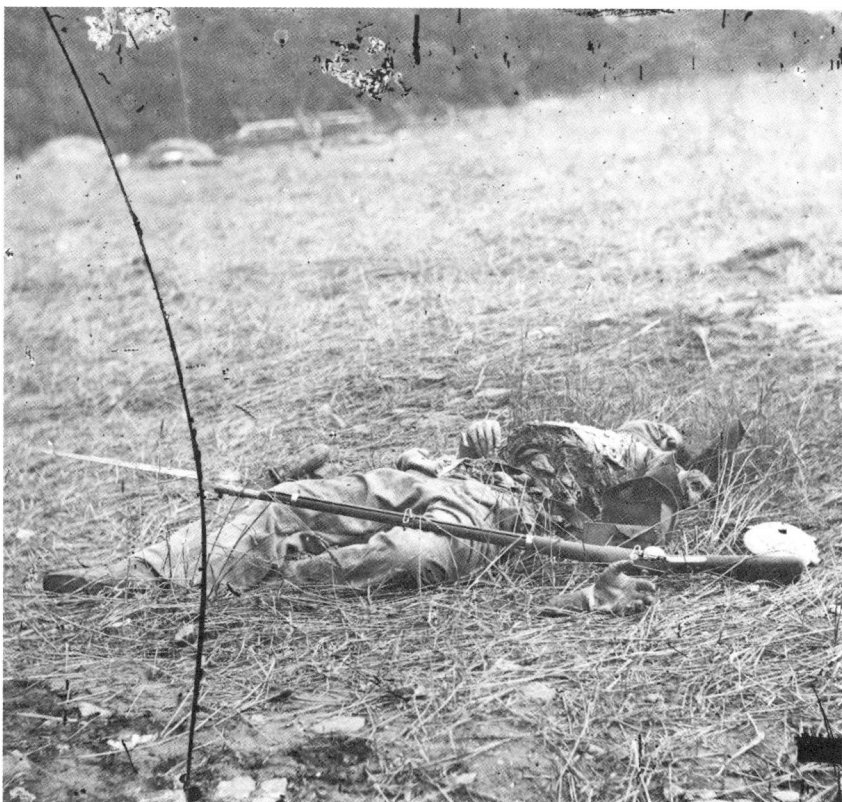

Dead soldier near Rose Farm, Timothy H. O'Sullivan, July 5-6, 1863. Courtesy of Library of Congress, Prints and Photographs Division

Little Round Top. Assistant Surgeon James Groves, 16th Mississippi in Posey's Brigade, was mortally wounded at the Bliss Farm on July 2nd.

As the fight for Little Round Top ended around sunset with the Confederates repulsed, Ewell's Corps launched an attack on the Union right flank to the east. Charging up the slopes of Cemetery Hill and Culp's Hill, Johnson's and Early's troops were not able to dislodge the remaining Twelfth Corps forces, reinforced by Eleventh and First Corps regiments. During the evening attack, Assistant Surgeon Matthew Butler, 37th Virginia, in Steuart's Brigade of Johnson's Division, had his horse shot out from under him while he tended to the wounded, but he was able to limp off the field with only a foot wound.

The fighting on July 2nd continued until 9 or 10 P.M., but the work of the surgeons at aid stations on the battlefield went on through the night. Assistant Surgeon Francis Wafer, 108th New York, was on the field at an aid station, under intense fire during the fighting July 2nd.

> About 10 o'clock [P.M.] all firing ceasing, the rattle of firearms was succeeded by sounds not so exciting but more melancholy the familiar creaking of ambulances collecting the wounded—for which the night was favorable—a beautiful moonlight one. Having shown Lt. Sullivan, 7th West Virginia in charge of our Division [Second Corps 3rd Division] ambulance train any wounded I knew not already removed I then tried to obtain a little rest—which I needed as the excitement of spending the day under fire was followed by much depression.[23]

Assistant Surgeon Albert Vander Veer, 66th New York, described a temporary hospital, probably located at the Peter Frey House along Taneytown Road. "The wounded were brought back and our temporary hospital was located in a farm house that had been built for many years, of stone. We worked through the night with the aid of candles and oil lamps."[24] Assistant Surgeon James Beverly Clifton, 16th Georgia, was on duty on the battlefield at an aid station on July 2nd at the George Rose Farm. In his diary for July 2nd he wrote:

> Our men slept on the "field" that night, which was black with the Enemy's killed and wounded. After attending to all the wounded in the rear, I have concluded to ride over to the Brigade and see how the Men are getting on. It is now after midnight. In riding over the field I can hear nothing but the groans of the wounded which the enemy has not been able to remove, in consequence of our holding the ground. The Moon is shining beautifully, and the ground in front is almost black with Yankees . . . Near the Brigade is a large stone Barn at which I find a great many of our wounded who have not been cared for. I immediately go to work to send them off to the rear.[25]

George A. Bruce, in his history of the 20th Massachusetts, described the aftermath of the second day:

What was a time of rest and sleep to the larger part of the army was a busy period for those whose duty it was to bury the dead and care for the wounded . . . Then was heard the rumblings of wagon wheels, and soon hundreds of ambulances were drawn up in rear of the lines, and with them come surgeons, hospital stewards and stretcher bearers without numbers. With their lighted lanterns they passed to the front and settled over the valley seeking out the wounded, and everywhere finding a full harvest.[26]

Assistant Surgeon Simon Baruch, 3rd South Carolina Battalion, described his experiences caring for the wounded of McLaws's Division following the battle on July 2nd.

Kershaw's Brigade, to which my command belonged, was deployed opposite the peach orchard, preparing to charge a battery of artillery, the shells from which I saw and felt in uncanny proximity, when I received orders to proceed to the field hospital, the Black Horse Tavern, on the Hagerstown road. We had scarcely opened our battle field supplies and hurriedly set up operating tables, constructed of doors laid upon dry goods boxes and barrels, when the ambulances began to bring their sad loads, the result of the charge on the battery in the peach orchard. Wounded men related how the battery had been captured and a Wisconsin brigade supporting it put to flight, when an order to close a gap on the right of the line deflected the charging column and enabled the retreating artillerymen to return and send a destructive enfilading fire of grape into their flank. Nearly all the wounds were on the left side. All day and all night the work continued at the field hospital, and throughout the following day also the wounded came pouring in, many on foot, among them several captured Union soldiers, on two of whom I operated, attending them like our own.[27]

At the 2nd Division hospital of the U.S. Second Corps, J. Franklin Dyer had had a long day. He explained in his journal:

In the early part of the battle of Gettysburg, I was engaged in locating and preparing the hospital, after which I went to work attending to wounded, but frequently had occasion to go to the front, to see that all in my department was going on right—that those surgeons who were ordered to examine the wounded and dispatch them to the rear were at their posts and that the ambulance officers were doing their duty.[28]

On the evening of July 2nd he wrote, "I have sat down in the little kitchen of the house near which we have our hospital to write a few words. The family have fled . . . I have here about five hundred or six hundred in the house, barn and under the apple trees . . . It is now one o'clock . . . I must get a little sleep and be up at daylight."[29]

July 3rd

Assistant Surgeon James Beverly Clifton, 16th Georgia, spent the night at an aid station at the Rose Farm and recorded in his diary that "I did not sleep a moment last night but remained at the old barn trying to get the wounded off. At daylight this morning the artillery commenced firing and finding myself in a critical place, I attempted to make my way to the rear."[30] Assistant Surgeon Francis Wafer, 108th New York, recounted that "Cannonading commenced on our right at 4 AM. This was soon followed by . . . sustained musketry fire occasionally mixed with cheers indicating charges of infantry, and then several hours of relative quiet except for occasional guns testing range and sharpshooters aimed at the artillery stationed along Cemetery Ridge."[31] The cannons Wafer heard were probably Union artillery bombarding a position at the foot of Culp's Hill still held by Steuart's Brigade following the previous night of intense fighting. The Confederate infantry attacked Culp's Hill but after six hours of fighting were forced to withdraw. The occasional artillery fire aimed at Cemetery Hill proved deadly for Assistant Surgeon William Moore, 61st Ohio, who was stationed behind the Union line along the Taneytown Road around 11 A.M. trying to move wounded back from the front. While mounted on his horse, he was struck in the right thigh and died of his wound on July 6th. He was the only fatality in the Union medical corps at Gettysburg.[32]

The Fifth Corps hospitals had been moved back out of range of Confederate cannons earlier that day. John Billings described how

On July 3d, at seven o'clock A.M., I was ordered by Surgeon Milhau, medical director of the corps, to remove the hospital to a point about one mile to the rear. This was done as rapidly as possible. A few shells began to drop in as the first train of ambulances moved off, and by eleven o'clock A.M., the fire on that point was quite brisk. Little or no damage was done, however, and by four o'clock P.M., all the wounded were safely removed. The new site was a grove of large trees, entirely free from underbrush, on the banks of a little creek, about half a mile from the Baltimore turnpike.[33]

Surgeon Justin Dwinelle, 106th Pennsylvania, in charge of the Second Corps hospitals, described the decision to move from the Granite Schoolhouse area to the rear of the George Bushman farm in anticipation of an attack on July 3rd. "Preparations were being made for the removal when the enemy commenced their attack upon the left centre at one o'clock. We were literally Shelled out and compelled to hurry forward our movements with all possible dispatch."[34]

Although there is some disagreement about the exact time, Professor Michael Jacobs at Gettysburg College precisely recorded the beginning of the Confederate cannons at 1:07 P.M. All accounts agree that the colossal exchange of artillery that ensued and lasted for two hours was like nothing they had ever experienced. At the Catholic church in town, Assistant Surgeon James Fulton, 143rd Pennsylvania, remarked, "Of all that I have seen in war this Exceeded in grandeur And Solemnity—about 300 guns playing the earth as it seemed to us would tremble. Shells bursting in air as they went Screaming over us, an occasional Striking in town . . ."[35]

Assistant Surgeon Francis Wafer, 108th New York, had spent the morning with his regiment, but after accompanying a wounded officer to a temporary hospital, he found more than enough to do and remained there for the rest of the day. Described as a small stone farmhouse on the Taneytown Road, probably the Frey House, "This temporary hospital was merely a place where some surgeons who were on duty on the field, assembled to apply light dressings to the wounded and superintend the removal of the wounded in ambulances to the operating hospital further in the rear."[36] Located in the center of the Union line, it received heavy fire. "While the heavy cannonade lasted it became impossible for the Surgeons to do anything—but patiently await the result. The hum of fragments of shells around us was incessant."[37] Assistant Surgeon Edward Heckel, 27th Pennsylvania of the Eleventh Corps, stationed near the Cemetery, likely was wounded during the heavy bombardment on July 3rd.

Then came the now famous attack of Pickett's Charge, and Wafer and the other surgeons of the Second Corps were soon overwhelmed with casualties.

> As soon as the firing had abated a little, the wounded began to arrive in vast numbers & in the course of an hour fully a quarter of an acre about the house where it was—was pretty thickly covered with victims of the struggle . . . The few bandages in our Medical Knapsacks were already exhausted. We found many homespun linen sheets in the house that were torn into strips & made a good substitute while they lasted. Our assistants exhausted the only well there giving them water, as that & some Morphine . . . was all we could do until [they were] removed to the large field hospital."[38]

At the Second Corps Field Hospital, Surgeon William W. Potter, 57th New York, had managed to sleep for a few hours but was up by daylight on July 3rd.

> After assisting at many operations, as well as making a number myself to spell the chief operator, I once again repaired to General Zook's side . . . until near two o'clock. . . . The famous cannonade, the prelude to Pickett's heroic charge, was in full blast at this hour, and Zook breathed out his life amidst the uproar and mad clamor of two hundred guns—the grandest combat of field artillery the world ever beheld. As soon as the general breathed his last I made haste for the front where I knew my services were needed. I arrived at the hospital not a moment too soon. After the sound of the cannon died away there was a short interval of comparative silence. Then came the infantry battle. The 2nd Corps received the weight of the shock, and our hospital was soon overflowing with wounded men in the care of whom we were busy all

night. I took a short nap near morning, but began work again soon after daylight [on] the 4th.[39]

Among the many wounded of the Second Corps was Assistant Surgeon Frederick Dudley, 14th Connecticut, positioned near the center of the line defending Cemetery Hill. He was wounded in the shoulder and later treated at the Corps hospital.[40]

At the Twelfth Corps hospital, at the George Bushman Farm, Surgeon John J. H. Love, 13th New Jersey, described how,

> During the cannonade on the afternoon of July third, the surgeons and attendants became so excited that all, for a time, left their work and crowded the top of a knoll in rear of the hospital, from which a view could be had toward our line of battle. The roar was terrific; the ground under us trembled . . . the cannonade begins to slacken and die out, and in a little while come the rattle and steady roar of musketry. Which side holds its own? No ambulances come in; no messages from the front . . . The moments seem hours. Presently an orderly is seen hurrying across the fields, "The union lines stand firm," he shouts. Each man breathes a silent prayer of thanks to God and then with three cheers for General Meade and the Army of the Potomac, all return to work.[41]

In approximately one hour, the Confederate assault on Cemetery Hill had been repulsed with devastating results. Assistant Surgeon William H. Taylor, 19th Virginia, later described the casualties in Garnett's Brigade of Pickett's Division. Sixty-five percent of his brigade was lost and every officer of his regiment was killed or wounded on July 3rd. He had been with the brigade during the charge.

> As the troops advanced we kept with them and closely scrutinized the locality in the search for places suitable for stations, noting trees, fences, straw-stacks, depressions of the surface, or whatever offered a show of shelter, and especially looking for gullies, which were the most desirable of all. It was necessary for these stations to be near the engaged men, and we could not always find a satisfactory place; and sometimes our

only protection while ministering to a wounded man was by sitting or even lying, with him on the ground.[42]

He recalled that their aid station was located in a "little dell in a grove conveniently in the rear of the troops, where they waited for the battle which began "with that furious cannonade which is remembered as the most thunderous that has ever shaken the earth." Finding himself in the line of fire, he fled, but was struck in the leg, losing three or four inches of tissue from his gluteus maximus muscle. Assistant Surgeon Robert Worthington, 7th Virginia with Kemper's Brigade, was also wounded during the charge.

Chaplain Peter Tinsley, 28th Virginia, described the scene at Garnett's brigade hospital that afternoon in his diary on July 3rd:

> The scene at our hospital is horrid beyond description & by far the worst I have ever seen. Friend after friend comes and gives the most dreadful account of the slaughter of his comrades so that, that which we hear of is worse almost than what we see . . . After all the men are sent off to Division Hospital at Breams Mill I go there also to attend to the wounded, taking with me the body of Maj. Wilson to bury it.[43]

During the night while ambulances continued to bring wounded to the hospitals, the Confederate army pulled back from the town of Gettysburg and consolidated its position along Seminary Ridge. Asa Hardman, attending to the wounded at the Sheads house, recalled that, on July 3rd,

> As night approached, we tried to gather any information as to the condition and intentions of the enemy. As fast as any news was gained it would be brought in and reported to the wounded officers and to our surgeons, who were supposed to know more about the situation than we did . . . By the time it became fully dark, it was evident to us that Lee was preparing to retreat.[44]

CHAPTER 6

Aftermath, July 4–6

"The whole army is like a great monster panting for breath," Assistant Surgeon William Child, 5th New Hampshire, wrote home after a battle.[1] Thomas Galwey of the 8th Ohio used similar language when he wrote that on the night of July 3rd, "Both armies were now utterly exhausted. The one defeated and taking breath before beginning a general retreat; the other now confident yet compelled by reasons of humanity to nurse the thousands of wounded and to bury the numberless dead of both armies that now strewed the ground in all directions."[2] The men of the two armies that had clashed for three days at Gettysburg were indeed exhausted, but the surgeons had little opportunity to rest and recuperate. A flood of wounded continued to pour into the various hospitals from the battlefield. Surgeon Henry Janes, U.S. 6th Corps, described the cruel aftermath of battlefield wounds that he and other surgeons faced. He contrasted the pageantry of "an army marching past in well aligned platoons, with colors floating, bands playing . . . arms polished and shining in the sunlight," with the stark reality of

> The wounded at the field hospital during and after the battle as they are brought on the long lines of stretchers and ambulances. This man in the deep coma has concussion of the brain; see the pitiful expression of this boy with both eyes shot out; the horrible appearance of this officer whose nose, jaw, and almost all his face has been torn off by a shell; here is a boy with both legs torn off by a shell; another with both arms completely shattered; this one with the distressed breathing and frothy

blood oozing from mouth and nose is wounded in the lungs; observe the ghastly pallor and faintness of the man with blood-soaked clothes, he is dying of hemorrhage; notice the apathetic dullness of some and the agonizing pain of others of these poor filth-covered creatures shot through the abdomen.[3]

The image of the surgeons at their tables, swiftly amputating arms and legs, was frequently described with horror by non-medical observers. For the surgeons, however, amputation offered their patients the best option for surviving compound fractures and mangled limbs, even without modern antiseptic conditions. Those with mortal wounds, especially to the torso, could only be given morphine to alleviate their pain. Decimus et Ultimus Barziza, a wounded Confederate prisoner treated at the U.S. Twelfth Corps hospital, witnessed the streams of blood and piles of arms and legs as surgeons performed amputation after amputation in full sight. But his graphic description of the sights and sounds of suffering among the wounded is even more harrowing.

> He who has never seen the rear of an army during and immediately after a battle, can form no idea of the scene, while the mere mention of a Field Hospital to a soldier, brings up recollections of blood and brains, mangled limbs, protruding entrails, groans, shrieks and death. And when night comes upon them, and their wounds begin to grow chill, and pains shoot piercingly through them, then the deep and agonizing groans, the shrill death-shriek, the cries for water, opium, any thing, even death, make up the most horrible scene that can be conceived of.[4]

It was a scene repeated throughout the hospitals of both armies where surgeons worked to alleviate suffering and save lives, amputating limbs, removing bullets, binding up wounds and administering morphine to the dying. The current estimate of more than 30,000 wounded overwhelmed the hospitals and surgeons of both sides. The American Battlefield Trust cites the total number of wounded as 14,529 Union and 18,735 Confederate.[5]

CONFEDERATE RETREAT

The Confederate medical staff was still dressing wounds and performing operations on the evening of July 3rd when General Lee began issuing orders for surgeons to prepare the wounded for evacuation in the retreat from Gettysburg. His goal was to remove as many wounded as possible along with the large wagon trains of supplies and livestock plundered from the farms and towns of Pennsylvania. The destination for the Confederate wounded was the General and Receiving Hospital at Staunton, Virginia, 200 miles away; from there they could be transported by railroad to the hospitals of Richmond. First the long Confederate wagon trains had to make their way through mountain passes and across the Potomac River back into Virginia. Even as the wounded from July 3rd were being brought into the Confederate hospitals to be treated, surgeons had already begun to sort the wounded into those who could walk on their own, those well enough to be transported in the available ambulances and wagons, and those too badly injured to travel who must be left behind as prisoners. Every available vehicle was loaded with wounded for the long and painful journey back to Virginia.

Ewell's Second Corps divisions were the first to receive orders to remove as many wounded as possible from the field hospitals farthest east along Hunterstown Road at the same time that their forces were withdrawing from battle positions north and east of Gettysburg. The ambulances and wagons carrying the wounded continued toward Fairfield where they waited until they could begin the arduous journey over the mountains on July 4th through pouring rain and darkness. The surgeons in charge of each division made the arrangements for the wounded in their hospitals. Assistant Surgeon Thomas Fanning Wood, 3rd North Carolina, was assigned to report on the number of wounded in Johnson's Division and identify those who were able to walk or be transported. "The men were not slow to find out that we were preparing to fall back and leave them as prisoners."[6] As Wood surveyed his patients, he recalled how he "knew the men well by this time, and they greatly desired that I remain with them." Instead, Surgeon Dabney Herndon, 15th Louisiana, a more senior surgeon, was ordered to remain with the wounded. Wood described how "Every empty wagon was loaded with wounded men, and the roads leading toward the Potomac were full of troops, stragglers, slightly wounded men, making their way as they could. But there was no panic."[7]

The other divisions of Ewell's Corps received similar orders to remove as many of the wounded as could travel. Surgeon Isaac Scott Tanner, 21st North Carolina, a brigade surgeon in Early's Division, recorded casualties of the dead and wounded of his regiment and noted the names of the wounded "left in hospital near Gettysburg."[8] Assistant Surgeon Abner Embry McGarity, 21st Georgia, accompanied the train of retreating wounded from Rodes's Division. "On the evening of July 4th, I was sent back [to] Williamsport with the wounded of our Brigade that were able to travel—those that were not were left at Gettysburg. That night, a very dark and rainy one, some Yankee Cavalry broke in upon us and captured a good many of our ambulances and wagons with a good many of our wounded."[9]

While Ewell's ambulance and baggage trains were assembling at Fairfield to begin the arduous journey through Monterey Pass toward Hagerstown on the way to Williamsport under Major Harman, Ewell's quartermaster, Gen. John Imboden, was tasked with organizing the First and Third Corps trains to travel by way of Cashtown Pass. The Third Corps ambulance trains of Heth's Division were ready to move before dawn on July 4th and Anderson's Division was ready to leave at 6 A.M.

Longstreet's First Corps was the last to leave Gettysburg. Assistant Surgeon James Clifton, 16th Georgia, wrote in his diary for July 4th: "No fighting today. It has been raining very hard today. It is reported that our Army will fall back tonight . . . There is some foundation for the rumor, as we have distinctly heard artillery or wagons moving all day."[10] Clifton noted on July 5th, "Left the battle-field of Gettysburg last night about midnight, and marched over the worst roads I ever saw."[11] Before leaving, Erwin James Eldridge, Wofford's brigade surgeon, left $75 in cash with Acting Assistant Surgeon David H. Ramsaur, 18th Georgia, to purchase supplies for wounded left with him at the Cunningham Farm.[12]

LEFT IN THE HANDS OF THE ENEMY

Louis C. Duncan's history of the battle estimated that 5,000 Confederate wounded were left behind in the Confederate field hospitals, and an additional 1,800 were held as prisoners in Union hospitals. Approximately seventy Confederate surgeons were left behind and remained on duty in Confederate field hospitals in Gettysburg on July 5th, becoming prisoners of war "left in the hands of the enemy."[13]

Hunter Holmes McGuire, medical director of Ewell's Second Corps, ordered Surgeon William Riddick Whitehead, 44th Virginia, to stay behind to oversee the hospitals of Johnson's Division and the rest of the Second Corps. According to Whitehead's account, "About eight o'clock PM of July 3rd, the Corps Surgeon, Dr. Hunter McGuire called to see me and told me of General Lee's preparations for retreat that night and selected me to take charge of all the wounded of Ewell's Corps who could not be conveniently removed."[14] Although he was promised four additional surgeons from Johnson's Division, Whitehead recalled that only Surgeon Frank Lavigne Taney, 10th Louisiana, reported to him.[15] Chief surgeon of Early's Division, Samuel B. Morrison, selected one surgeon from each brigade to remain at a ratio of approximately one surgeon for every sixty-five wounded. This was consistent with patient/surgeon ratios in other divisions ranging between fifty and one hundred patients for each surgeon left behind.[16] General Rodes reported that he left half of the wounded in his division, about 760 patients, with four surgeons, six assistants, ninety-seven attendants, and ten days' rations, but Federal records indicated as many as 800 wounded and only two surgeons at each of the three hospital locations for Rodes's Division.[17]

Of the approximately 4,400 wounded of Hill's Third Corps, about 1,761 wounded were left at Gettysburg. Surgeon John Henry McAden, 13th North Carolina, was left in charge of 700 wounded of Pender's Division with four other surgeons, one from each brigade.[18] Seven surgeons of Heth's Division were left behind with more than 900 wounded at various locations.[19] In the hospital at Butt Farm, 111 wounded were left with Surgeon Henry de Saussure Fraser, chief surgeon of Anderson's Division and seven other surgeons.[20] Some of Hill's wounded had previously been moved to the rear in hospitals set up in Fairfield. Duncan reports that 871 wounded were left in Fairfield in the care of Surgeon John Wilson, 11th North Carolina, and Surgeon Benjamin Franklin Ward, 11th Mississippi; both were captured at the hospital on July 5th.

In Longstreet's First Corps, McLaws's Division left 576 wounded with ten surgeons, two chaplains, and seven nurses and cooks.[21] Division Surgeon Francis William Patterson, 17th Mississippi, remained in charge. Hood's Division reportedly left 515 out of a total of 1,542 wounded at the division hospital located at the John Edward Plank Farm with Surgeon Thomas Alexander Means, 11th Georgia, in charge of eight other surgeons.[22] Pickett's Division left about 280 of its 1,200 wounded at Francis Bream's Mill and the Myers and Currens farms. At the John S. Crawford farm, Acting Assistant Surgeon Robert Leonidas Knox, 17th Mississippi, and Acting Assistant Surgeon C. H. Brown, 18th Mississippi, remained with the wounded there. Assistant Surgeon Simon Baruch, 3rd South Carolina, had been assigned to McLaws's division hospital at Blackhorse Tavern during the battle where he performed operations on Union and Confederate wounded from July 2 to 4. Having received "a command from General Lee for Drs. Pearce, Nott and Baruch to remain at the Black Horse Tavern field hospital 'until further orders'" the night before, Baruch recalled the scene on July 5th: "The morning found us amid novel surroundings. The slightly wounded had been removed, most of them being able to march, The field hospital contained two hundred and twenty-two seriously wounded men, ten orderlies, and three surgeons, The demands of hunger claimed paramount attention, for we had not eaten a meal in three days."[23] In his diary, Chaplain Tinsley of 28th Virginia left a detailed description of Pickett's division hospital at Bream's Mill where he remained with the surgeons on July 4th.

We take leave of our friends who had been lingering around the Hosp. Dr. E. Rives of 28th Va is left in charge of the Division Hosp. & with him are Grigsby Mayo of Kemper's Brig. Nowlin of Armistead's & Harrison of Garnetts & myself as Chaplain. (Chaplains however have an option in this matter.) We have our tents pitched in Curren's yard & take our meals in his house, we ourselves furnishing the raw material

& Mary (the servant girl) preparing the two meals for us. Mrs. C. was absent.[24]

About two o'clock on July 5th, Gen. John Sedgwick's U.S. Sixth Corps troops took possession of the Bream's Mill hospital and promised to send medical staff and supplies. Tinsley spoke highly of Sedgwick's men: "In other uniforms they might pass for southerners if they could only tell the straight truth. They are halted in front of our Hosp. & from the free and friendly conversations between them & our wounded, you would suppose they were friends and acquaintances."[25]

THE UNION HOSPITALS

Residents, Union surgeons, and the wounded in the town of Gettysburg woke on July 4th to the realization that Confederate troops had left during the night. The wounded of July 1st and their surgeons were no longer prisoners, but neither side was completely sure what might happen next. Confederate sharpshooters along Seminary Ridge held back any further attack by Union forces and helped shield the continuing retreat.

The Union surgeons at work in the corps hospitals behind the lines had more than enough to do to care for their own and the captured Confederate wounded and had little opportunity to assess the military situation. Surgeon Benjamin Rohrer, 10th Pennsylvania, wrote in his diary for July 4th from the 3rd Division, Fifth Corps hospital: "We were busy attending to the wounded, and heard little of what was going on at the front. Our division left Gettysburg on the 7th."[26] Assistant Surgeon Cyrus Bacon, 2nd U.S., described his work in the 2nd Division 5th Corps Hospital:

Independence day. We celebrate by the retiring of Lee's army. They have gone . . . At the hospital we are early at work. Good day. Colton and Brenneman assist me at the operating table. Colton is "tiffed." Rain in afternoon and we doctors showed the men that we were exposed to it as well as they.[27]

Assistant Surgeon Alfred Thorley Hamilton, 148th Pennsylvania, was still working in a field hospital when he wrote in his diary for July 4th:

> This national day was enlivened by our patriotic airs by the bands inspired the troops—an occasional shell passed over us during the day [.] Skirmishing was kept up most of the day by pickets—Our brigade still supported the batteries in the same position they held during the whole fight—I had charge of about thirty rebel wounded, in a house of Jacob Hummelbaugh . . .[28]

U.S. Surgeon Daniel Garrison Brinton described his experiences as division surgeon, 2nd Division, 11th Corps, during and after the battle.

> From the 1st of July till the afternoon of the fifth, I was not absent from the hospital more than once and then but for an hour or two. Very hard work it was, too, & little sleep fell to our share. Four operating tables were going night and day. On the 4th of July, which in its surroundings gloomy enough, was enlivened by our belief that we had gained a victory, the number in the hospital was 1000. A heavy rain came over in the afternoon and as we had laid many in spots without shelter some indeed in the barnyard where the foul water oozed up into their undressed wounds, the sight was harassing in the extreme. We worked with little intermission, & with a minimum amount of sleep. On one day I arose at 2 AM & worked incessantly till midnight. I doubt if ever I worked harder at a more disagreeable occupation.[29]

Surgeon Jonas W. Lyman, 57th Pennsylvania, provided a report on his work at the 1st Division Third Corps hospital.

> operating staff of the division, placing their tables near each other, were constantly employed, while the remaining officers were no less busily engaged in dressing and supplying the general wants of the hundreds of wounded men who continued to increase our numbers during that day and the succeeding night. As usual, a large proportion of the graver cases of injury were the last to be brought from the field, and the cases for operation on the night of the 3d and morning of the 4th accumulated, occupying the entire operating force without intermission.[30]

REMOVAL OF THE WOUNDED

Letterman's new ambulance corps had made significant improvements in the capacity of the Army of the Potomac to remove wounded from the battlefield. Some Union wounded who remained inaccessible in areas under Confederate control through July 4th were left unattended on the battlefield from July 1st to 3rd. Assistant Surgeon William Breakey, 16th Michigan, working at the 1st Division Fifth Corps hospital, described how "On the morning of the 4th of July, when we hardly knew whether the battle was ended or we had been victorious, I was sent with ambulances and attendants with stretchers to look for wounded still on the field."[31] According to Jonathan Letterman's official report, Union wounded had been removed from the field within Union lines by July 4th.

> The ambulance corps throughout the army acted in the most commendable manner during those days of severe labor. Notwithstanding the great number of wounded, amounting to fourteen thousand one hundred and ninety-three, I know, from the most reliable authority and from my own observation, that not one wounded man of all that number was left on the field within our lines early on the morning of the 4th of July. A few were found after daylight beyond our farthest pickets, and these were brought in, although the ambulance men were fired upon, when engaged in this duty, by the enemy, who were within easy range.[32]

Assistant Surgeon Francis M. Wafer, 108th New York, described that by July 4th, the wounded left on the field were mainly Confederates.

> Our stretcher bearers had removed most of their wounded from our front during the night, but some unfortunates had escaped observation, or were in the hurry of the occasion considered too hopelessly injured to remove. On our men attempting to remove these during the day they were deliberately fired at by the enemy sharpshooters. Consequently they were doomed to lie there another day by the recklessness or barbarity of their comrades . . . Although the night was wet, it was one of rest & as such appreciated by the weary Army of the Potomac.[33]

Union surgeons clearly understood the medical consequences of removing the wounded from the battlefield as quickly as possible. Surgeon William B. Chambers, 97th New York, left in charge of the First Corps 2nd Division hospital, reported, "we had in our Hospital 4 cases of Tetanus, 3 of which were confined to Confederates who all died. One of which is a Union Soldier who I believe ultimately got well, the only reason that can be given for this improportionate mortality was the fact that the Confederates after being wounded were exposed for two nights on the Battle Field."[34]

BURIAL OF THE DEAD

Meade reported that "July 5 and 6 were employed in succoring the wounded and burying the dead."[35] Responsibility for burials and the proper handling of dead bodies often came under the direction of the medical corps. Those who died in hospitals were buried as soon as possible for sanitary and health reasons, while burial of those left slain on the field often fell to members of regimental details who made every effort to identify the dead, but many were buried as "unknown." The sorting of both dead and wounded was aided by the Union's system of corps, division, and brigade badges sewn to caps and uniforms. Thomas Galwey of the 8th Ohio described the work of the regiments in burying the dead July 4th and 5th.

> As for us we have been attending to our wounded and have been picking up such of our dead as we could recognize. Each regiment selects a suitable place for its dead and puts a head-board on each individual grave. The unrecognized dead are left to the last, to be buried in long trenches.[36]

As always, the army gave priority to the wounded and dead of its own ranks. Burial of Confederate dead continued for several days following the battle, sometimes by details of Confederate prisoners.

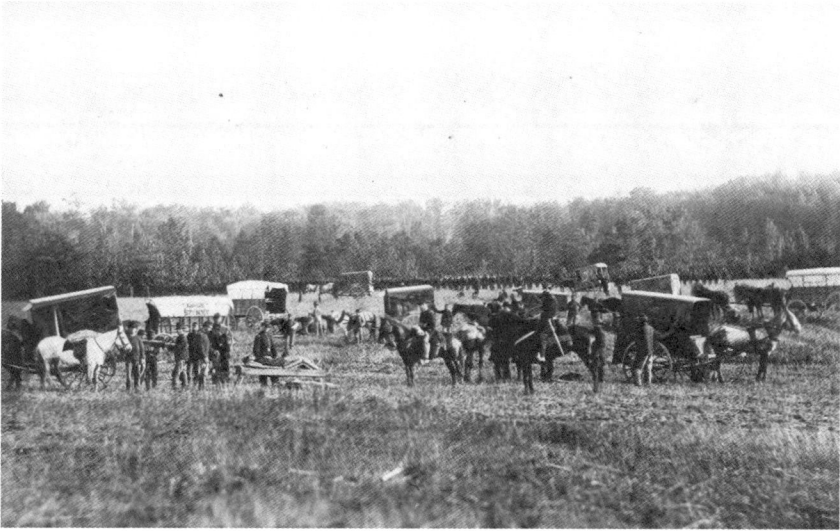

Ambulance corps removing wounded from battlefield. The ambulance corps of the Army of the Potomac worked throughout the battle to remove wounded to hospitals as quickly as possible. Courtesy of U.S. Army Heritage and Education Center, Carlisle, Pennsylvania

FOOD AND SUPPLIES

General Meade's military decision to hold back hospital supplies during the battle created additional hardships for the wounded in the immediate aftermath of the battle. Jonathan Letterman complained that:

> Its effect was to deprive this department of the appliances necessary for the proper care of the wounded, without which it is as impossible to have them properly attended to as it is to fight a battle without ammunition. In most of the corps the wagons exclusively used for medicines moved with the ambulances, so that the medical officers had a sufficient supply of dressings, chloroform and such articles until the supplies came up, but the tents and other appliances which are as necessary were not available until the 5th of July.[37]

John McNulty, medical director of the Twelfth Corps, who had disobeyed or ignored Meade's orders, could smugly report, "It is with extreme satisfaction that I can assure you that it enabled me to remove

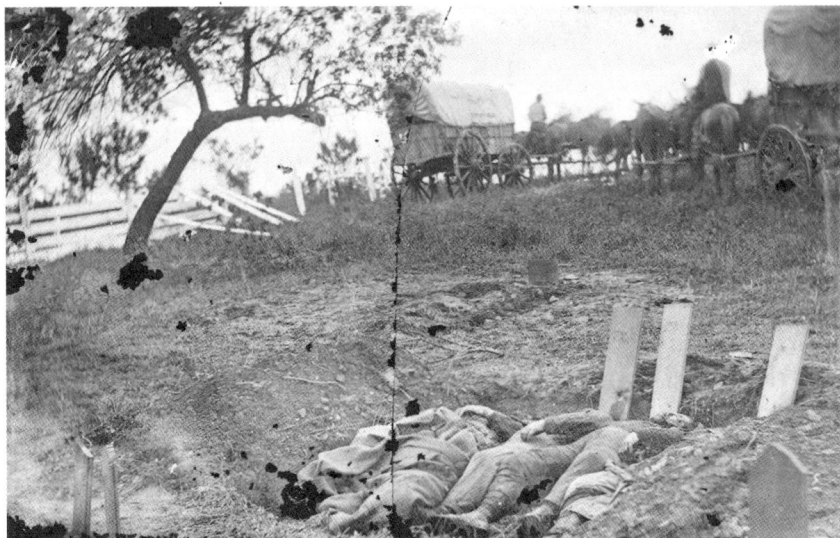

Unfinished Confederate graves near the center of the battlefield. These burials show the U.S. Army practice of positioning a board to identify graves. Timothy H. O'Sullivan, July 5-6, 1863. Courtesy of Library of Congress Prints and Photographs Division.

the wounded from the field, shelter, feed them and dress their wounds, within six hours after the battle ended; and to have every capital operation performed within twenty-four hours after the injury was received."[38]

John Shaw Billings's experience at the Fifth Corps hospital reflects the situation facing the medical officers of the other corps hospitals whose medical supply wagons had been held back during the battle. Needed supplies had to be transported by wagons until the damaged railroad tracks to Gettysburg could be repaired.

> On the morning of July 5th, the regimental medical supply wagons came up, and from them I removed all the hospital tents and tent flies, with two hospital mess chests. On this day, the Division moved. I was left behind in charge of the hospital, which then contained about eight hundred wounded. Twenty men were detailed from the division to act as assistants about the hospital. I was also given two ambulances and two six mule wagons. The ambulance train, which had up to this time been engaged in collecting the wounded of the Division from the

various corps hospitals to which some of them had been carried, and in hauling straw for bedding, accompanied the Division, as did also the Autenreith wagons . . . By this time Surgeon Brinton had reached White Church with a special medical supply train, and from him I procured such supplies as were most needed . . . The greatest want which I experienced was that of tools. I had not a shovel or pick with which to bury the dead or construct sinks and no axes. I was compelled to send out a foraging party in procuring two shovels and an axe. Seventeen hospital tents were pitched.[39]

The destruction of railroad bridges and tracks by the invading Confederates interrupted the delivery of much-needed supplies to Gettysburg and delayed the evacuation of the wounded to hospitals in major cities. Until service was restored to the outskirts of Gettysburg on the evening of the 6th, the closest rail service located 25 miles away in Westminster, Maryland, meant that supplies to Gettysburg had to travel by wagon over muddy roads. Wagons from Harrisburg and the east faced difficult ferry crossings due to the strategic burning of the Wrightsville bridge over the Susquehanna.

Letterman's official report maintained that there were sufficient medical supplies during the battle provided by the ambulances and the Autenrieth wagons equipped with anesthetics, dressings, drugs, and instruments. Individual surgeons also reported that they had sufficient medical supplies during the battle. Except for the Twelfth Corps, the rest of the army lacked the tents, bedding, clothing, cooking utensils, and food normally transported in the hospital supply wagons. Although Letterman requested that the hospital trains be brought up immediately, Meade at first allowed only half the wagons, because he was still concerned about Confederate cavalry raids. U.S. Medical Purveyor Jeremiah Bernard Brinton arrived with his auxiliary supply wagon train from Westminster on the evening of July 4th. The remainder of the army supply wagons arrived July 5th.

Without railroad access, food was in short supply by July 4th. The two armies had already consumed most of the food available from townspeople in Gettysburg. On July 4th, Chief Commissary of Subsistence Henry F. Clarke was able to distribute 30,000 army rations to hospitals

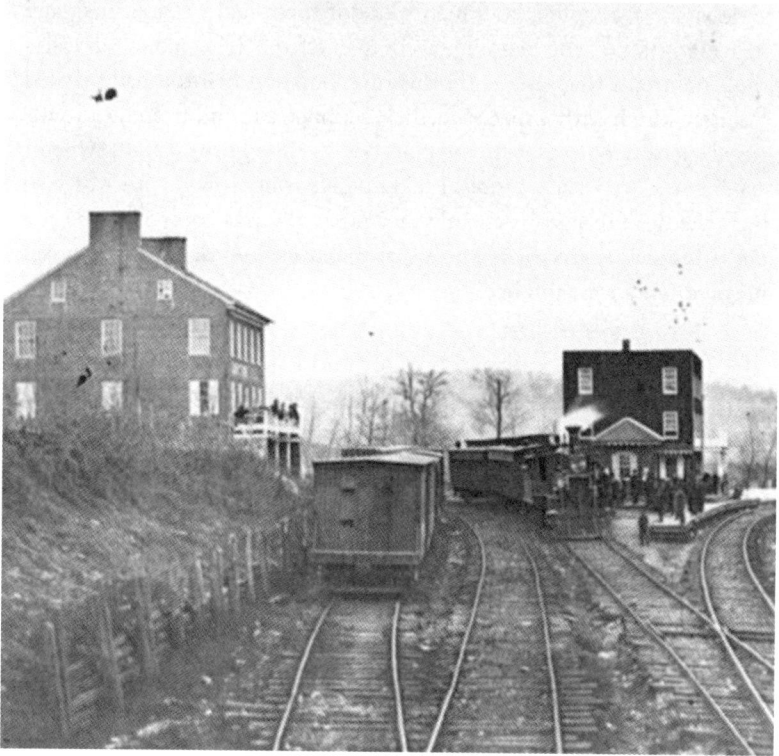

Hanover Junction, November 1863. Gen. Herman Haupt was able to restore service to Gettysburg by July 4th after bridges and tracks between Hanover Junction and Gettysburg were destroyed by Confederates on June 27, 1863. Eventually, more than 15,000 wounded were transported through Hanover Junction en route to major cities.
Courtesy of Library of Congress Prints and Photographs Division

then containing about 16,000 wounded.[40] Surgeon Justin Dwinelle, 106th Pennsylvan' erving as medical officer in charge of the Second Corps hospi ed that on July 4th, "I received this day delivered at the H. ix thousand rations of Tea Coffee sugar crackers S t Pork and three thousand six hundred pounds of n July 4th Surgeon Alexander Jackson Ward, 2nd nedical officer in charge of the First Corps hospi ns of milk, 350 pounds of mutton, 100 pounds of pork from Peter Conover for a total of $60.20 to help feed the First Corps hospital.[42] By July 6th Billings was able to write to his wife from the Fifth Corps hospital, "It has rained steadily for four days but I have got all the wounded under cover at last and have all got soup and coffee, but many of them cannot have their wounds dressed oftener than once in two days."[43] Surgeon Jonas Wellman Lyman, 57th Pennsylvania, reported from the Third Corps hospital "that, notwithstanding the obstructions met with in procuring supplies from the commissary department, owing to the supplies in ambulances and supply wagons, and the energetic and faithful labor of Assistant Surgeon Albion Cobb, 4th Maine, in charge of the cooking department, the wounded of the division suffered but slight inconvenience from want of food."[44]

In addition to the army supply wagons that arrived on July 4th and 5th, several wagon loads of supplies reached Gettysburg from citizens and relief organizations who had anticipated the battle in Pennsylvania and made preparations for supplementary supplies and assistance. Despite the lack of railroad access and the continued threat of Confederate Cavalry for the first several days, both the U.S. Sanitary Commission (USSC) and the U.S. Christian Commission (USCC) successfully delivered several loads of much-needed supplies. One Christian Commission shipment arrived at Westminster by rail on Saturday July 4th, accompanied by delegates Andrew Boyd Cross and Jerome B. Stillson. Using an army wagon supplied by General Buford they hauled these supplies to Gettysburg through the night and rain, arriving on July 5th. Other Christian Commission delegates also found their way to Gettysburg. I. O. Sloan and Walter Alexander, unable to secure other transportation, reportedly walked most of the way from Westminster to Gettysburg in driving rain.[45]

VOLUNTEERS

Volunteers from surrounding areas began to arrive even before train service to Gettysburg resumed. Residents of Gettysburg had been assisting with the care of the wounded since the beginning of the battle. Some, including Robert Grier McCreary, belonged to a local branch of the Christian Commission and had already gathered medical supplies in anticipation of a battle; others simply volunteered to help with wounded as individuals, opening their homes and churches. Ellen Orbison Harris, Secretary of the Ladies' Aid Society of Philadelphia, already an experienced battlefield nurse, left Washington on July 3rd with chloroform and stimulants that she could carry with her. Stopping at Baltimore, she left there at 5 P.M. and arrived at Westminster at 4 A.M. on July 4th after ten hours on the train. There she met wounded Gen. Winfield Scott Hancock and received permission to ride to Gettysburg in the ambulance that had brought him.[46] Mary Morris Husbands, another experienced nurse, left Philadelphia on July 3rd. From Westminster, she traveled with Isabella Fogg, a nurse from Maine, and together they made their way to Gettysburg by riding in General Meade's mail wagon. Husbands arrived July 4th and went to work at the Second Corps 3rd Division hospital. Fogg, after consulting with Dr. Letterman, went to the Fifth Corps Hospital.[47]

A group of Catholic sisters from the Daughters of Charity at Emmitsburg, Maryland, 10 miles away, arrived in Gettysburg on July 5th, accompanied by their chaplain, Father Francis Burlando. Establishing themselves at the Gettysburg Hotel, they quickly went to work at the Court House and St. Xavier Catholic Church. By July 6th, eleven sisters were at work and more soon joined them with additional supplies.

Residents of nearby York, Pennsylvania, provided supplies and volunteers. The *Philadelphia Inquirer* reported,

> On Sunday morning, and long before daylight, light buggies, double carriages, and market wagons began to make their appearance and were driven into the points where our hospitals are located. These vehicles were all loaded with substantials and delicacies for the sick, brought and distributed by the fair hands of the ladies of York and adjoining counties, many of which ladies are now doing duty as volunteer nurses.[48]

Mary Sophia Cadwell Fisher and her eldest son Robert were among those who responded quickly to the news of the battle on the morning of July 4th:

> The public square in York was rapidly filled with wagons packed with provisions, clothing, blankets and hospital stores waiting the arrival of the banished horses which had been sent across the river before the

occupation of the town. About 3 pm I started with two ladies and my son in a two-horse wagon loaded with necessaries of every kind.[49]

Arriving early Sunday morning, July 5th, they could hear the occasional report of gunfire as they approached Gettysburg and reached the Fifth Corps hospital about 7 A.M. They spent the first night in Gettysburg assisting at the Court House, and on Monday moved to the Second Corps hospitals where she found Dr. Dwinelle, the head surgeon "most courteous to the volunteer nurses."[50] While most Union surgeons rejected the need for civilian volunteers, Dwinelle's Second Corps hospitals continued to accept more volunteer help than the other corps hospitals, either by personal preference or because of the large number of both Union and Confederate wounded under his care. Mrs. Fisher summarized the situation she found at Gettysburg:

> The long continued and severe fight had exhausted both men and means. The surrounding country had been depleted by the demands of both armies, draining every available source. The lack of horses to transport provisions and the panic of the rural population in the vicinity rendered it impossible to procure the wherewith to supply the necessities of the immense number of wounded men, more than twenty thousand in the immediate neighborhood. The army moved at once, taking the medical stores and leaving behind a very inadequate corps of surgeons and nurses.[51]

THE ARMY OF THE POTOMAC MOVES ON

When Jonathan Letterman left Gettysburg with the Army of the Potomac on July 6th, he placed Henry Janes in charge of the hospitals with a reported 106 surgeons or approximately one for every 100–150 Union wounded. Janes had previous experience working in military hospitals and had served for two years as surgeon of the 3rd Vermont before his promotion to surgeon of U.S. Volunteers in the Sixth Corps on April 20, 1863. While the number of surgeons assigned to the various corps hospitals at Gettysburg, per Letterman's orders, might have seemed adequate in theory, the large number of Confederate prisoners in addition to the large numbers of Union wounded, the temporary lack of supplies, transportation difficulties, and the initial lack of railroad service to evacuate patients to other hospitals all added to the severity of the situation that Janes and the remaining surgeons faced. Union surgeons who remained, like their Confederate counterparts, had been among those serving in the various field and corps hospitals. As some of these surgeons left to rejoin their regiments, those who remained had to care for the same number of wounded. Some regimental surgeons who were assigned to staff the corps hospitals stayed for only a few days to complete operations; others remained weeks or months.

Surgeon Alexander Jackson Ward, 2nd Wisconsin, stayed in Gettysburg until August 18th. A veteran of the Mexican War and the California Gold Rush, he was responsible for more than 2,300 wounded in the First Corps hospitals located near White Church along the Baltimore Pike.[52] Altogether, First Corps wounded numbered approximately 3,200. A third of the wounded from the first day of the battle remained in public and private buildings throughout the town. Surgeon John Beech, 24th Michigan, remained at the Express Office hospital along with Surgeon Abram William Preston and Assistant Surgeon John C. Hall, of the 6th Wisconsin; Preston left in mid-September after the hospital closed. Surgeon James Farley, 84th New York, remained at the Washington Hotel. Surgeon Charles J. Nordquist, 83rd New York, remained at Christ Lutheran Church. Surgeon Pascal A. Quinan, 150th Pennsylvania, and Assistant Surgeon James Fulton, 143rd Pennsylvania, remained at the Catholic and Presbyterian churches. At the Lutheran Seminary, Surgeon Robert Loughran, 80th New York, remained with Assistant Surgeons Abram Brower Haines, 19th Indiana, and Warren Underwood, 151st Pennsylvania. Loughran remained in charge of the Seminary hospital until August 17.

On July 5th Alexander N. Dougherty, medical director of the Second Corps, issued orders to organize the three division hospitals under the overall direction of Surgeon Justin Dwinelle, 106th Pennsylvania. One third of the operating staff was to remain with fifty nurses, attendants, etc. In fact, reports of the Second Corps indicate that more than half of the operating teams (twenty surgeons in all) were left to care for an estimated 3,200 patients. The 1st Division alone reported 800 Union and

200 Confederate wounded and a total of 230 operations.[53] Surgeons had little choice in the matter of who stayed with the wounded and who left with the regiments; that decision was made at the corps level. Assistant Surgeon James Dana Benton, 111th New York, welcomed the opportunity to remain at the Second Corps Hospital and assist with operations:

> When the "Army of the Potomac" moved in pursuit of Lee, I was detailed to remain as an assistant to Dr. McAbee with one other of our Division forming an operating board. Dr. McAbee is the Chief Surgeon of our Division and for over a week I had the opportunity of assisting in hundreds of very important operations and in consequence my mind is impressed with many items relating to surgery that I should not have gained had I gone on with the Regt.[54]

The reduced staff at other corps hospitals was similarly organized. At the Third Corps hospitals, Surgeon Thaddeus Hildreth, 3rd Maine, was left in charge.[55] Surgeon Augustus M. Clark, 4th U.S., remained in charge of the Fifth Corps hospital until August 3rd.[56] Surgeon Cyrus Nathaniel Chamberlain, U.S. Volunteers, was placed in charge of the Sixth Corps hospitals with the fewest number of wounded.[57] The Eleventh Corps division hospitals were consolidated at Spangler farm on July 6th with Surgeon James A. Armstrong, 75th Pennsylvania, as medical officer in charge. Remaining with him were nine medical staff.[58] The Twelfth Corps hospitals remained at the George Bushman House with Surgeon H. Ernest Goodman, 28th Pennsylvania, in charge.[59]

Surgeon William H. Rulison, 9th New York Cavalry, took charge of cavalry surgeons who remained in Gettysburg. Surgeon Elias W. H. Beck, 3rd Indiana Cavalry, and Assistant Surgeon Hiram Dana Vosburgh, 8th New York Cavalry, remained with wounded at the Presbyterian church in Gettysburg. Surgeon Theodore Tate, 3rd Pennsylvania Cavalry, was left in charge of the wounded at the Public School. Assistant Surgeon Perrin A. Gardner, 1st West Virginia Cavalry, was left in charge of the cavalry wounded at Hanover.[60]

Surgeon William Warren Potter, 57th New York, was still hard at work at the operating tables of the Second Corps 2nd Division hospital when his regiment left Gettysburg on July 5th. He continued at the hospital until the majority of operations had been completed before he left to rejoin his regiment.

> During the 4th, in the midst of a heavy shower, I amputated the thigh of a rebel captain whose name I have forgotten. He belonged to a NC regiment and was full of hope and courage. I have no doubt that he recovered. So the work went on for the next three days until the 7th when we were relieved by surgeons from Washington and the North.[61]

Assistant Surgeon Daniel M. Holt, 121st New York, was glad to leave Gettysburg with the Sixth Corps, preferring to stay with his regiment,

> for the reason that when an action is over and you have sent your wounded away provided for, it is the end of the matter; whereas in a Division Hospital your work has only just begun. Here amputations and operations of every kind with subsequent treatment is to be given—the very worst part of the business. If there is one thing more disagreeable or more dirty than another, it is the dressing sloughing, stinking gun shot wounds.[62]

For the surgeons who remained, along with the additional military staff and volunteers who arrived to assist them, the long arduous work of caring for the wounded was just beginning.

CHAPTER 7

Relief for the Wounded, July 7–22

BY JULY 7TH THE ARMY OF THE POTOMAC AND MOST OF ITS MEDICAL staff had moved on in pursuit of General Lee and the Army of Northern Virginia. The military battle at Gettysburg had ended, but the medical battle to save lives was just beginning. Both armies, anticipating additional casualties, left only the limited number of surgeons and supplies that could be spared. Placed in charge of the hospitals at Gettysburg, Henry Janes and the remaining surgeons now faced the daunting task of transforming the chaotic remains of a battlefield into an efficient, functioning hospital with thousands of wounded, limited supplies, and reduced staff. If exhaustion was the term most often used to describe the immediate aftermath of the battle, confusion seemed to best describe the next few weeks. Sophronia Bucklin, a volunteer nurse traveling from Baltimore with Rebecca Stanley Caldwell of the Sanitary Commission, described her first impressions of Gettysburg on July 18th, two weeks after the battle: "On Saturday we entered the battle town. Everywhere were evidences of mortal combat, everywhere wounded men were lying in the streets on heaps of blood-stained straw; everywhere there was hurry and confusion, while soldiers were groaning and suffering."[1] The *Philadelphia Inquirer* for July 10th reported, "Colonel Smith, the Provost Marshal, is doing all he can to systematize matters, but still affairs are in the greatest confusion."[2]

Transportation delays caused by the destruction of railroad lines created food shortages and delayed the ability to evacuate patients to general hospitals in nearby cities. To further complicate the situation, the wounded were spread out over a large area of several miles—from churches and houses in the town of Gettysburg, to barns and tents extending for miles in every direction. The large number of captured Confederate wounded in Union hospitals and those left behind in Confederate hospitals presented an additional and unanticipated burden. With wells drained dry and overflowing streams polluted with dead bodies and the carcasses of slain horses, clean water was scarce and both the wounded and their caregivers often fell sick. The smell of death and decay was overpowering.

Provost Marshal Marsena Patrick, who had been supervising prisoners and burial of dead, left Gettysburg to rejoin the Army of the Potomac on July 7th, and Capt. Willard Smith, an assistant quartermaster, was sent to Gettysburg to oversee the cleanup of the battlefield and secure government property. Responsibility for policing the battlefield, securing government property, issuing passes, guarding prisoners, and burying the dead was assigned to Pennsylvania state militias. It would be weeks before civilian authority could be restored. Col. Hiram Alleman of the 36th Pennsylvania Militia arrived July 9th to take over command of the battlefield as military governor. G. R. Frysinger of Company A, 36th Pennsylvania Militia, wrote home on July 17th that "Gettysburg cannot be called a town, but a large collection of hospitals."[3]

The Medical Department in Washington continued to discourage civilian volunteers, despite the limited capacity of 175 military surgeons, both Confederate and Union, left to care for the more than 20,000 wounded that remained in Gettysburg. One volunteer nurse described how "The few surgeons who were left in charge of the battlefield after the Union army had started in pursuit of Lee had begun their paralyzing task by sorting the dead from the dying, and the dying from those whose lives might be saved; hence the groups of prostrate, bleeding men laid together according to their wounds."[4] As volunteer relief workers arrived they were shocked to see so many wounded men, still lying on the bare, muddy ground without shelter and, in many cases, wearing dirty, torn, or no clothing at all.

Jonathan Letterman's report to the Medical Director's Office dated October 3, 1863, expressed his frustration at not having hospital supplies on hand during the battle and the lack of railroad transportation after the battle, but he staunchly defended his decision to leave only 106 Union surgeons.

> The time for primary operations had passed, and what remained to be done was to attend to making the men comfortable, dress their wounds, and perform such secondary operations as from time to time might be necessary. One hundred and six medical officers were left behind when the army left; no more could be left, as it was expected that another battle would within three or four days take place, and in all probability as many wounded thrown upon our hands as at the battle of the 2d and 3d, which had just occurred . . .[5]

While Letterman reported that most primary operations had been performed by July 7th, firsthand accounts suggest that he overestimated that number and certainly neglected to include the large number of Confederate wounded still untreated. Bennett Augustine Clements, assistant medical director of the Army of the Potomac, and author of a *Memoir of Jonathan Letterman*, later defended Letterman's reluctance to accept civilian help:

> It came soon to be known that the Medical Officers of the Army of the Potomac could care for their wounded without the uncertain aid of surgeons and nurses from civil life. . . . He knew his corps could do the required work, and he desired to add to their self-reliance. For similar reasons he did not at this period, when his Department was in good working order, encourage the Sanitary Commission to apply their noble means of relief to the service of that Army . . . Many inexperienced persons represented that on many battle-fields the wounded were not well cared for, yet such complaints scarcely ever were heard from the wounded. Straw to lie on, food and water, and the skillful attention of his surgeons, are all that the tried soldier desires or the experienced medical officer would demand on the battle-field.[6]

Not everyone agreed with this optimistic view that the Army of the Potomac's remaining surgeons could meet the needs of the wounded after the battle of Gettysburg. Dr. John Hancock Douglas, associate secretary of the U.S. Sanitary Commission, arrived on July 7th and described the work of the surgeons in stark terms, echoing other accounts that confirmed the lack of staff to care for the large number of wounded during the first weeks after the battle.

> Another difficulty, inseparable from the campaign, was the small number of medical officers left upon the ground to take charge of the large number of wounded . . . Those left behind had to divide their attention among our own wounded and those of the enemy who had fallen into our hands, the number of Confederate surgeons left behind being inadequate to their care. In previous battle there has always been a full quota, if not the entire medical corps of the army, to attend to the wounded. The labor, the anxiety, the responsibility imposed upon the surgeons after the battle of Gettysburg were, from the position of affairs, greater than after any other battle of the war . . . The battle ceasing, their labors continue. While other officers are sleeping, renewing their strength for further efforts, the medical are still toiling. They have to improvise hospitals from the rudest materials, are obliged to make "bricks without straw," to surmount seeming impossibilities. The work is unending, both by day and night, the anxiety is constant, the strain upon both the physical and mental faculties unceasing. Thus after this battle, one operator had to be held up while performing the operation and fainted from exhaustion, the operation finished. One completed his labors to be seized with partial paralysis, the penalty of his over exertion.[7]

Bushrod Washington James, a volunteer physician from Philadelphia, arrived on July 7th and worked for five days in the Second Corps hospitals before falling ill. He described how

> Every surgeon in the hospital was kept busy nearly a week amputating limbs, probing for and removing bullets, or sewing, bandaging and dressing the wounds . . . I saw men, some officers among them, feverish and bleeding or weak almost to death because there were not then surgeons enough to operate upon the vast multitude in time to save them all ere gangrene set in, for the regimental surgeons had to join

their commands on the march . . . we were such a pitiable few among so many wounded.[8]

One Union surgeon, Harry McAbee, 4th Ohio, resigned his commission after the battle protesting,

After the battle of Gettysburg, with but three assistants, I was left in charge of a thousand badly wounded men, not a few of whom, I fear, absolutely died for want of appropriate and good professional care. It is my deliberate opinion that the failure to furnish a sufficient number of medical officers on that occasion has cost the country more good men than did the charge of any rebel brigade on that severely contested field.[9]

UNION SURGEONS

Most of the military surgeons were too busy to update their diaries or write letters immediately following the battle. Assistant Surgeon Cyrus Bacon, 2nd U.S., left a rare perspective since he kept his diary current during his work at the 2nd Division, Fifth Corps hospital located near the Michael Fiscel farm. On July 6th he reported performing a large number of operations and working on the hospital registers for the wounded of the 2nd and 14th U.S. regiments. Two days later, he recorded that the men were better protected with tents, but "The camp is quite a scene. People now beginning to come in with supplies for the wounded. I work hard at dressing today. This has been continuous from [the] first. The surgeon's work is after the battle."[10] Like many other surgeons he was too busy to leave his hospital post until July 11th, a full week after the battle ended. On July 12th he made his first visit to town for supplies, stopping at the Adams Express office for ice, the Christian Commission for books, and the Sanitary Commission for *charpie*, a lint used for dressings. He recorded that there were six surgeons operating at the 2nd Division hospital. At least three, including Bacon, became sick with dysentery or were "poisoned" from treating infected wounds. It was not until July 20th that he could report that he was getting his camp "ship shape."[11]

Surgeon William Watson, 105th Pennsylvania, wrote letters home during his work at the 1st Division, Third Corps hospital at the nearby

Trostle farm. On July 9th he wrote home to his physician father, "I am so very busy that I have time to write but a few lines. We have eight hundred wounded in our Div. Hospital and only eight Medical Officers to attend them."[12] He hoped to complete operations for his division so that he could turn his attention to the one hundred Confederate wounded still needing treatment.

Confederate Surgeons

Confederate surgeons who remained with their wounded faced similar issues of supplies and staffing. Assistant Surgeon Simon Baruch, 3rd South Carolina Battalion, in Kershaw's Brigade, described the six weeks he spent in the field hospital at the Black Horse Tavern.

> On the morning of the second day of our captivity I was called to the flap door of my tent and was surprised to be greeted by an officer in a chaplain's uniform. His face beamed with kindness as he said: "I am Dr. Winslow, of the Christian Commission. I have come to offer you any assistance in our power and to furnish you some supplies . . . Two hours later I was on the way to Gettysburg, accompanied by an orderly, who had hired two horses by paying a shoulder of bacon, of which our commissary had left a needlessly abundant supply. At the office of the Christian Commission two bags were filled with supplies for the wounded. Being advised to apply to the sanitary commission, I walked to this large warehouse filled with hospital supplies which extended over the neighboring sidewalk . . . I was advised also to apply to Dr. Letterman, medical director of the Army of the Potomac, and found in him a true soldier, magnanimous to his enemy, and a true physician, considerate of the wounded. Handing me a blank requisition, he instructed me how to fill it, approved it, and sent it to the medical purveyor for execution.[13]

Baruch's account of Gordon Winslow misidentifies him as representing the Christian Commission rather than the Sanitary Commission, but otherwise matches Winslow's account of the assistance provided to Confederate hospitals. Winslow served as chaplain of the 5th New York until he mustered out in May 1863 to become Sanitary Commission inspector with the Army of the Potomac. Arriving soon after the battle, he was assigned to oversee the Confederate hospitals and reported back to the Sanitary Commission on July 22nd on the 5,452 Confederate wounded that he found in twenty-four separate hospitals over a twelve-mile area.

> The Corps of Confederate Surgeons are, as a body intelligent and attentive. The hospitals are generally in barns, outhouses, and dilapidated tents. Some few cases are in dwellings. I cannot speak favorably of their camp police. Often there is a deplorable want of cleanliness.[14]

Winslow was not alone in his criticism of the Confederate hospitals. Reporter John Y. Foster spent four days at Gettysburg with a delegation from Philadelphia under the auspices of the Christian Commission. Arriving on July 10th with supplies, Foster had harsh words for the Confederate surgeons: "much in this distressing condition of the rebel wounded was owing to the neglect and indifference of their own surgeons. Many of these surgeons seemed altogether destitute of those sensibilities which lend a softening influence to the rugged necessities and always forbidding duties of this important office. Some were almost brutal in their treatment of the men left to their care."[15] Foster and other Northern volunteers often compared Confederate surgeons and patients unfavorably to their Union counterparts, but surgeons of both sides were criticized for lack of empathy and concern for the wounded by nurses and volunteers who sympathized with the suffering of the wounded on a more personal and emotional level.

CONTRACT SURGEONS AND MEDICAL OFFICERS

Jonathan Letterman had little use for civilian physicians, but he grudgingly acknowledged the need for additional surgeons when he "asked the Surgeon-General, on July 7th, to send 20 medical officers to report to Dr. Janes, hoping they might prove of some benefit, under the direction of the medical officers of this army who had been left behind. I cannot learn that they were ever sent but it is not clear how many were on duty in the first weeks after the battle."[16] There is no known official list of the medical officers dispatched to Gettysburg in response to Letterman's request, but contemporary accounts help document who they were and what roles they played. By July 11th at least seventeen contract surgeons and seven Union army medical staff had arrived in Gettysburg.[17] The medical staff who arrived after the battle included a mix of high-ranking medical officers, regular army U.S. Volunteers assigned to nearby hospitals, and contract surgeons already employed in military hospitals in Baltimore, Philadelphia, and Washington. When Medical Inspector Edward Perry Vollum arrived on the evening of July 8th, he focused his efforts on expediting the evacuation of wounded at the railroad depot by assisting Surgeon Joseph Osborne, 4th New Jersey, who "was using his best endeavors to work through the confusion and crowds of wounded with which he was surrounded."[18] By July 22nd more than 10,000 wounded had been evacuated from the Gettysburg hospitals in just over two weeks.[19] U.S. Surgeon John H. Brinton, curator of the newly established Medical Museum in Washington, DC, provided a firsthand account of his work in Gettysburg in his published memoir.

> Immediately after the battle of Gettysburg, I was ordered by the Surgeon-General to go there on special duty. There was, then, two or three days after the battle, some difficulty in reaching Gettysburg from the south, the Washington side . . . My duty at this time was twofold, first to render what help I could surgically, and secondly to collect specimens and histories for the museum.[20]

Physicians dispatched from Philadelphia and Baltimore hospitals included both U.S. Volunteers and contract surgeons. Assistant Surgeon William Fisher Norris, U.S. Volunteers, arrived July 11th traveling with Dr. Thomas Forrest Betton, a contract acting assistant surgeon who was already working in Philadelphia military hospitals. It is sometimes assumed that the contract surgeons, officially designated as "acting assistant surgeons," were less qualified than their commissioned colleagues, but this was not necessarily the case. A graduate of the University of Pennsylvania in 1832, Betton taught surgery at Franklin Medical College in Philadelphia from 1846 to 1848 and was a respected member of the medical community of Philadelphia. William Norris, on the other hand, was just beginning his career after graduation from the University of Pennsylvania in 1861. He served as resident physician at Pennsylvania Hospital until he received a commission as assistant surgeon in the U.S. Volunteers in June 1863. The twenty-four-year-old wrote his first letter home to his father, Dr. George W. Norris, professor of clinical surgery at the University of Pennsylvania, expressing William's dismay at the conditions he found compared with his experiences in Philadelphia hospitals.

Dear Father

I was so busy yesterday that I was unable to write. I arrived here yesterday at 11 am, delivered my stores and reported for duty and was immediately assigned to the Hospital of the 3rd division 1st Army Corps wch occupies at present a Catholic Church and that of some Protestant organization wch is located opposite. A Dr. Quinan U.S.V. is Surgeon in charge. The Hospital contains 200 patients and is in a state of utter confusion. Men with serious wounds lying about with very little attention. There are no intelligent assistants or Surgeons. The only man who seems to know anything at all is the Surgeon in charge. Even the food was insufficient. When I came I was at once put in charge of the Commissary & cooking & of the police [cleanliness] of the Hospital in fact made executive Officer with a general oversight of everything subject to the Surgeon in charge, I have nothing at all to do with the treatment.[21]

Norris, a newly enlisted U.S. Volunteer, was initially impressed with Quinan's previous army experience, but Quinan proved so overbearing and ineffective that he was eventually dismissed. After four days Norris's next letter acknowledged the difficulties of transitioning from a makeshift battlefield hospital to a well-organized general hospital and described his duties, "in a newly organized Hospital with few supplies at command" more realistically.

I draw and superintend the distribution of rations to the men, the cooking, the cleanliness of the wards, the outside police and guard—digging of sinks, burial of the dead, supplying the establishment with medicines sheets, etc. My greatest difficulty is that I am unable at present to get the dirty shirts, blankets, sheets, etc. washed.

By July 15th, he could see improvements.

The Hospital is now getting into very fair condition we have arranged beds on top of the alternate pews thus leaving a space between each bed; and our nurses, ward masters and police force are becoming more efficient. The Sanitary and Christian Commissions are a vast assistance to us, supplying quantities of needful articles wch cannot be got from the Government. . . . I have at my command 26 men as police, six surgeons 22 nurses, 1 teamster with a six mule team, a Hospital Steward and two clerks.[22]

Assistant Surgeon William Williams Keen, U.S. Volunteers, was working at Satterlee Hospital in Philadelphia when he was ordered to Gettysburg after the battle. His description makes clear that the work of the surgeons continued long after the primary operations had been completed.

Secondary hemorrhage began to appear even before the end of the first week, but during the second week they occurred with dreadful frequency. When I was on duty for twenty-four hours as officer of the day, and it was my duty to attend to all emergency night calls, I had five cases of secondary hemorrhage in a single night about two weeks after the battle.[23]

Medical Inspector John Meck Cuyler, U.S. Volunteers, arrived on July 11th and diplomatically concluded in his report to Surgeon General Hammond:

The number of medical officers detailed by Medical Director Letterman to remain with the wounded was thought to be sufficient and probably might have been had not the thousands of the enemy's wounded been thrown unexpectedly on our hands. For some days after the battle, many of the rebel wounded were in a most deplorable condition, being without shelter of any sort, and with an insufficient number of medical officers and nurses of their own army.[24]

A Georgian by birth, Cuyler pitched in to assist the understaffed Second Corps hospital, operating on Confederate wounded until he cut himself during an operation on a patient with gangrene and immediately amputated his own finger to avoid infection.[25]

The Second Corps hospital, with large numbers of both Union and Confederate wounded, was in no position to turn down qualified volunteers. Surgeon Justin Dwinelle, left in charge of the hospital, reported that on July 7th three-quarters of amputations had been completed: "There also reported to me for duty on the seventh Eight or nine contract surgeons; [Army] surgeons Walker, Norris and Morris; Asst. Surgeon Barry of the eleventh corps; several Confederates; and about Thirty volunteer Surgeons."[26] Most Union surgeons resisted volunteer medical help, agreeing with Letterman's after-battle report that clearly restated negative assessments of non-military surgeons.

> No reliance can be placed on surgeons from civil life during or after a battle. They cannot or will not submit to the privations and discomforts which are necessary, and the great majority think more of their own personal comfort than they do of the wounded. Little more can be said of those officers who have for a long period been in hospitals. I regret to make such a statement, but it is a fact and often a practical one. Dr. [Henry] Janes, who was left in charge of the hospitals at Gettysburg, reports that quite a number of surgeons came and volunteered their services, but "they were of little use." This fact is so well known in this army that medical officers prefer to do the work rather than have them present, and the wounded men, too, are much better satisfied to be attended by their own surgeons.[27]

Dwinelle, however, was cautiously willing to accept extra help: "If good Surgeons of undoubted reputation can be sent to us in time, stay with us while their services are needed, conform to the same rules and regulations and put up with the same inconveniences without fault finding that the corps Surgeons have too, Their Services will be appreciated."[28] Based on his own personal observations working at the Second Corps hospital, Medical Inspector Cuyler afterwards praised both the medical officers and citizen surgeons, adding that he "never saw men work harder and complain less of the difficulties that surrounded them."[29]

Civilian Volunteers

Despite the Medical Department's official disdain for volunteers, relief for the wounded in the various field hospitals for the next few weeks relied heavily on the additional supplies and assistance provided by a wide variety of civilian sources, mostly operating independently of one another and with little or no central coordination. On the night of July 6th, the railroad lines reopened to within a mile of town, bringing carloads of supplies as well as volunteer doctors and nurses. Communities throughout the North responded to local newspaper accounts of the battle and calls for "relief for the wounded" with an outpouring of supplies and volunteers. Among the first on the scene were representatives of the two national organizations—agents of the U.S. Sanitary Commission and delegates of the U.S. Christian Commission. By 1863, both organizations had assigned representatives who traveled with the Army of the Potomac and were among the first on the scene during and after the battle. They were soon joined by many more volunteers anxious to distribute the hospital supplies and food stockpiled and waiting to be shipped from depots in Washington, Baltimore, and Philadelphia. While the two organizations maintained a cautious rivalry, competing for donations and volunteers and distributing supplies independently of one another, they often worked side by side in the field. Other relief efforts were organized by the Adams Express Company, agents sent by various states, local relief organizations, and individual volunteers. The overlapping efforts of so many organizations added to the confusion and made it difficult to confirm affiliations or determine under whose auspices individual volunteers may have worked.

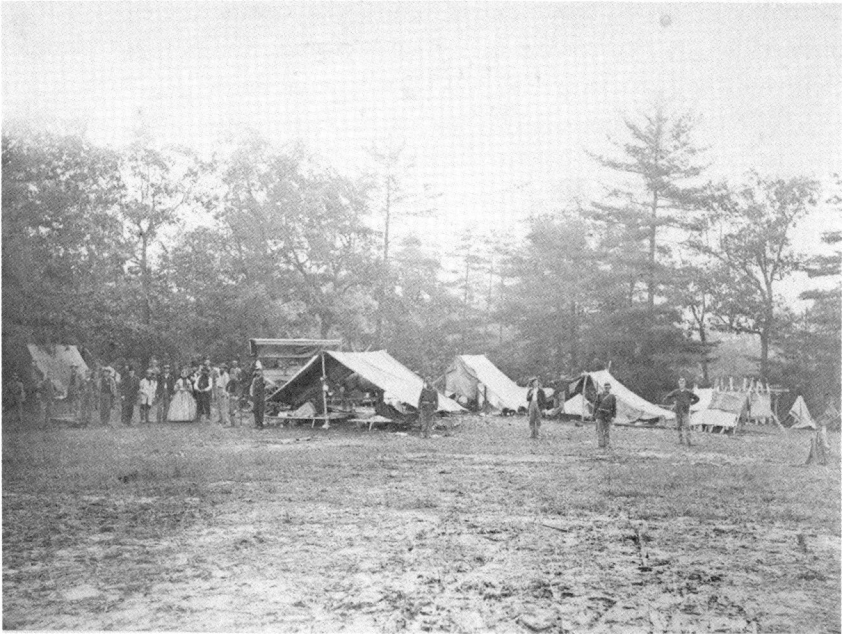

Second Corps Hospital Frederick Gutekunst, July 11–15, 1863 Identified surgeons include Surgeon J. Wilson Wishart, 140th Pennsylvania, and Medical Director Alexander N. Dougherty. Identified Christian Commission delegates include the Reverend Jerome B. Stillson from Rochester, New York, and the Reverend Robert Matlack of Philadelphia, wearing a white shirt. Courtesy of Special Collections and College Archives, Musselman Library, Gettysburg College

U.S. SANITARY COMMISSION

Founded on June 9, 1861, as "A Commission of Inquiry and Advice in respect of the Sanitary interests of the United States Forces," by an order of the secretary of war, the U.S. Sanitary Commission set out to "inquire with scientific thoroughness" the subjects of diet, cooking, clothing, tents, camping ground, and transportation. It soon expanded its work to include relief "to organize, methodize, and reduce to serviceableness, the vague and haphazard benevolence of the people toward the Army."[30] The Commission approached its work as a "national" effort serving all federal forces and criticized individual state relief efforts that only provided for their own sick and wounded for what it called "state-ish spirit," the "heresy of state sovereignty" and "local jealousies."[31] The Sanitary

Commission prided itself on its centralized organizational structure, businesslike practices, paid professional staff, and close working relationship with the U.S. Army Medical Department. The Relief Department oversaw feeding stations, lodges and transportation for wounded, and the needs of wounded immediately following a battle.

Arriving on July 6th Dr. John Hancock Douglas took charge of operations at Gettysburg and established storehouses to distribute supplies. By July 8th a Gettysburg building owned by Fahnestock & Co. had boxes piled from floor to ceiling.[32] The number of supplies was impressive. In his report Dr. Douglas listed supplies of 7,143 pairs of drawers, 10,424 shirts, 4,000 pairs of shoes and slippers, 1,200 crutches, and 110 barrels of old linen for bandages. Among the food items delivered to Gettysburg were 8,500 dozen eggs, 6,430 pounds of butter, 12,900 loaves of bread, 400 gallons of pickles, and 3,566 bottles of brandy, whiskey, and wine.[33]

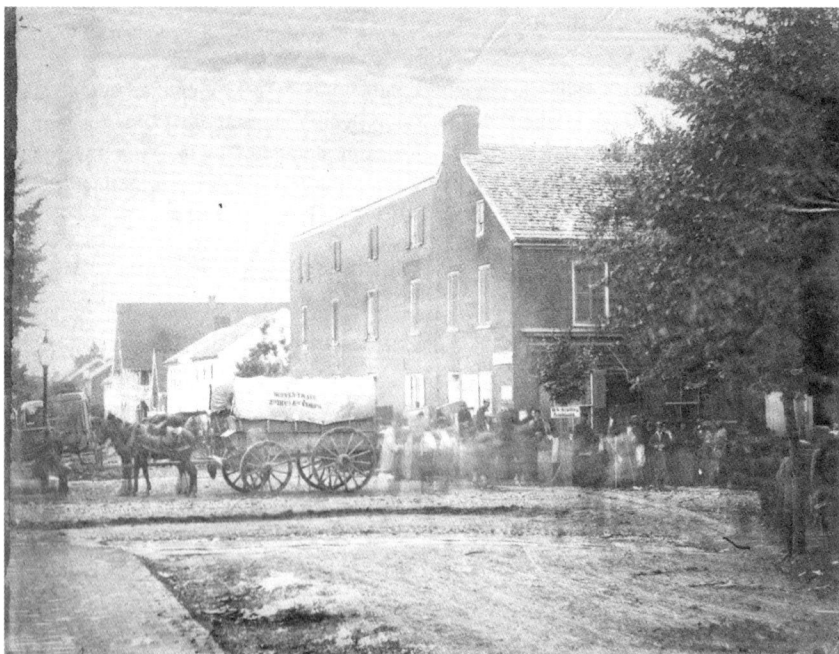

Headquarters U.S. Sanitary Commission, Gettysburgh [sic] with wagon from "Supply Train 2nd Divn 6th Corps." Courtesy of New York Public Library

The first railroad depot lodge was set up by members of the Sanitary Commission on July 7th with tents sent from Baltimore.[34] Georgeanna Woolsey and her mother, Jane Eliza Newton Woolsey, arrived on one of the first trains to the outskirts of Gettysburg on July 7th. "There stood the temporary lodge and kitchens and here hobbling out of their tents came wounded men who had made their way down from the Corps hospital expecting to leave at once in the return cars."[35] The two women helped feed the wounded at the first lodge along the railroad tracks and later at the railway depot in town after July 10th when the railway tracks into town were fully repaired. Sanitary Commission members working at the first lodge included Dr. Robert Hooper of Boston, Joshua B. Clark from New Hampshire, and Joseph Shippen from Pittsburgh.[36] A group from Canandaigua, New York, headed by Dr. William Fitch Cheney, managed the operation at the second lodge in town until it closed at the end of July.[37]

Sanitary Commission agents also assisted with record keeping for the Medical Department. In addition to daily visitation to hospitals and consultation with medical officers about supply needs, "A list of names and wounds of all inmates in each hospital was taken and forwarded to the office of the Hospital Directory in Washington. This work was performed by Mr. Dooley from the Directory Office, assisted by Stille, Struthers, Hazlehurst, Dullus, Beitler, and Tracy from Philadelphia; Hosford, Myers, Braman from NY."[38]

U.S. CHRISTIAN COMMISSION

Although the work of the two commissions sometimes overlapped, their roles and methods differed significantly. While the Sanitary Commission endeavored to support the Medical Department with increased efficiency, improved medical practice, and supplementary supplies, the Christian Commission's goal was to support the work of regimental chaplains and provide direct assistance to individual soldiers. The Christian Commission began its work in 1861 as an offshoot of the YMCA, at first focusing exclusively on conversations, conversions, and religious tracts to support the spiritual needs of soldiers. By 1863 it had expanded its mission to meet the physical needs of wounded by distributing donated supplies collected by church groups and sewing circles and providing volunteers to help nurse the wounded. While the Sanitary Commission prided itself on its professional full-time, paid agents, the Christian Commission relied on untrained volunteers, "armed with both stores and publication for all wants of body and mind,"[39] who only had to make a commitment of six weeks to receive a commission as a Christian Commission delegate.[40] John Calhoun Chamberlain, a theological student on his way to Virginia to visit his brothers Lawrence and Thomas serving in the 20th Maine, stopped off at the headquarters of the Christian Commission in Philadelphia in June 1863. He received his commission papers the same afternoon, providing him with a military pass and free passage on the railroad.[41] The Christian Commission did not accept women as delegates, but the Maryland Christian Commission provided independent nurses with credentials needed to reach wounded in the field.[42] The Commission later admitted that lack of vetting sometimes led to abuses, admitting that "some came as delegates of the Commission, who ought not have been there, and some professing to be, who were not commissioned."[43]

The Christian Commission may have been referring to some of the Confederate sympathizers from Baltimore who sent supplies and volunteers to assist Confederate wounded. Simon Baruch described how "Two young women belonging to a historic Maryland family came to the hospital, under the chaperonage of an elderly English nurse, and remained with us, occupying garret rooms, until the hospital closed. They administered to the wounded, prepared the food and dressings, and read the burial service over those who succumbed. Their services were inestimable. Now and then sympathizing friends from Baltimore appeared in carriages, bringing supplies and good cheer for our wounded boys."[44]

Some of the Baltimore women who came to nurse Confederate wounded were involved in clandestine efforts on behalf of the Confederate cause. Best known is Euphemia Mary Goldsborough, who arrived July 12th and worked for nine weeks caring for Confederate wounded at the Pennsylvania College and later at Camp Letterman. After her return to Baltimore, she was indicted for treason and banished to Richmond for the remainder of the war. Another Baltimore nurse at the College hospital, Margaret Branson, formed a relationship with patient Lewis

Thornton Powell, who later attacked William Seward as part of the Lincoln assassination plot. Two sisters who were forced to leave Gettysburg by U.S. authorities, Martha Louise Loane Banks and Annie G. Loane Parr, were staunch supporters of the Confederacy along with their husbands William Emmett Banks and David Preston Parr. David Parr has been identified as one of the Confederate sympathizers who assisted the Lincoln assassination conspirators.[45]

The report of the Christian Commission's Maryland Committee praised the work of women nurses, although they were not officially delegates: "The hospitals that were favored with their presence presented a home-like attraction that was often envied by the less fortunate sufferers."[46] They cooked special diets for the wounded, kept patients clean and clothed, wrote letters for them, and sometimes assisted with medical care and dressings. Clarissa Fellows Jones, a young teacher from Philadelphia, and Mrs. Jane C. Moore and her daughter Jane Boswell Moore from Baltimore, were among the women nurses who received passes from the Maryland Christian Commission. Other women who volunteered at Gettysburg coordinated their efforts with Christian Commission delegates to distribute supplies.

While the Sanitary Commission distributed their supplies to surgeons through formal requisitions submitted by the surgeons of the Medical Department, the Christian Commission preferred personal distribution from delegate to soldier, avoiding what they viewed as unnecessary red tape. At Gettysburg the work was organized by three paid Christian Commission agents.[47] A building on the central square owned by Martin Stoever and rented to merchant John Schick was quickly readied to receive supplies. A second storehouse across the street was soon added to accommodate the large volume of goods arriving for distribution.

> Cars were to be unloaded, boxes to be unpacked and repacked, transportation to be obtained, telegraphy to be done, invoices to be verified, the books of the Commission to be kept, letters of acknowledgment to be written, those of inquiry from friends of the wounded to be answered.[48]

By July 8th the Christian Commission had also established a station in each Corps hospital with an experienced manager overseeing the work of five or six volunteers. The Commission supplied meals to both delegates and the wounded at "an eating saloon" managed by Louis Muller of Baltimore.[49]

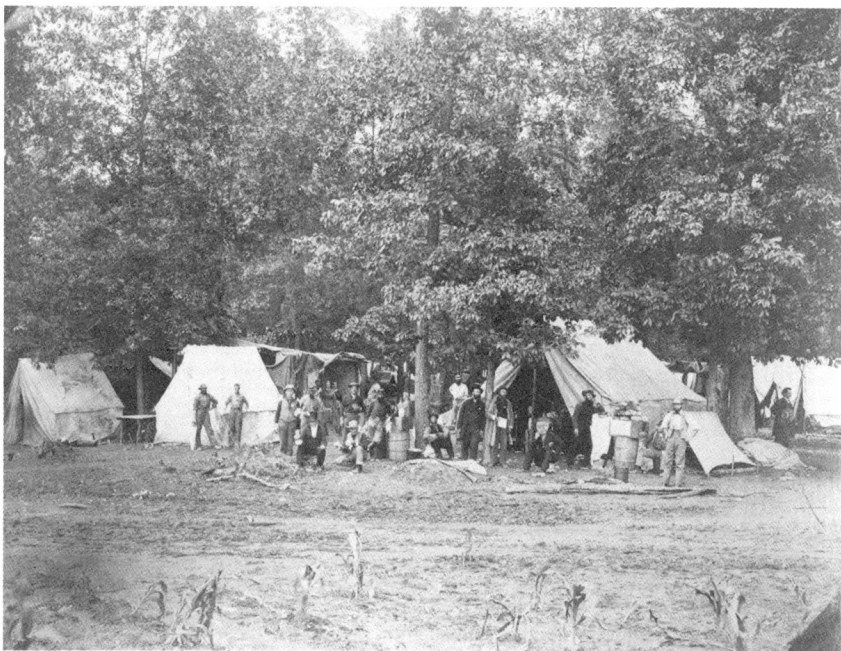

Christian Commission at 2nd Corps Hospital Frederick Gutekunst, July 11–15, 1863 Jerome B. Stillson in a patterned coat stands in front of the Christian Commission supply tent wearing the identifying badge of the U.S. Christian Commission. Next to him is Surgeon Justin Dwinelle, 106th Pennsylvania, wearing what appears to be the trefoil badge of the Second Corps. Nurses can be seen in the background along with other volunteers.   Courtesy of Special Collections and College Archives, Musselman Library, Gettysburg College

ADAMS EXPRESS COMPANY

Founded in 1854, Adams Express provided a range of services throughout the Civil War, delivering packages, documents, messages, and even serving as paymaster for both Union and Confederate soldiers. Following the battle of Gettysburg, the Baltimore-based company organized its own ambulance corps, providing doctors, nurses, wagons, hospital stores, clothing, and food, and earning high praise for their efforts. Daily shipments from Baltimore began on July 5th and by July 7th they had established a storehouse in Gettysburg to receive and distribute supplies valued at $5,000 per day.[50] John Q. A. Herring supervised the efforts of forty people organized in three companies to work in the hospitals at Gettysburg.[51]

STATE AGENTS

States sent "agents" to Gettysburg to inspect conditions and assist the wounded of their regiments as an example of the "Stateism" deplored by the Sanitary Commission. Assistant Surgeon John Shaw Billings, 7th U.S., described how this placed the regular army regiments at a disadvantage.

> Various State auxiliary associations brought fresh bread, mutton, fruits, etc., for their State regiments, but there were none for the regular troops. Finally there came along a wagon from the Fire Department of Baltimore. They said "this is just the kind of place we want to find, that don't belong to any State." Baltimore was rather neutral. After the wagon had been unloaded they informed me that they had packed one box for the surgeon. I got the benefit of that box, and it was most judiciously packed.[52]

Presbyterian minister Isaac Monfort was commissioned as military agent for Indiana and opened the Indiana Agency in Washington, DC, in February 1863, to assist men on the battlefield and in the hospitals. "In times of need after a battle . . . he would start with twenty or thirty nurses and helpers with lint, bandages and clothing and food for the sufferers, and personally tender them aid in the field."[53] Similarly, New Hampshire maintained a Soldiers' Aid Association headquartered in Washington, DC, and Governor Joseph Gilmore dispatched a number of volunteers to help care for men of New Hampshire regiments.[54]

Michigan's efforts to provide relief for the wounded illustrate the sometimes-conflicting agendas of multiple political and volunteer organizations. Michigan governor Austin Blair appointed Dr. Joseph W. Tunnicliff Jr. and his wife to a paid position as assistant state military agent headquartered in Washington, DC, in 1863. Tunnicliff visited the Gettysburg battlefield and reported on the care of the wounded but drew criticism for holding a paid position in contrast to the Michigan relief association that operated with unpaid volunteers. Judge James M. Edmund, Lincoln's appointee to the General Land Office, served as the chairman of the volunteer Michigan Soldiers' Relief Association also headquartered in Washington, DC. That organization dispatched physicians and volunteers from Washington to Gettysburg following the battle.[55] The Common Council of Detroit decided to launch its own efforts. The *Detroit Free Press* of July 9th reported an appropriation of $2,500 divided between a newly formed Common Council Committee and the "Michigan Aid Society" at Washington. Members of the Detroit committee, including the mayor, three aldermen, and Dr. Moses Gunn, also visited Gettysburg.[56]

New York's governor Horatio Seymour appointed his brother John F. Seymour as general agent to look after the needs of New York regiments at Gettysburg. The *New York Tribune* of July 15 reported,

> Mr. John F. Seymour, General Agent of State of NY for the relief of the State Soldier; Gen [John] Quackenbush, surgeon General of the state with a large and efficient corps of couriers, surgeons, and assistants are at Gettysburg and ministering to the wants of the wounded New York soldiers under the direction and with the sanction of the US Army authority.[57]

When Seymour became ill and had to leave Gettysburg, he asked Dr. Theodore Dimon to act as state agent in his place on July 16th.[58] Like many of the civilian physicians who volunteered at Gettysburg, Dimon had previous battlefield experience as a regimental surgeon. Arriving July 12th, he first reported to Medical Inspector Cuyler and was assigned to the Second Corps Hospital to oversee Confederate wounded. When no one at headquarters was able to give him directions, he instead made his way to the hotel serving as a hospital for New York wounded, where he found that "every part and parcel of the premises were disorderly and filthy" and the supervising surgeon spent his time "concocting iced drinks for himself and visiting friends and in exclaiming against the women's nursing staff."[59] Dimon worked to get the hospital in order. As state agent he inspected various hospital sites and reported on the needs of New York State wounded. His report to Seymour dated August 1st provides a detailed description of each Corps hospital, comments on amputations, burials of the dead, and suggests the need for a national cemetery at Gettysburg.[60]

Not surprisingly, the battle of Gettysburg, fought on Pennsylvania soil, elicited a vigorous response from Pennsylvanians. On July 5th Governor Andrew Curtin wrote to Surgeon General William Hammond, "Our people over the State are exceedingly anxious to render aid and assistance to the wounded at Gettysburg. Will you say how many volunteer surgeons I may send."[61] The response from James R. Smith, Assistant Surgeon General, was immediate: "The Medical Director of the Army of the Potomac has plenty of surgical aid."[62] Curtin was no doubt responding to the many offers of assistance coming from Pennsylvania communities. On July 6th, a contingent from the Sanitary Committee of Pittsburgh was in Harrisburg with twenty surgeons, trying to get to the battlefield.[63] On July 9th, Mrs. Harris of Philadelphia, already in Gettysburg, telegraphed the governor that "surgeons are greatly needed."[64] Communities across the state did not hesitate. Local Gettysburg physicians volunteered their services to care for the wounded and young women from Gettysburg, many of them teachers who were home for summer holiday, worked in the hospitals alongside other volunteers.[65] Groups from nearby Lancaster and York were among the first to arrive. A group from Phoenixville, organized as the Phoenixville Union Relief Society by Rebecca Lane Pennypacker Price, had obtained a pass from Governor Andrew Curtin through the intercession of Phoenix Iron Company owner David Reeves. Despite credentials from Governor Curtin, they were able to travel to Gettysburg only by securing an additional

Christian Commission pass in Maryland. Price and other volunteers from Phoenixville worked at the 11th Corps hospital.[66]

The *Philadelphia Inquirer* of July 6th reported under the heading of "Relief for the Wounded" that a "Committee of Ladies intend starting out from this city to Harrisburg, and if necessary to the scene of the late battle, to minister to the sick and wounded soldiers, having full authority to act in this capacity from Gov. Curtin."[67] Local groups in Philadelphia—Ladies' Aid Society, Soldiers' Aid, and Penn Relief—all responded to the call for volunteers as well as individual churches. Emily Bliss Souder wrote in her memoir of Gettysburg that "Many clergymen and citizens as well as surgeons and physicians of every grade hastened to the relief of the wounded and dying and many ladies made speedy arrangements to go to the field."[68] Most of the volunteers that Souder mentions by name were socially connected through family, women's aid societies, churches, and civic organizations like the Union League associated with Philadelphia's elite mercantile class.[69]

Another group of volunteers, who left Philadelphia on July 6th with Dr. Henry Teas Child, included women associated with radical ideas of spiritualism and dress reform, some of whom who had formal medical training. Child was accompanied by a group of volunteer nurses organized by Eliza Wood Burhans Farnham, a dress reform advocate and former matron at New York's Sing Sing prison, who had studied medicine in New York City. Farnham, Cornelia Hancock, and others in their group were probably supported by Penn Relief, a predominantly Hicksite Quaker organization, that also included Harriet Painter, an 1860 graduate of Pennsylvania Women's Medical College and dress reform advocate, who was traveling with her husband in the 7th New Jersey. Volunteer surgeon, Dr. Mary Edwards Walker, another dress reform advocate, was traveling with the Painters.[70] Accounts of the unconventional Philadelphia nurses and women doctors appear in the diary of Confederate chaplain Peter Tinsley, 28th Virginia, when he described Northern "she doctors."

> We meet many "she doctors" who amuse us very much in spite of our
> disgust. In going from one hospital to another we fall in with one of

these creatures, & walk along with her a mile or two, as she & her party are our guides. She is young, pretty, intelligent, & but for a grain of modesty would be a charming creature . . . Others that we meet have bloomer costumes encroaching more or less on male attire. They seem very assiduous & well pleased to examine & dress all sorts of wounds (perhaps) occasionally to amputate a leg.[71]

A letter from Sanitary Commission Secretary Frederick Law Olmsted on July 15th includes an explicit reference to "'The hermaphrodite Medico' means 'Miss Walker, M.D.' 'Doctoress Walker,' 'Walker, M.D. on the warpath,' as one of ours describes her."[72]

Many of the caregivers at Gettysburg, including civilian volunteers, fell ill and were forced to leave; few volunteers lasted more than a week or two before succumbing to dysentery, exhaustion, and the unhealthy environment. Both Dr. James and Dr. Child returned home sick after a week in Gettysburg. Eliza Farnham left sick and exhausted after four days at Gettysburg and died six months later from consumption.[73]

By July 22nd conditions at the field hospitals had improved considerably. Thanks to volunteer efforts, ample food and supplies were available in addition to government rations and supplies. Cornelia Hancock wrote home that the Second Corps field hospital was "in first rate order now."[74] On July 22nd, Christian Commission delegate Isaac Oliver Sloan wrote to the chairman of the Maryland Commission in Baltimore:

My dear friend-We are getting relieved in a measure from the pressure following the first 10 days or two weeks after the battle. Many of the wounded have been sent off and arrangements for the comfort of the sufferers remaining in the hospitals are so systematized and perfect that the work of the delegates is now comparatively easy . . . There is not so great a demand for attention to the physical wants of the men now as during the first two weeks after the battle.[75]

Two weeks after the Army of the Potomac departed, leaving 20,000 Union and Confederate wounded on the battlefield, the situation at Gettysburg was beginning to improve. The number of patients had been reduced by at least half through evacuation to nearby cities; others had died from their wounds. As military surgeons at the Corps hospitals gradually left to rejoin their regiments, they were replaced by additional contract surgeons. Plans to close the Corps hospitals and consolidate medical care for the wounded in a new general hospital at Gettysburg were already underway.

CHAPTER 8

Camp Letterman, July 22–November 20

On July 22, 1863, the General Hospital at Camp Letterman officially opened, ushering in the next phase of care for the wounded and the surgeons who remained in Gettysburg.[1] The first stage in the treatment of the wounded focused on emergency treatment of binding wounds and amputating shattered limbs to save lives, even as many continued to die in the field hospitals from disease, infection, and the severity of their wounds. The next goal was to remove as many surviving patients as possible to military hospitals in nearby cities. Thousands of wounded were transferred to hospitals in Baltimore, Philadelphia, Washington, New York, and New England. Medical Inspector Edward Vollum reported that, as of July 22nd, 11,425 wounded (7,608 Union and 3,817 Confederate) had been removed from Gettysburg. Nearly 5,000 wounded still remained (1,995 Union and 2,922 Confederate) who could not be safely evacuated.[2] The last phase of care involved closing the corps hospitals and consolidating the remaining patients in general hospitals at Gettysburg until they either died or recovered enough to be safely moved.

CAMP LETTERMAN

The original locations of the various Union corps hospitals and the corresponding Confederate hospitals had been chosen in haste during the battle, based on proximity to battle lines or immediate availability of buildings to shelter the wounded. Both military surgeons and civilian volunteers preferred well-ventilated tent hospitals to crowded buildings with poor ventilation, as Dr. Theodore Dimon explained in his report to New York State Agent John F. Seymour.

> It was plain to be seen, however, that the wounded in the town were not doing as well as those under tents in the field. The confinement of odors from wounds treated in rooms, accumulations of soiled straw and dressings in the enclosures about the buildings, free circulation of air obstructed by surrounding houses, and the town crowded with visitors, all must have proved unfavorable influences.[3]

As the number of patients at Gettysburg decreased through evacuation or death, pressure mounted to return public and private buildings being used for hospitals to civilian use. Weeks of occupation, rain, mud, surgery, and hasty burials of the dead raised concerns about camp hygiene in the existing field hospitals. The Second Corps moved its hospital tents at the end of July before relocating to the new General Hospital. Dr. Dimon's report explained that the wooded location of the Second Corps Hospital proved undesirable because "The trees kept out the sun and obstructed the circulation of the air. The space was too small rendering it necessary to crowd the tents and narrow the streets and the ground continued wet after rains."[4] Emily Bliss Souder, a nurse at the Second Corps hospital, left a similar account: "On Thursday (July 23) . . . the camp was changed to another location, known as 'the clover field,' a change which was very needful on every account."[5] She also noted that the trees had prevented "sun and wind from exerting their purifying influences."[6]

Plans for a general hospital began immediately after the battle. On July 5, 1863, a circular issued by Seth Williams, Assistant Adjutant General, had ordered, "The Medical Director will establish a General Hospital at Gettysburg for the wounded that cannot be moved with the army."[7] After Medical Director Jonathan Letterman left Gettysburg with the Army of the Potomac on July 7th, leaving Surgeon Henry Janes in charge, Janes continued to report to him for the first two weeks. On July 9th he wrote to Letterman that "We have been short of nurses, surgeons, and transportation, both ambulance and railroad. I shall be able to begin the permanent hospital soon if I can get the hospital tents. There are not enough in the corps hospitals for the purpose."[8] Five days later he reported to Letterman that a "fine site" had been selected and he was anxiously awaiting the tents.[9] The next day on July 15th, Capt. William G. Rankin, depot quartermaster in Gettysburg, confirmed that "The Hospital tents arrived to-day, and are being put up."[10] By July 16th, 80 acres of George Wolf's farm, located along present-day Route 30, were being prepared for the hospital under the supervision of Surgeon Cyrus Nathaniel Chamberlain, U.S. Sixth Corps.[11] Unlike the earlier hospitals, located behind battle lines or in buildings temporarily appropriated for the purpose, Camp Letterman was designed to provide the most healthful and convenient environment possible for recuperating patients. The site was situated on high ground, conveniently adjacent to the railroad tracks, with plenty of fresh air and clean water.

Accounts of Camp Letterman often cite "convenience" and "order," in contrast to the decentralized and improvised nature of the battlefield hospitals. Christian Commission agent Andrew Boyd Cross wrote a particularly detailed description of this transition.

> As the men at the different hospitals became fit for removal, they were sent away to hospitals in different parts of Maryland and Pennsylvania, and the District of Columbia. Then a general hospital was established near the town, about 1¼ miles east on the York turnpike, while the Seminary was also retained. The general hospital of tents was in a very excellent situation, a beautiful spot, with a skirt of woods on north-east and also on south-west, a good spring of water very near, the ground gradually rolling so that water did not remain after a rain. There were from 125 to 150 tents. Those for the wounded were large, well-built and capable of containing comfortably from twelve to sixteen persons, were on good bedsteads with mattresses. The arrangements were such as to make everything convenient, so much so that, after observing those in tents and such as were in our large and well-constructed buildings, we were fully persuaded that the tents, until severely cold weather, were the most healthy and convenient for the patients, and as convenient for surgeons and nurses.[12]

Cornelia Hancock wrote home on August 8th from the General Hospital, describing the new location. "Our hospital is on rising ground, divided off into six avenues, and eighteen tents holding twelve men each on each avenue. We call four tents a ward and name them by letter, mine is ward E." Compared to conditions at the Second Corps hospital, she could report that "The water is excellent and there is order in everything. I like it a great deal better than the battlefield, but the battlefield is where one does most good."[13]

Various accounts differ on the number of tents, from nurse Sophronia Bucklin's inflated estimate of 500 to more realistic estimates of between 125 and 150, but all agreed on the military precision of the rows of tents arranged into divisions and wards. Assistant Surgeon William Norris's description provides a detailed contemporary account at the time when the camp was first established:

The Hospital consists of Hospital Tents on the slope of a hill near Gettysburg & on the railroad; plenty of good water & woods on two sides of the encampment. Dr. Goodman (Surg to Geary's regt [28th Pennsylvania]) formerly resident at the Alms house is in charge. He has put me in charge of the row of tents appropriated to the 1st Corps. 16 tents holding 192 beds. These are subdivided into wards 48 beds to the ward, each under charge of an assistant surgeon.[14]

Assistant Surgeon William Breakey, 16th Michigan, recollected,

We had one of the finest field hospitals of the war named in honor to the medical director of the Army of the Potomac, Camp Letterman, The open ground—about sixty acres—sloped to the west, offering excellent surface drainage. They were accurately laid out into streets which were graded, giving sufficient room between for double hospital tents, leaving ample space between the tents, the earth under each tent leveled and packed, making a smooth hard floor. The quarters of the medical director, surgeons, medical purveyor, quartermaster, commissary, sanitary and Christian commissions and mess hall, were in a grove on the north side.[15]

Photographs of Camp Letterman taken by the Tyson Brothers in 1863 document the arrangement of tents. The photographs show rows of double tents, spaced about 10 feet apart, and measuring approximately 15 feet x 28 feet, each designed to hold twelve beds, as described by both Norris and Cross. Six avenues, roughly 30 feet wide, separating seven rows of tents would correspond to seven divisions and twenty-eight wards.[16] This configuration could accommodate 112 double tents housing 1,344 patients. This corresponds to Breakey remembering that during the three months he was on duty, the total number of patients treated at Camp Letterman totaled about 3,000, and the average was probably 1,200–1,500 patients at one time.[17]

CONSOLIDATION

When Sophronia Bucklin and Rebecca Stanley Caldwell arrived in Gettysburg on Saturday, July 18th under the auspices of the Sanitary Commission, they were first directed to the Seminary hospital, but the next day proceeded to the new general hospital. On Sunday "we took our way up to the hospital ground, where five hundred tents had already been erected . . . The hospital lay in the rear of a deep wood in a large open field, a mile and a half from Gettysburg, and overlooking it, the single line of rail which connected the battle town with the outer world sweeping it on one side. . . . "[18] Bucklin reported that they were the first women at the general hospital and that patients were already being brought from other locations.

The move to the general hospital took several weeks, and patients continued to be moved there from other locations until early September. William Norris, placed in charge of the First Corps, 3rd Division hospitals at the Presbyterian and Catholic churches in town, described the process of moving his patients in a letter to his father on July 26th from the General Hospital near Gettysburg:

> On Thursday afternoon I received orders to break up the Hospital & move all the men out to the General Hospital . . . This however would have been impossible to execute and it was finally countermanded our departure fixed for the next morning [July 24]. At 4 o'clock AM

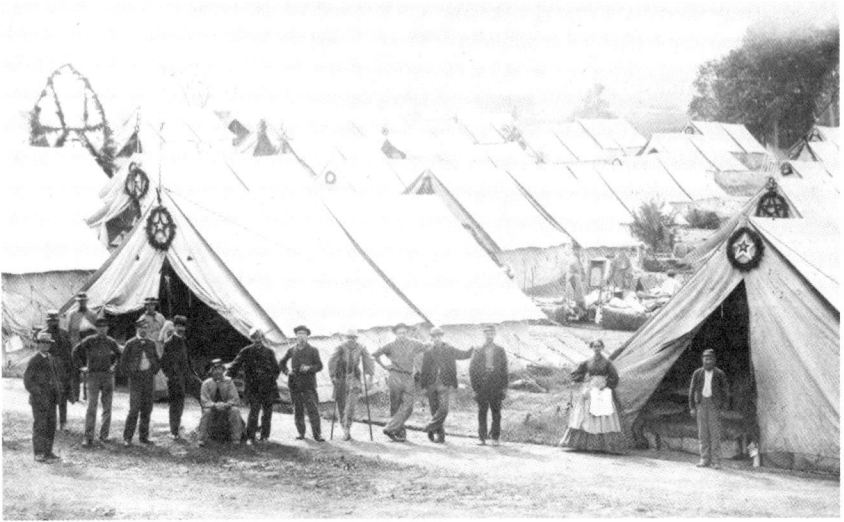

Letterman General Hospital tents with patients and attendants. Tyson Brothers Photographers, Gettysburg, September 1863. Courtesy of Library of Congress, Prints and Photographs Division.

the Hospital was astir, and by 8 AM all wards had been dressed, the patients had had their breakfast and we were beginning to move. I sent those cases capable of transportation to Harrisburg and most of our stumps [amputees] by ambulance to the Genl Hospt. Our comp fracts of thigh and leg I had carried in stretchers and as the distance was a mile and a quarter, it was a considerable undertaking. By stirring up the Provost Marshal for a detail of men & keeping every available man steadily at work I succeeded in having everything moved out by 7 pm. I then started & walked out myself. Our patients bore the journey better than I had anticipated, those carried in stretchers did not appear to have suffered at all.[19]

The new hospital was still being set up when he arrived on July 24th. "Everything here is yet up side down we are building proper kitchen, oven, etc. Last night I occupied one of the vacant hospital tents it rained here all the night. The night previous I slept in a stretcher."[20]

On July 27th Emily Souder wrote home to her husband that "the Second Corps is being moved to the General Hospital with all convenient dispatch" since "the surgeons were wanted with their regiments, which made concentration necessary."[21] She reported,

> The sick have been removed from several of the churches; and the process of purifying is going on very energetically. The Third and Fifth Corps are being brought into the General Hospital, which is near the railroad. The Twelfth Corps is entirely removed; the Eleventh Corps nearly so. The ambulances and litters are constantly passing through the town.[22]

Dr. Dimon also reported that by July 30th, the general hospital at Gettysburg was nearly completed and the Eleventh, Twelfth, and Sixth Corps hospitals had been relieved of all their patients and others were in process of being transferred.[23] The Fifth Corps hospital reportedly moved on July 31st.[24] Dr. Dwinelle, Surgeon, 106th Pennsylvania, in charge of the Second Corps hospitals predicted that some of his patients could not be removed for two weeks.[25] By August 5th Clarissa Jones wrote, "We are packed up ready to leave this camp at an hour's notice. Many of the men have been removed and by this hour tomorrow we expect all but a few cases will have gone."[26] Cornelia Hancock wrote to her sister on August 6th, "We have all our men moved now to General Hospital."[27]

Consolidation of Confederate wounded also accelerated following the construction of the general hospital. Writing from "Camp Letterman near Gettysburg" on July 27, Norris reported that "Our camp presents a very bustling scene constant arrivals of patients today. A considerable number of Rebs."[28] Chaplain Peter Tinsley, 28th Virginia, chronicled the removal of patients from the Confederate hospital at Bream's Mill. On July 24th he reported, "The usual routine—A Yankee Surgeon Tate [Theodore Tate] accompanied by a citizen Dr. from Pittsburgh visit our hosp., examines patient &c with reference to sending them off. He is extremely ungentlemanly—entirely ignores our Surgs & goes through the ward pointing out to his Sergt those to be sent off next day."[29] When the Confederate hospitals were closed down at the beginning of August, Tinsley, other chaplains, and most of the Confederate surgeons were transferred to the provost marshal in Baltimore as prisoners; only nine Confederate surgeons remained at Camp Letterman until October.[30]

The buildings of Pennsylvania College (now Gettysburg College) mainly housed Confederate wounded after the battle. Captain Decimus et Ultimus Barziza, 4th Texas, wounded and taken prisoner on July 2nd, was taken to the field hospital of the Twelfth Corps during the battle. "This Field Hospital soon became very filthy, and the wounded were moved as fast as possible to Gettysburg. There was a college building in the town, which had been used by the Confederates whilst they occupied the place. To this building most of the Confederates were carried."[31] The remaining Pennsylvania College patients were moved to Camp Letterman by July 29th so that college classes could resume in mid-September.[32]

The Lutheran Seminary served first as an aid station during the morning of the first day's battle, and later as the U.S. First Corps, 1st Division, hospital. By the end of July, it was selected to serve as a second general hospital for both Union and Confederate wounded to take advantage of the healthy environment provided by its higher elevation and adequate water supply. Franklin Fayette Pratt, 76th New York, served as a nurse in the Court House in town from July 1st until his patients were moved to the Seminary on August 3rd. He wrote home,

> We moved all the wounded from the Court House yesterday to the Seminary, and put the most of them in large tents, which are very comfortable. We have 6 wounded men in a tent, which is too many. There should be four in each tent. It is too crowded. There is one tent here yet with some Rebel wounded in it. They have just as good care as our own men. I think it a much better place here than in town. It surely is more quiet, and there is a better air, for it is on high ground.[33]

He described his shift from 6 p.m. until midnight "sitting up with the wounded men . . . I am always on hand, when on duty, to attend to their every want."[34] Pratt described the work of the Sisters of Charity, the abundance of good food, and the extras still furnished by private contributions. Pratt continued at the Seminary hospital until September

5th, when all patients except James McFarland were moved to the Camp Letterman general hospital or to other cities.

One Union cavalry surgeon resisted orders to consolidate and at first refused to close his hospital. Local complaints against Assistant Surgeon Perrin A. Gardner, 1st West Virginia Cavalry, in charge of the Union Cavalry hospital in Hanover, Pennsylvania, prompted Henry Janes to investigate. He reported, "The Doctor was remarkably successful in gaining the dislike of the inhabitants of the town and the men under his command."[35] Dr. Gardner acknowledged that he threatened to burn the houses of liquor drinkers, wrote an article forbidding a young woman from visiting the hospital because she had spoken disrespectfully to him, and admitted that he had made $1,000 since the battle by embalming bodies of the dead. Despite his claims that he took orders only from the medical director of Kilpatrick's Cavalry Division, the hospital was broken up around August 15th, and Gardner was ordered to rejoin his regiment.

By mid-August the *Adams Sentinel* reported that there were 1,600 patients at the general hospital and an additional 400 divided among the Seminary, public school, and Shead's and Buehler's Hall (also referred to as the Express Office).[36] A few patients remained in private residences. The Public School and Express Office hospitals closed in August, allowing the military surgeons working there to return to their regiments, and the patients were either evacuated or moved to Letterman.[37] When James McFarland, the last patient at the Seminary, left for home on September 16th the Seminary hospital closed and the process of consolidation to the Camp Letterman General Hospital was completed.

STAFF CHANGES

Consolidation was not the only change taking place at the end of July. On July 18th Jonathan Letterman reported that the hospitals at Gettysburg "were taken from under my control."[38] While Henry Janes remained in charge of the Gettysburg hospitals, he now reported to Surgeon William S. King, medical director of the Department of the Susquehanna.[39] On assuming responsibility for the Gettysburg hospitals, King's first orders were to hire additional contract surgeons to relieve the remaining regimental surgeons so that they could rejoin the troops.

Joseph R. Smith, senior assistant in the Office of the Surgeon General in Washington, DC, made it clear that King should "make contracts with such doctors as you may be able at $112.83 per month and to thus relieve with all practible dispatch the Medical officers of the Army of the Potomac who will be sent to their regiments when so relieved . . . it is desirable as soon as possible to close the hospitals at Gettysburg."[40] King lost no time securing contracts with three Gettysburg physicians who had been assisting with the wounded since the battle. On July 23rd he signed contracts for Dr. Charles Horner (July 23–September 8) and Dr. Henry Huber (July 23–September 8) and on July 24th for Dr. Robert Horner (July 24–October 23), all at the rate of $100.[41] A few days later, the Surgeon General's Office wrote to King that "a number of contract Physicians have been employed by this office and ordered to report to you for duty, and others will be engaged as the proper material presents itself. Should any of these Surgeons prove incompetent, you will please annul their contracts at once and report the fact to this office."[42] Other contract surgeons were being referred from medical directors in Philadelphia and Harrisburg. Dr. James Potter Wilson, serving at Camp Curtin in Harrisburg, telegraphed Henry Janes on August 1st: "More Surgeons here than required. Shall I send them to Gettysburg." One of those surgeons, Henry K. Neff, described how he was recruited to return to Gettysburg.

> I then went to Harrisburg PA where my Regiment was to be mustered out on the 24th of July—Dr. JP Wilson, Medical Director at Harrisburg informed me he had just had a dispatch from the Surgeon Genl. at Washington, ordering him to send ten (10) surgeons for duty to Gettysburg and wished me to go as one, which I did. I remained there in charge of the Div No 3, General Hospital (Drs. Oakley and Emanuel having charge of Division No 1 & 2) until relieved by Dr. Janes on the 27th of August 1863.[43]

Another of Dr. Wilson's recruits, James Ross Reily, former surgeon of the 179th Pennsylvania, was not at the battle of Gettysburg but mustered out with his regiment in Harrisburg on July 25, 1863, and was "Assigned to duty after the battle of Gettysburg as Surgeon in Charge of 1st Corps hospital by Surgeon Janes, US Vols in charge hospitals about Gettysburg."[44] Prior service created confusions with some contracts. Neff wrote in December 1863 that he had not been paid for his work at Gettysburg and, even after his death, his widow tried to confirm his service at Gettysburg to receive payment. On August 29, 1863, Janes and King were still sorting out how to pay Dr. Reily since "If Dr. Reily's Regiment is mustered out it would be proper to relieve him at once as I do not know how he could be paid after the mustering out of his regiment."[45]

During August changes in medical staff continued as regimental surgeons left Gettysburg to be replaced by contract physicians. Nurse Cornelia Hancock wrote from Camp Letterman on August 17th, "We no sooner get a good physician than an order comes to remove, promote, demote or *something*. Everything seems to be done to aggravate the wounded."[46] On August 5th, King wrote to Janes that "I will write to Dr. Wilson and stress to send no more contract physicians to you. Relieve all the Regimental Medical Officers you may not deem indispensable for the proper and skillful treatment of your wounded."[47] On August 18th Janes reported that all remaining medical officers of the Army of the Potomac were released except for four surgeons and four assistant surgeons. He reported 1,600 patients remaining and added, "I have moved to Camp Letterman to take personal charge but have little time for anything but official business."[48] Correspondence between Janes and King provides a sampling of the paperwork involved in staffing the general hospital with contract surgeons. On August 17th Janes wrote to King, "Acting Assistant Surg Thos Smith requests to be relieved as he feels unwilling to report to a younger man. I think his request should be complied with as his loss will not be irreparable."[49]

Concerns about the qualifications of some contract surgeons also resulted in dismissals. King made it clear to Janes that "it is not desired that our wounded should be left in the hands of any but those fully competent. Those not deemed fully competent among the contract physicians, no matter with whom the contracts were made, should be reported at this office at once that their contracts may be annulled and they relieved from duty."[50] Henry Janes duly reported that Dr. J. B. Carpenter of Theresa, Jefferson County, New York, who had contracted with the surgeon general July 28, 1863, was relieved from duty at Camp Letterman for appropriating money from patients for his own use while on duty at the Confederate hospital of the Third Corps and for other irregularities.[51]

At the Seminary hospital, contract surgeons also replaced the departing military surgeons. James Ross Reily, now mustered out and serving as a contract surgeon, took charge of the hospital from Surgeon Robert Loughran, 80th New York, and as many as nine other contract surgeons served there until the beginning of September when the remaining patients were moved to Camp Letterman.[52]

At Camp Letterman, Assistant Surgeon Breakey recalled, "The work was systematized and professionally interesting and agreeable. Medical Director Hanes [Janes] of Vermont, and Surgeon-in chief Chamberlain of Massachusetts and the staff generally were able men, with whom it was a pleasure to be associated."[53] On duty at Camp Letterman from July 31st when the 5th Corps hospital moved, until October 26 when he left due to illness, Breakey would have known and served alongside most of the medical staff at Letterman. Sources suggest that the medical staff at Letterman totaled between thirty-five and fifty surgeons at any one time. Two members of the Maryland Christian Commission visited Gettysburg at the end of August and reported that Dr. Janes, superintendent or medical director, and Assistant Superintendent Dr. Chamberlain were in charge of seven division and twenty-six ward surgeons. They found the surgeons "to be of very communicative talent, and bland and attractive manners," and contrasted the "tenderness" of the surgeons they met in the General and Seminary Hospitals with the "roughness and brutality" they had witnessed earlier among the surgeons in the battlefield hospitals.[54] An undated source recorded that Surgeon Cyrus N. Chamberlain oversaw twenty-eight acting assistant surgeons, seven assistant surgeons, and four surgeons plus nine Confederate doctors.[55] Various lists, records, signed testimonials, and other reports suggest that these numbers represent an accurate assessment of the medical staff of Camp Letterman in full operation in mid-August.

The hospital staff was a combination of military surgeons, contract acting assistant surgeons, and Confederate medical officers. Altogether, at least sixty-six physicians were on duty there during its four months of operation. Of the twenty Union military surgeons and assistant surgeons who served at Camp Letterman, seven of them, including Henry Janes, were from the Sixth Corps, which had been held in reserve during the battle and experienced the fewest casualties. The rest were regimental surgeons and assistant surgeons drawn from the other corps, including cavalry, the medical purveyor, and two of the additional U.S. assistant surgeons who had been sent to assist after the battle.[56]

At least thirty-seven contract surgeons eventually served at Camp Letterman before it closed.[57] The medical backgrounds of these acting assistant surgeons did not differ significantly from the military surgeons who served at Gettysburg. Most had graduated from the same medical schools as their commissioned colleagues. Fifteen graduated from the University of Pennsylvania, seven from Jefferson, and seven from Pennsylvania Medical College. Others graduated from Georgetown Medical College, DC; Victoria College, Toronto; University of Maryland, Baltimore; and Castleton Medical College, Vermont. At least two had studied in Europe. One graduated from an eclectic medical college. The oldest, Thomas Tucker Smiley, born in 1795, was probably the elderly doctor that Cornelia Hancock describes in charge of Ward E on August 6th.[58] Thirteen of them, still in their twenties, were either recent graduates or had taken time off from their studies to serve as contract physicians. The remainder had between five and twenty years of medical experience. While some contract surgeons were newly recruited, others had served in Philadelphia and Washington hospitals or had previous experience as regimental surgeons. Some of the contract surgeons who served in the Corps hospitals moved to Camp Letterman with their patients. These included James Shivers from College Hospital; Henry Leaman, Robert Horner, and William Miller Welch from Seminary hospital; Benjamin Butcher from the Presbyterian church; and Henry Neff from the 11th Corps hospital.

The Dregs of Battle
The patients who remained at Camp Letterman in August were described by the Sanitary Commission as

only the desperate cases of amputation, compound fracture, and penetrating wounds of the chest and pelvis. These were collected with the utmost care, many of them on stretchers, from miles around, and placed under the three hundred tents which constitute Camp Letterman Hospital; which contained, in truth, the very dregs of battle from two armies.[59]

The patients at Camp Letterman represented the most serious cases. Assistant Surgeon Breakey later estimated from memory that the cases of gunshot and shell wounds included: 1,000 amputations divided equally among forearms, legs and thighs; seventy penetrating wounds of the chest, and forty of the abdomen; twenty skull fractures; and 200 knee injuries.[60] The surgeons continued to treat wounds with dressings, splints, and secondary amputations. Many patients suffered from life-threatening hemorrhages, diseases, and infection. Thirty-five-year-old Andrew Cheever of the 16th Massachusetts was wounded July 2nd and had his thigh amputated on July 18th in the Third Corps hospital. After admission to the General Hospital on August 1st, his wound was infected and treated with tincture of iodine. He also had a cough, urinary difficulty, and diarrhea, but he survived and was eventually discharged.[61] Confederate F. W. Smith, twenty-two, of the 14th Virginia, was wounded July 3 and admitted to the general hospital on July 24. He had compound fractures of the right thigh and flesh wounds in his left forearm and shoulder but was also suffering from prostration and tetanus, unable to eat solid food because of muscle rigidity in his jaw. Treated with "morphia administered freely with beef tea and milk punch," he died on August 8th from tetanus.[62]

Women nurses frequently described the condition and suffering of their patients in their letters and memoirs. Cornelia Hancock wrote in mid-August that "not one of the men under my care that can get up yet! How patient they are though never complain and lay still from day to day."[63] Nurses Sophronia Bucklin and Anna Holstein both described the painful deaths of patients slowly wasting away with disease or dying suddenly from a hemorrhaging stump, and often commented on their stoic acceptance of death. Sophronia Bucklin among other nurses observed

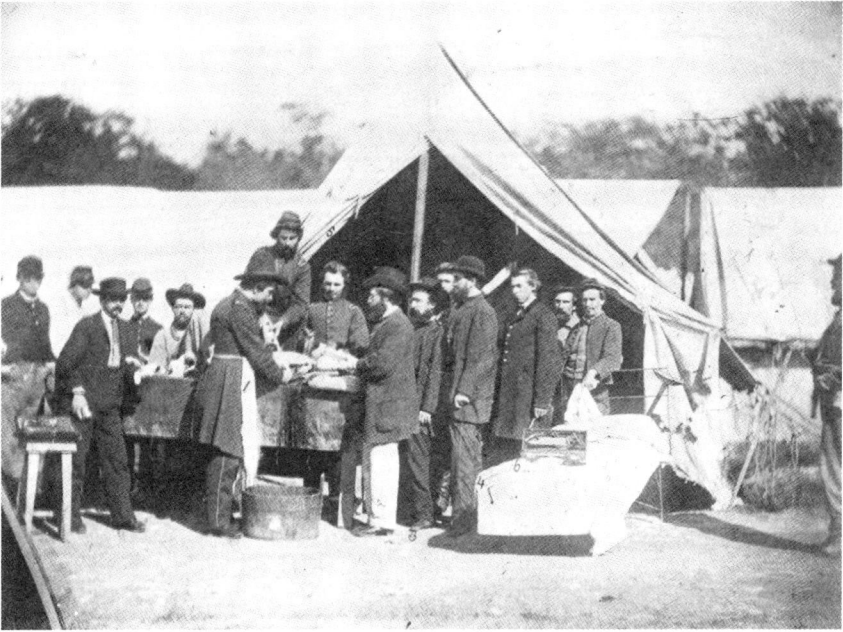

Operating tent at Camp Letterman Hospital, Gettysburg, Pennsylvania. Dr. Henry Janes is shown operating on twenty-one-year-old Peter Brock, 28th Massachusetts, wounded on July 2nd. The operation was described by Sophronia Bucklin and in a case report submitted to the *Medical and Surgical History of the War of the Rebellion* (Vol. II of Part II, 591). Brock survived and received a disability pension September 1873. Peter S. Weaver, photographer, October 20, 1863. Courtesy of U.S. Army Heritage and Education Center, Carlisle, Pennsylvania.

that "many more of the rebels died than of our own men—whether from the nature of their wounds, which seemed generally more frightful, or because they lacked courage to bear up under them."[64] The more likely reason was that, as prisoners, they had received treatment later than the Union wounded and suffered more from the consequences of infection, gangrene, and tetanus.

A PRISON HOSPITAL

By mid-July the number of Confederate patients consolidated into the general hospitals at Letterman and the Seminary created new concerns about their status as prisoners. During the first weeks after the battle, the provost responsible for policing the battlefield was occupied with protecting government property left on the battlefield from curious visitors and thieves and left the supervision of the wounded to the medical staff and volunteers. Immediately following the battle, Union medical staff treated Confederate wounded as patients rather than prisoners. By the end of July, high-ranking Confederate patients like generals Isaac Trimble and James Kemper were transferred from private homes to the Seminary hospital and placed under constant guard. Fears about prisoner escapes from the hospitals were not unjustified. The *Adams Sentinel* of July 21 reported that "Thursday night last (July 16) a number of rebels who were connected with the hospitals in this place managed to get hold of Federal uniforms, arms and horses and in this disguise made their escape towards Dixie. They have since been retaken."[65] Emily Bliss Souder wrote on July 28th that "Some *ladies* from Baltimore made themselves a name and a fame, a few days since, by furnishing citizens' clothes for some rebels to flee in. They stole several horses, and made their escape, but most of them were retaken."[66] Additional steps were taken to tighten security with General Order No. 2 issued July 30th by the Department of the Susquehanna and signed by Col. Hiram Alleman, 36th Pennsylvania Militia, the appointed military governor of Gettysburg. In addition to halting the disinterment of dead until cold weather for health reasons, the order restricted visitors to Confederate wounded. Passes were now required to visit Confederate hospitals; extra food and supplies for Confederates were to be distributed through surgeons and divided equally among all patients; and no citizen clothing was allowed in any hospitals.[67]

Cornelia Hancock encountered these new protocols when she first came to Camp Letterman:

> No citizens are allowed in Camp without a pass only after four o'clock. The militia go around after dark and pick up strangers to take them out of camp. The other night they asked me if I was a detailed nurse. As it was before I was sworn in, I had to say "No." They said their orders were peremptory, so I would have to go, but Steward Olmstead appeared and told them that I was all right, so they went away.[68]

Franklin Pratt at the Seminary also noted, "There has been changes made here since I last wrote you. The Rebels and Union was in tents side by side all mixed up. Now, we have got the Rebels all in one row of tents, and our men all in another, so that visitors can tell us apart. At our tent, we had a small National flag raised to distinguish us from the Rebels, as they were in the tent next to us. Some of the visitors took us for Rebels and passed us by, before we raised the Stars and Stripes."[69]

Dr. Janes came under increasing pressure to enhance security and remove as many Confederate wounded as possible to more secure prison hospitals. On August 27th a letter regarding Confederate wounded, signed by Col. William Hoffman, Commissary General of Prisoners, requested that all Rebel officers among the sick and wounded be forwarded to Johnson's Island near Sandusky, Ohio, as soon as possible, "None must be permitted to escape by being detained there [at Gettysburg] beyond the proper time for their removal."[70] The Surgeon General's Office was also anxious to transfer the expenses for Confederate patients from the Medical Department to the Office of Prisoners. On September 19th Janes was asked to forward reports of daily averages for Confederate and Union soldiers under his care between July 1 and September 1. "The report is needed to estimate the amount due the Medical Department from the appropriation for the Prisoners of War."[71] Requests for information on Confederate wounded continued until December 5th, when a frustrated Janes replied that he had only privates pulled from the ranks to handle the paperwork from treating 20,000 wounded.[72]

RELIEF ORGANIZATIONS

Relief organizations also consolidated and reorganized as their work shifted from emergency support on the battlefield during the first weeks to a more centralized presence at the general hospitals. Dr. John H. Douglas, previously in charge of U.S. Sanitary Commission efforts, left Gettysburg and placed Dr. Gordon Winslow in charge of operations at Camp Letterman where "the Sanitary Commission established its more permanent and systematic methods of relief at that place."[73] The Sanitary Commission station consisted of large tents "spread beneath tall oaks and hickorys"—a lodging tent for thirty persons and six or eight other tents for stores and offices. Samuel Bacon Jr. continued to act as Sanitary Commission store-keeper. "A kitchen to prepare the lighter diet prescribed by the surgeons was under the direction of ladies, two of whom remained there for several months."[74]

As patients from the various Corps hospitals were moved to Camp Letterman, the Christian Commission formally ended its special field operations on August 7th and turned over the hospital stores and store-rooms to the local Gettysburg Army Committee of the U.S. Christian Commission with Robert G. McCreary of Gettysburg as chairman. "A store tent, sleeping tent and eating tent with some 12 delegates formed the Christian Commission establishment at the general field hospital."[75] "At the general hospital we had our tents and delegates, continuing from the commencement of the encampment to its close. The labors here were systematic and regular, because we had gotten things into one place, and under regular order. The services of ministers and laymen from different denominations, were here rendered with diligence and fidelity."[76]

HOSPITAL ROUTINE

Regular order governed the daily functioning of the hospital. Sophronia Bucklin described how each attendant had specific work. "First the surgeon in charge, next the hospital steward, then the ward surgeons, next women nurses, ward masters, men nurses, wound dressers, and night watch. The officer of the day made his rounds every two hours, day and night, ascertaining that no watchers were asleep. . . . and to administer medical aid, if required."[77] With order came regulations and plenty of the dreaded "red tape." Cornelia Hancock and Sophronia Bucklin both reported run-ins with Mrs. Kate Duncan, the matron responsible for hospital supplies of linens, pads, and pillows.[78]

Food preparation and distribution were tightly regulated and sometimes a point of contention. Hospital patients, weakened from wounds and disease, required special "low diets" of broth, toast, rice, custards, lemonade, flavored water, and milk punch. Cornelia Hancock wrote home to describe the scale of the main cook house that prepared meals for 1,300 men.[79] Sophronia Bucklin described how

We soon had a government kitchen, a low diet kitchen, and an extra diet kitchen, with several large stoves, and large cauldrons in which to make the soup which was always served for dinner. One set of men were detailed for soup-making, another for roasting beef, another for cooking vegetables, and when the great oven was prepared, the bread for the whole hospital was baked in its heated depths.[80]

Bucklin and Hancock both complained that Mrs. Anna Holstein, in charge of the special diet kitchen, often made it difficult for them to fill orders for their patients. Hancock vowed that "I *will* get the things for the men without orders and she is a great respector of order."[81] Bucklin described how Mrs. Holstein forbade the nurses to prepare extra food or go inside the kitchen, even "deeming it necessary to keep a guard, with fixed bayonet, at the entrance."[82] The surgeons were often called on to intercede. Acting Assistant Surgeon Elias P. Townsend, officer of the day on August 19, reported that Mrs. Holstein complained about bogus orders to the kitchen for those that shouldn't receive rations.[83] Although food was plentiful, eggs and butter were sometimes in short supply, and patients routinely complained about not getting enough to eat. When Medical Inspector John Cuyler returned to Gettysburg to visit Camp Letterman on August 30th, he talked with patients and specifically asked them if they got enough to eat. He then turned to Surgeon Chamberlain and told him that "The first thing to set your self about is feeding these men . . . feed them till they can't complain . . . clean avenues and clean tents [will] not cure a man."[84]

Sophronia Bucklin outlined the daily care required by so many seriously ill and disabled patients as the "summer days glided swiftly away." The daily routine for the nurses included distributing beef tea, stimulants and extra diet three times a day, wound dressing, washing faces, combing hair, shaving beards, seeing to clean bedding and clothing, and delivering extra drinks ordered by the surgeons. She compared the regular routine of hospital life to "the methodical operations of a thorough housekeeper: except that men died, and in their empty beds others were speedily laid to recover or die also."[85]

Trivial Pursuits

Despite the hard work, the suffering and death, the hospital staff still found opportunities to relax and socialize. The Reverend Franklin J. F. Schantz, on his second visit to Gettysburg, July 22–27, found the surgeon-in-chief of the Seminary hospital with "a party of men in his room, drinking and singing negro melodies."[86] Col. George McFarland of the 151st Pennsylvania, a patient at the Seminary, wrote in his diary in early September that "some noisy drunken attendants and doctors . . . took part in a general jollification—a regular drunk, in which rumor says all or nearly all were engaged, even many of the patients down stairs waiting for transportation." Several days later, he recorded, "There are some rowdies here with their chief Dr. R. who keep everyone awake with their revelries."[87] Not surprisingly, Reily and the four acting assistant surgeons on duty at the beginning of September were all young men in their twenties, only a few years out of medical school, where parties and drinking had been commonplace.

Other pursuits were less boisterous and disruptive. Assistant Surgeon Breakey described his time at Letterman as "among the happiest days of my life." In fact, "once the general affairs were so well in hand that it was practicable for part of the staff to get off duty in the afternoons, and we walked, rode in ambulance or on horseback over the field, becoming familiar with most parts of this famous battleground." Breakey's young wife joined him in Gettysburg after a year of separation following their marriage the year before. She was one of several wives, including the wives of Lewis Oakley and Henry May, who visited the wounded, wrote letters, and provided other nursing services. The living arrangements for the Breakeys included "two nine feet square wall tents, a reception and bedroom next door to Dr. Winslow's. A canvas carpet, a barrel chair, a tanbark sidewalk. We went to the headquarters' mess for meals and had none of the ordinary cares of housekeeping that detract so much from the enjoyment of modern civilized social life."[88]

Anna Holstein wrote in her memoir, "Hospital life, with its strict military rule, is so wearisome and monotonous, that what would be the most trivial pleasure at other times and places, is *here* magnified into a matter of great importance."[89] She described two special events in addition to occasional tours of the battlefield and visits to town. On

September 23rd a banquet was held at Camp Letterman for the remaining 1,183 patients. Holstein described how "In September, while the hospital was still crowded with patients, a festival was given for their amusement." The surgeons and "their ladies," Christian Commission, friends in Philadelphia, and ladies of the town all participated in arrangements, with committees appointed for different wards so that none would be neglected. The streets and tents were decorated with evergreen arches and patriotic designs, bands played, a dinner was served, and in the evening "an entertainment of *negro* minstrels, the performers being all *white* soldiers in the hospitals," was deemed the crowning pleasure of the day.[90] On October 20th Mrs. Holstein, Mrs. May, and "a few patriotic friends from Montgomery County obtained a large flag and organized a ceremony to place it on Round Top."[91]

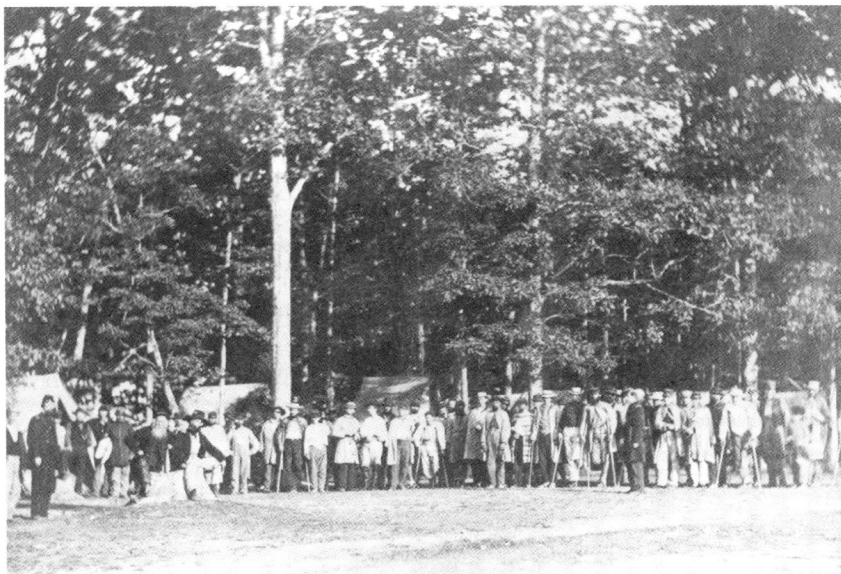

Wounded Confederates at Camp Letterman. This photograph was probably taken September 23rd during the picnic for Camp Letterman patients. Gordon Winslow and Henry Janes are seated in the left foreground. Courtesy of U.S. Army Heritage and Education Center, Carlisle, Pennsylvania

Closing Camp Letterman

By the end of October Holstein reported that the "work of reducing the number of patients now began in earnest. Sixty were at one time sent in the cars, who had each but one arm apiece; the next train took the same number with one leg apiece, and one little cavalry boy who had lost both at the knee."[92] The *Adams Sentinel* reported on November 10th that the number of wounded was rapidly diminishing to less than a hundred, "and a week or two will probably witness the breaking up of the Camp as they are being removed as fast as their situation will allow."[93]

During October, reduced numbers of patients meant that fewer surgeons were required. Contract surgeons relieved from duty included: W. L. Hayes (October 8); William B. Jones (October 10); Daniel R. Good (October 9); Charles S. Gauntt (October 12); and James Newcombe (October 29). Surgeon Oakley was ordered to rejoin his regiment October 28 and Assistant Surgeon Breakey left sick for Washington.[94]

The Sanitary Commission reported that on November 17th the last carload departed for Pittsburgh in the railway ambulance, ending the Sanitary Commission relief operations at Gettysburg.[95] Sophronia Bucklin and Judith Plummer, the only remaining government nurse, were allowed to stay on for the cemetery dedication on November 19th. Bucklin recalled,

> The hospital tents were removed—each bare and dust trampled space marking where corpses had lain after the death-agony was passed, and where the wounded had groaned in pain. In their place, Gettysburg was full to its utmost capacity, and again the white tents were spread on the hospital ground, to accommodate the crowds of people, who had journeyed hither from all points.[96]

For nurses like Anna Holstein who attended the ceremonies, it "had to us a deeper interest than to many of the lookers-on: many of the quiet sleepers, by whom we were surrounded, we had known, and waited upon until care was no longer needed . . . There was now, November, 1863, nothing more to be done at Gettysburg, and we gladly turned our faces homeward."[97]

For Henry Janes the paperwork of dismantling the hospital continued. The last of the surgeons were relieved November 20–21; Surgeon Chamberlain, Assistant Surgeon May, and Acting Assistant Surgeons Stonelake and Welch were ordered to report to the medical director in Philadelphia on November 20th; the contracts of Acting Assistant Surgeons Townsend and Sutton were annulled. Dr. Janes was left on duty with only Acting Assistant Surgeon Egon A. Koerper to help complete the records of the hospital, two stewards to inventory hospital property, and three attendants to assist them. By October 23, he had turned over 159 iron bedsteads, twenty-eight bales of hair pillows, and bedsacks to the Medical Purveyor of Baltimore. Additional supplies of medicines and hospital stores were returned on December 21, 1863.[98] The *Adams Sentinel* provided a fitting tribute to the closing of Camp Letterman:

> The arrangements of the Camp Hospital were so perfect, and such constant and prompt attention given to the wants of the wounded, that the sufferings incident to those terrible results of war have been very much ameliorated, and the brave soldiers, who were the sufferers, with tearful eyes acknowledge the kind attention that they have experienced from all about them, both male and female—and will never forget Gettysburg.[99]

CHAPTER 9

Left in the Hands of the Enemy

ON NOVEMBER 19, 1863, AS PRESIDENT ABRAHAM LINCOLN DELIVERED his now famous address at the dedication of the national cemetery in Gettysburg, Pennsylvania, Union and Confederate surgeons taken prisoner after the battle were still held at Libby Prison in Richmond, Virginia, and Fort McHenry in Baltimore, Maryland, waiting to be exchanged. While the experiences of the Gettysburg surgeons fit into a larger history of prison policies and practices, the specifics of their imprisonment and eventual release provide important insights into the often-confusing status of surgeons taken prisoner during the Civil War and later described by S. Weir Mitchell as "an irregular business." "In some cases, they were returned, and in others were held by the enemy . . . In many cases surgeons on both sides remained with their own wounded after defeat."[1] Surgeons of the defeated army who remained to care for their wounded after battles found themselves left "in the hands of the enemy." Although it was generally accepted in principle that surgeons, as noncombatants, should not be held as prisoners of war, the reality on the battlefield was much less certain. Harvey Ellicott Brown in the *Medical Department of the United States Army from 1775 to 1873* described how one surgeon left with the wounded after the first battle of Bull Run was released in a few days while another was taken to Richmond to attend Union wounded and released the following year.[2] Louis C. Duncan, in his account of the first battle of Bull Run, provided historical context, explaining,

The making prisoners of medical officers at Bull Run seems to have been due to the general ignorance of the laws and customs of war of nearly every one at that time. Immunity from capture for medical officers and protection for the wounded had been practiced at various times for three hundred years. It was a regular custom in the time of Frederick the Great and also in the Napoleonic Wars. After the fall of Napoleon everything military declined and with the rest this custom fell somewhat into disuse. The suffering of the wounded at Solferino in 1859 led directly to the Geneva Convention of 1864. That the custom was known in 1861 is shown by the clamor made by the captured surgeons. On being taken to Manassas they managed to make their complaints known to General Beauregard. He, being conversant with the military usages of Europe, wrote a letter to the Secretary of War at Richmond recommending that these medical officers be set at liberty. That this was not done was probably due to the civil authorities.[3]

While both sides claimed that they followed the "customs of war among civilized nations," and blamed mistreatment of prisoners on the other, both sides used noncombatants—civilians, chaplains, and surgeons—as political and military pawns. Duncan probably correctly attributed inconsistent treatment of surgeons to political rather than military policies. Both the surgeons and the commanders in the field understood the scale and importance of medical care immediately following a battle. Surgeons of the losing side expected to remain on the field until their wounded could be exchanged or removed to prison hospitals. Military authorities supported treating surgeons as noncombatants because they feared surgeons might be unwilling to remain with the wounded if they faced long imprisonments after their work on the battlefield was completed. Union surgeons held in Libby Prison complained that "if our government expects us to stay with our wounded, when we are liable to capture by the enemy, then it is their duty to keep us from suffering so long in prison . . . we are often left unprotected with our unfortunate wounded, entirely at the mercy of the enemy."[4]

Without clear and consistent guidelines, captured surgeons frequently found it necessary to advocate on their own behalf. After the battle of Winchester in May 1862, seven Union surgeons taken prisoner with their wounded refused a conditional parole. Assistant Surgeon Josiah F. Day Jr., 29th Maine, wrote "We are all non-combatants, we have nothing to do with the fighting; our duties are to alleviate the suffering of the sick and wounded, and I for one will never consent to tie my hands by any promise written or otherwise, so that I cannot attend to the duties of my profession among the sick and wounded until regularly exchanged as you ask."[5] Phillip Adolphus, later assistant surgeon with the 8th U.S. Infantry at Gettysburg, was one of the surgeons who negotiated with Hunter H. McGuire, medical director of Gen. Stonewall Jackson's Corps, to sign an agreement that came to be known as the Winchester Accord.

> We surgeons, and Asst. Surgeons, United States Army, now prisoners of War in this place do give our Parole of Honor on being unconditionally released to report in person, singly or collectively To the Secretary of War in Washington City as such and that we will use our best efforts that the same number of medical officers of the Confederate States Army now prisoners or may hereafter be taken to be released on the same terms. And furthermore we will on our honor use our best efforts to have this principle established viz the unconditional release of all medical officers taken prisoners of war hereafter.[6]

The Union surgeons apparently fulfilled their promise and on June 6, 1862, U.S. Secretary of War Edwin M. Stanton issued Special Order No. 60 which simply stated, "The principle being recognized that medical officers should not be held as prisoners of war it is hereby directed that all medical officers so held by the United States shall be immediately and unconditionally discharged."[7] Gen. George McClellan, commander of the Army of the Potomac, then wrote to Gen. Robert E. Lee, commander of the Army of Northern Virginia, proposing an agreement between commanders that medical personnel, as noncombatants, were not subject to capture. Lee responded on June 17th that he concurred.[8] As General-in-Chief of the Armies of the United States, however, Henry Halleck voiced his concerns that the order went too far because captured medical officers were needed to assist after battles. Writing to Edwin Stanton on June 29, 1862, he wrote,

The principles recognized by the laws and usages of war and the one on which I have always acted in this department is that medical officers are not to be detained as prisoners of war when their services are not required to take care of their own sick and wounded. Paragraph IV of General Order No. 60, introduces an entirely new principle not recognized by the laws of war which will lead to great inconveniences. It is impossible for our medical officers after a battle to attend the sick and wounded prisoners, and usually it is impossible for some weeks to hire citizen surgeons for that purpose. In such cases humanity requires that captured medical officers be retained for that purpose. I respectfully suggest that the paragraph be changed so as to conform to the heretofore established rules as recognized in Europe.[9]

Until July 1862, most correspondence about prisoner exchanges referenced the precedents of the "cartel agreed upon between the U.S. and Great Britain in 1813."[10] This agreement cited the usage and practice of civilized nations to provide for humane treatment of prisoners, adequate nutrition, and a system of paroles and exchanges based on rank. It explicitly stated that all noncombatants, including surgeons and chaplains, were exempt from capture.[11] For the first year of the war, this 1813 cartel provided the model for Union and Confederate prisoner exchanges. As the number of prisoners in Confederate and Union prisons overwhelmed the capacity of existing facilities, both sides reached an updated formal agreement in July 1862, known as the Dix-Hill Cartel.[12] Under this agreement prisoners were to be paroled within ten days of capture, delivered to specified locations, and returned home until notified of their official exchange. The agreement established a system of exchanges and communications through designated agents for each side.[13] The Dix-Hill Cartel notably made no reference to imprisonment of surgeons or the status and treatment of noncombatants, perhaps assuming that the policies established in June 1862 sufficiently addressed that issue. Surgeons who remained behind enemy lines to care for the wounded after battles continued to be released through the end of 1862, following the processes outlined by the Dix-Hill Cartel and the principles of the Winchester Accord.

By 1863, the Dix-Hill agreement began to unravel. President Abraham Lincoln remained reluctant to participate in any agreement that recognized the Confederate states as a separate nation. Jefferson Davis and the Confederate government accused Union generals of mistreating civilians, notably Gen. Benjamin Butler's execution of William Mumford of New Orleans as a spy. The situation further deteriorated with the Emancipation Proclamation of January 1863 and the recruitment of U.S. Colored Troops. The Confederacy made clear that they would refuse to exchange Black soldiers and would instead turn them over to local authorities to be treated as former slaves and returned to servitude. White officers of Colored Troops would be prosecuted by local authorities for breaking existing Southern laws against fomenting slave insurrections. The United States responded by suspending exchanges of all officers and threatening retaliation for mistreatment of U.S. Colored Troops and their white officers.

General Order No. 100, issued on April 24, 1863, attempted to present a comprehensive statement on the rules of war that the United States intended to follow. Compiled by noted legal expert Francis Lieber, and often referred to as the Lieber Code, it confirmed the status of medical staff as noncombatants and seemed to address General Halleck's earlier concerns about medical care on the battlefield.

> The enemy's chaplains, officers of the medical staff, apothecaries, hospital nurses, and servants, if they fall into the hands of the American Army, are not prisoners of war, unless the commander has reasons to retain them. In this latter case, or if, at their own desire, they are allowed to remain with their captured companions, they are treated as prisoners of war, and may be exchanged if the commander sees fit.[14]

Equally important, it recognized the necessity of retaliation as "the sternest feature of war" and defined the status of hostages as prisoners of war.[15] Various methods of retaliation, including hostages, were used by both governments to force the other side to discontinue behaviors or practices that threatened individuals or groups.

Surgeons taken prisoner during the spring and summer of 1863 became hostages in retaliation for the holding of a high-profile political prisoner by Confederate authorities. Dr. William Parks Rucker of Covington, West Virginia, graduated from Jefferson Medical College in 1855. A slave owner loyal to the Union, his confrontational style involved him in numerous lawsuits and controversies. With the outbreak of war, he refused to take an oath of allegiance to the Confederacy and assisted the Union forces in burning bridges and appropriating horses. In July 1861, he stabbed a man who had attacked him and called him a traitor, was tried, and found innocent by self-defense. On July 25, 1862, he was captured by Confederate forces and accused of murder, horse stealing, and spying—charges that he and Federal authorities denied. At first, he was held at Castle Thunder in Richmond, but Confederate authorities could not decide whether to treat him as a civilian spy or a Union prisoner of war. Eventually he was turned over to Virginia state authorities to be tried in civil court for murder and larceny.

In retaliation William Ludlow, U.S. Agent for Exchange, recommended on January 25, 1863, "that some Confederate medical officer or prominent citizen of Virginia now in our hands (if we are so fortunate to have one) be immediately set apart as a hostage for Dr. Rucker."[16] Two days later Ludlow received orders to "retain Surgeon J.C. Green as hostage for Surgeon Rucker. Confederate officers will not for the present be exchanged for specific equivalents."[17] The son of Dr. Nathaniel Terry Green, from a prominent family of Danville, Virginia, James C. Green was held as a prisoner of war and a hostage for Dr. Rucker, first at the Old Capitol Prison in Washington, DC, then at Fort Norfolk, and he eventually joined the other surgeons at Fort McHenry before his release in November 1863. Confederates responded by holding three captured Union surgeons as hostages in Libby Prison.[18] By the summer of 1863, a growing number of surgeons on both sides were being held without exchange as negotiations for the release of Dr. Rucker continued and his trial was delayed multiple times. Both Union and Confederate surgeons taken prisoner during and after the battle of Gettysburg found themselves caught up in the controversy.

UNION SURGEONS TAKEN PRISONER AT GETTYSBURG

The treatment of Union surgeons after the battle of Gettysburg illustrates the lack of consistent policies. Most of the Union surgeons held as prisoners behind enemy lines during the three days of the battle were released when the Confederate army retreated, following the practice established by the 1862 agreements. Approximately thirty-five First Corps surgeons and a dozen Eleventh Corps surgeons remained prisoners with their wounded until July 4th. Those in town, under the control of General Ewell and his medical director Hunter McGuire, the negotiator of the Winchester Accord, were allowed to continue their work, while those at the Lutheran Seminary had their instruments and supplies confiscated and were unable to provide surgical assistance to the wounded until after July 4th. When Confederate general Robert E. Lee proposed an exchange of paroled prisoners on July 3rd, General Meade, following recent orders, refused the offer.[19] Against the advice of officers, about 1,500 Union prisoners nonetheless accepted the parole, including several surgeons of the First Corps.[20] Two assistant surgeons, William Henry Forwood and William M. Notson, both of 6th U.S. Cavalry, were taken prisoner with the wounded after the battle of Fairfield on July 3, 1863, but were released without incident. Only three Union surgeons were taken south with other Union prisoners after Gettysburg: Assistant Surgeons Charles E. Humphrey, 142nd Pennsylvania, Daniel Bishop Wren, 75th Ohio, and Lewis Applegate, 102nd New York.[21]

During the Confederate retreat on July 5th, Gen. J. E. B. Stuart's Confederate cavalry raided Emmitsburg, Maryland, and captured about one hundred prisoners, fifty horses, private property of the officers, surgical instruments, and medical supplies. According to a newspaper report, several Michigan cavalry surgeons were among those captured: Samuel Russell Wooster, Surgeon, and Amos Kendall Smith, Assistant Surgeon, 1st Michigan Cavalry; Addison Ray Stone and Sylvester L. Morris, Assistant Surgeons, 5th Michigan Cavalry; David C. Spaulding, Assistant Surgeon, 6th Michigan Cavalry; and George Rawson Richards, Assistant Surgeon, 7th Michigan Cavalry. "They desired to parole the surgeons who refused to accept by Dr. Wooster's advice and they were subsequently released, owing to the rebels being obliged to leave in haste."[22] Dr. Alexander McDonald, accompanying supply wagons of the Sanitary Commission through Emmitsburg on the way to the battlefield, was not as fortunate. On July 5th at 9:30 A.M. Confederate cavalry confiscated the horses, wagons, and supplies and held Dr. McDonald and the Reverend William George Scandlin as prisoners along with their driver, Leonard Brink, and African American Moses Gardner. McDonald's report to the Sanitary Commission describes their capture and the grueling march south with other prisoners from Gettysburg that ended on July 21st with their arrival at Libby Prison in Richmond.[23] Dr. McDonald and his party were not the only civilians taken prisoner. At least eight Gettysburg residents were taken to Richmond and imprisoned for twenty months, first at Libby and Castle Thunder and then in Salisbury, North Carolina.[24]

LIBBY PRISON, RICHMOND

When the Union surgeons from Gettysburg finally reached Richmond, about thirty other surgeons were already being held there. William Spencer, 73rd Indiana, captured during Col. Abel Streight's raid in Georgia, April 30th, and William W. Myers captured May 14th from the Steamship *Georgia*, were the first two surgeons to be formally designated as hostages. Thomas S. Morgan, 10th Missouri, captured at the battle of Raymond during the Vicksburg campaign, became the third hostage.[25] Twenty surgeons captured at the second battle of Winchester in mid-June were imprisoned at Libby along with other officers of Robert Milroy's command. Two surgeons were still held following their capture at Chancellorsville. The small number of only three Union surgeons retained as prisoners after the battle of Gettysburg suggests that the Confederate government already held a sufficient number of surgeons as hostages in early July. In October, five more surgeons were added after the battle of Bristoe Station, including four who had participated in the battle of Gettysburg: Assistant Surgeons Edward Kelley Hogan, 120th New York, John N. Miller, 120th New York, George W. Withers, 18th Pennsylvania Cavalry, and Surgeon Frederick Wolf, 39th New York.

After the battle of Chickamauga, September 19–20, 1863, a large number of captured Union surgeons were sent to Libby Prison in direct retaliation for the large number of Confederate surgeons from Gettysburg being held at Fort McHenry in Baltimore. On October 1, 1863, Confederate general Braxton Bragg wrote from Chickamauga that "Medical officers, except four exchanged for that number of our own, will be sent to Atlanta, as I learn ours are held in the East. We have about fifty."[26] The next day Union general William Rosecrans reported:

From the reports of four of our medical officers exchanged yesterday, those remaining in their hands, will, as soon as their services to the wounded can be dispensed with, be confined and held as prisoners of war. The rebel officers, assigning as the cause, state that seventy-two of their surgeons and assistant surgeons captured at the battle of Gettysburg in the legitimate discharge of their duties are now held by the United States Government as prisoners of war, and that the cartel has in this been violated on the part of the United States. They further state that they shall retain all U.S. medical officers captured, whether or not in the discharge of their duties as such, until the United States Government releases their medical officers captured at Gettysburg.[27]

Complaints about the treatment of surgeons continued in correspondence between Bragg and Rosecrans. On October 15th, Bragg replied to Rosecrans:

You are correctly informed in regard to the disposition made of your medical officers still in my hands. The apparently harsh treatment is the result of a necessity imposed by the action of your own Government. A large number of our medical officers and chaplains who have fallen into the hands of other commanders have long been and are still in close confinement in the East. This course has been pursued by your Government without giving mine any notice or reason. I am, therefore, instructed to hold those in my hands until some satisfactory explanation can be had with your Government . . . By an examination of the cartel for the exchange of prisoners, I do not find the stipulation in regard to medical officers which you think is violated. My own recollection is that the practice first originated in the action of my Government and was then continued under a special written agreement before the cartel for the regular exchange of prisoners was agreed on.[28]

Rosecrans, concerned about losing so many of his medical staff and apparently not privy to the political standoff over surgeons being held as hostages, forwarded Bragg's letter to Gen. Henry Halleck complaining that "we should suffer because officers elsewhere have carelessly or recklessly confined chaplains and medical officers without reporting the facts to the Govt."[29]

Meanwhile, the surgeons and other officers held at Libby endured months of overcrowding and worsening conditions further exacerbated by the increasing numbers of new prisoners during the summer and fall. By November, a report on Libby Prison issued by Confederate authorities described the conditions for the 1,044 officers held there as

> eight large rooms occupied by the prisoners, of which one is used as a hospital. These rooms are 103 by 42 feet. There is a water-closet on each floor. There is an ample supply of water on each floor, and there is also facility afforded for bathing, of which each prisoner can avail himself at will. The prison is thoroughly policed daily and is a cleanly condition. The officers are allowed to purchase such articles as they wish, not prohibited by the rules of the prison, and a competent person is employed whose sole business it is to make these purchases.[30]

Prisoner accounts provide a far grimmer picture of the conditions in the former warehouse situated along the James River. The surgeons received no special consideration and were housed along with other officers as prisoners of war. All prisoners entering the prison, including surgeons, were routinely stripped of overcoats, blankets, and personal possessions. Their money was confiscated and held by the prison authorities.

With over 1,000 men, the space allowed only about 6 feet square of living space for each prisoner. No bunks or chairs and few blankets were supplied, so prisoners sat and slept on bare floors. "Scrubbing day" may have helped with cleanliness, but it was torture for prisoners who spent their days and nights on the floor. Prisoners complained that the rooms were sometimes scrubbed in the evenings without time to dry, forcing men to sleep all night on damp floors. The daily ration per prisoner was consistently reported as three quarters of a pound of wheat bread, a

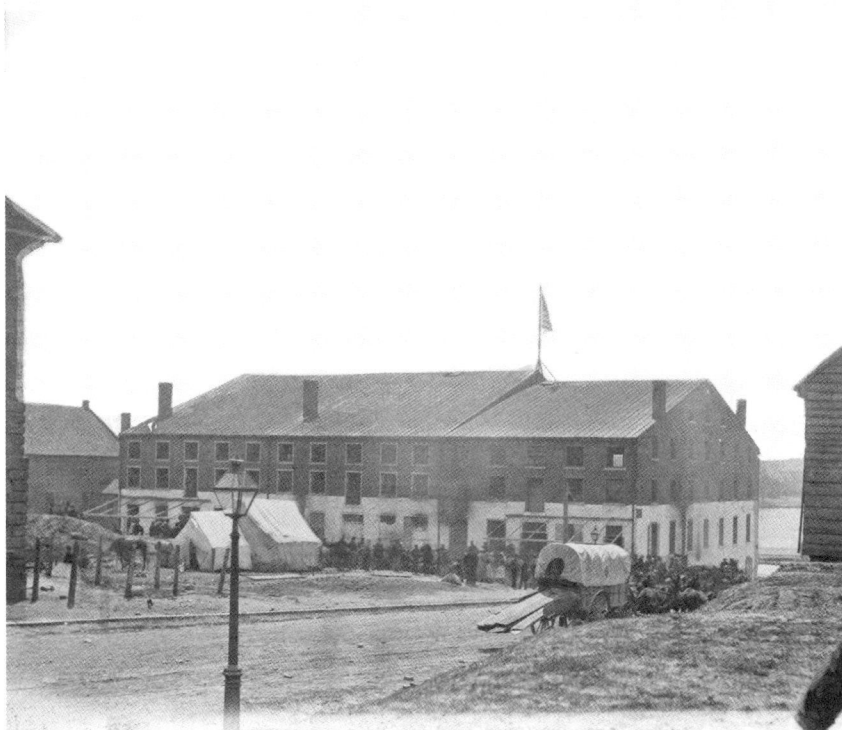

Libby Prison, Richmond, Virginia, 1865. Photograph by Mathew Brady. Courtesy of National Archives.

quarter pound of meat, and 2 ounces of beans, with later substitutions of cornbread for wheat, rice for beans, and two or three small, sweet potatoes instead of meat. Following their release, the imprisoned surgeons issued a report that "the rations furnished Union prisoners by the rebel authorities at Richmond, Va., are not sufficient to prevent these prisoners suffering from hunger and thus becoming debilitated and very susceptible to disease."[31] Dr. McDonald and Mr. Scandlin of the Sanitary Commission reported suffering from dysentery, a "scorbutic limb" attributed to drinking water drawn directly from the James River, and the lack of fresh vegetables. One surgeon, Harvey Lindsley Pierce, assistant surgeon of the 5th Maryland, was captured at Winchester in June 1863 and died in the Libby Prison hospital on November 5th of pneumonia.[32] Accounts left by surgeons detailed the unhealthy conditions that they endured.

The officers have to do their own cooking, and the supply of wood for this purpose is often insufficient, and occasionally for half a day none at all is sent in. A privy and sink render foul and disgusting one end of each room, polluting at times the air of the entire apartment. None are permitted to leave this building of accumulated and accumulating horrors till borne to the hospital or happily exchanged.[33]

Without access to fresh air or the outdoors, prisoners at Libby found it especially difficult to pass the time in the cramped, poorly ventilated quarters. Access to windows was so restricted that two of the surgeons, captured at Winchester, were fired on by guards for being too close to a window.[34]

Every day followed the same pattern—rising at 6:30 A.M., picking up blankets from the floor, checking clothes to kill lice which they referred to as "scrimmaging," preparing and eating meals. There was little or no reading material. A newspaper dubbed the *Libby Chronicle* was read aloud by Chaplain Louis Beaudry from notes he wrote on scraps of paper. To pass the time they played cards and chess, organized a lyceum of language classes, debates, and lectures, and held musical performances. A series of lectures on mesmerism by Maj. John Henry, 5th Ohio Cavalry, drew considerable interest and discussion. One prisoner recounted:

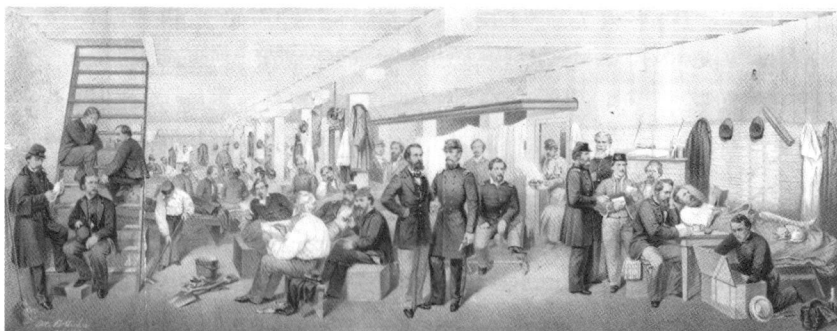

Libby Prison, Union prisoners at Richmond, Virginia. Lithograph of Sarony, Major & Knapp from drawing by Otto Rotticher, October 1862. Library of Congress Prints and Photographs Division

One of the officers lectures to us, on the subject of mesmerism. He tells us about the electric fluid which permeates all space, about clairvoyance, about the magnetic spheres, and about many other interesting facts connected with the mesmeric science. The fact, whether mesmerism be a science, however is caviled at by some of the medical faculty present, and at the succeeding meeting of the Lyceum, the all-important question: "Is Mesmerism a true science?" is discussed with much warmth, and at great length. . . .

The mesmeric excitement gains ground with alarming rapidity, and soon becomes general; all sorts of impromptu mesmerisers may be seen here and there about the room, surrounded by anxious and serious groups, and endeavoring with all the earnestness of mesmeric faith, to worry suspected mediums into an impossible sleep.[35]

Athletic exercise was restricted by the guards who intervened when the prisoners tried to fence, drill, dance, or walk because it made too much noise.[36] Some prisoners improvised by using a broom handle suspended from the cross beams as a trapeze for gymnastic exercises. William Spencer and the other surgeons at Libby took advantage of the opportunity to discuss medical topics among themselves: "There are many very scientific men amongst these surgeons, and we amuse ourselves, mostly apart from the other officers, discussing Hygea and Pandora and Esculpeus—hospital and field practice, surgical operations, medical theories, etc. etc."[37]

CONFEDERATE SURGEONS TAKEN PRISONER AT GETTYSBURG

The Confederate surgeons who became prisoners after the battle of Gettysburg were among those who remained with the wounded in the field hospitals or were captured with wounded during the retreat. Assistant Surgeon Simon Baruch, 3rd South Carolina Battalion, one of the surgeons left in Gettysburg with the wounded, was not overly concerned about the prospect of "capture by the enemy. Having been left in charge of the Disciples Church field hospital at Boonsboro, Md., under similar orders a year previous, and on that occasion having had six weeks of the most agreeable period of army life, I regarded this order into captivity with much more complacency than did my colleagues."[38] He described spending six weeks at the field hospital in Gettysburg, "replete with interesting ethical and surgical experiences."[39] Baruch and the other Confederate medical staff were free to move about town, visiting their wounded at various hospitals, gathering supplies from the Sanitary and Christian Commission stores, and were generally left undisturbed. Surgeon John Moore Hayes, 26th Alabama, caring for wounded at the Seminary Hospital and Camp Letterman until October, had his photo taken at Tyson Brothers Photographic Studio in Gettysburg. Some Confederate surgeons left Gettysburg to accompany convalescing prisoners evacuated to Baltimore, New York, and Philadelphia prison hospitals, but most remained in the Confederate field hospitals until they closed in early August. Nine Confederate surgeons moved to Camp Letterman and remained with Confederate wounded until October before being transferred to Fort McHenry.

Confederate surgeons captured during the retreat to Virginia were among those who accompanied the long trains of wounded or stayed with wounded in hospitals along the way. John Mutius Gaines and fifteen other Confederate surgeons were captured with the wounded at Williamsport on July 14. Gaines continued to take care of Confederate wounded in U.S. prison hospitals at Hagerstown and Point Lookout in Maryland and Chester and Fort Delaware in Pennsylvania before being exchanged on December 12, 1863.[40]

At the end of July, as Confederate surgeons left Gettysburg to accompany evacuated prisoners, they fully expected to be exchanged. Henry de Saussure Fraser accompanied a train load of wounded to Fort Delaware on July 20th and was headed to City Point on the *Flag of Truce* steamer when he was taken off and sent to Norfolk for further orders. He later joined other surgeons held at Fort McHenry.[41] An article in the *Baltimore Sun* on July 25, reported the arrival of Confederate surgeons and chaplains from New York expecting to be returned via Fortress Munroe, "They being noncombatants."[42]

On the night of August 7th, after the remaining patients in Confederate field hospitals had been moved to Camp Letterman, Simon Baruch and most of the remaining Confederate medical staff—both surgeons and chaplains—left Gettysburg in cattle cars and arrived in Baltimore. There they were detained by the provost marshal in a former hotel used as a prison. Surgeon William Riddick Whitehead, 44th Virginia, knew Baltimore well and realized that a famous restaurant was located opposite the prison. In a "bantering mood" and expecting to return to the Confederacy the next day, he and fellow surgeon Frank Lavigne Taney, 10th Louisiana, sent for a waiter and ordered soft shelled crabs and champagne which they ate "a la Turque" on a lap robe on the floor of the prison.[43] Surgeon Edward C. Rives, 28th Virginia, sent out for a more modest order of ice cream that he and his party ate with knives.[44] Whitehead received special treatment thanks to the efforts of Mrs. Bacon, a Baltimore resident who arranged for him to remain in Baltimore for several days to spend time with his "little cousin" and future wife, Elizabeth Flynn Benton, and her brother who were visiting Baltimore from New York.

The rest of the surgeons, still expecting to be released and returned to Richmond, were taken by boat to Fortress Munroe and then Fort Norfolk where Chaplain Tinsley was surprised to find Assistant Surgeon Harrison, who had left Gettysburg earlier and whom they assumed was already safely back in Richmond. The Gettysburg Confederate surgeons and chaplains, about fifty or sixty additional surgeons held at Fort Norfolk, and twelve additional chaplains returned to Baltimore and found themselves imprisoned at Fort McHenry as hostages.[45]

Fort McHenry, Maryland

"Among the first objects that meets the eye is new gallows—a very ominous sight as we are now supposed to be held as hostages," Chaplain Peter Tinsley wrote in his diary.[46] Simon Baruch recounted that they soon learned that they were hostages for Dr. Rucker. Fort McHenry was not a regular prisoner of war camp but was used primarily as a transfer point to house both military and civilian prisoners as well as Union troops. Chaplain Thomas Dwight Witherspoon, 42nd Mississippi, later recalled that "about a hundred surgeons, with some thirteen or fourteen chaplains, had been collected from various points and were incarcerated at Fort McHenry. As they constituted a somewhat anomalous class. . . . they could not be properly assigned to any of the permanent places of imprisonment . . ."[47] The accommodations for the surgeons at Fort McHenry consisted of a large wooden building fitted with double decker bunks large enough for two men on each level. The prisoners had full liberty of the grounds and were able to bathe in the Patapsco River, play "town ball" (an early form of baseball), and stage dress parades. To pass the time, they organized a debating society with subjects such as the comparative happiness of married or single life, and "Ought any Medical Colleges to admit Ladies to the degree of M.D." (decided in the negative). They held classes in French, German, and Spanish, read poetry, and gave lectures. The chaplains kept busy with a full schedule of prayers and sermons.

The normal prison fare consisted of three meals a day. Simon Baruch remembered:

> Breakfast consisted of hard-tack and sweetened black coffee. Each man dipped his coffee from the can and helped himself to hard-tack as he felt inclined. The quantity of food was more satisfactory than the quality. Dinner consisted of corned beef and potatoes, or pork and potatoes, or soup and soup beef, always with an abundance of hard-tack. Supper was a repetition of breakfast. We soon became accustomed to the rough fare and were glad enough to condone it when we realized the privileges we enjoyed.[48]

The rations were enhanced by a sutler on the grounds who provided ale, crackers, and cheese for those who could pay. Sympathetic ladies from Baltimore were allowed to visit and contributed baskets of food.[49]

Confinement took a toll as tempers flared and disagreements and bad behavior erupted among the prisoners. Simon Baruch reported,

> when Dr. DeG., of Georgia, disturbed a game of chess of Dr. N., of South Carolina. The latter, one of the quietest of men, but an earnest chess player, arose and slapped the face of the former. Immediately a challenge passed to fight a duel. From the "point of a needle to the mouth of a cannon" was the choice of weapons offered by Dr. DeG., who had spent too much of his scant money supply at the sutler's canteen. The duel was never fought.[50]

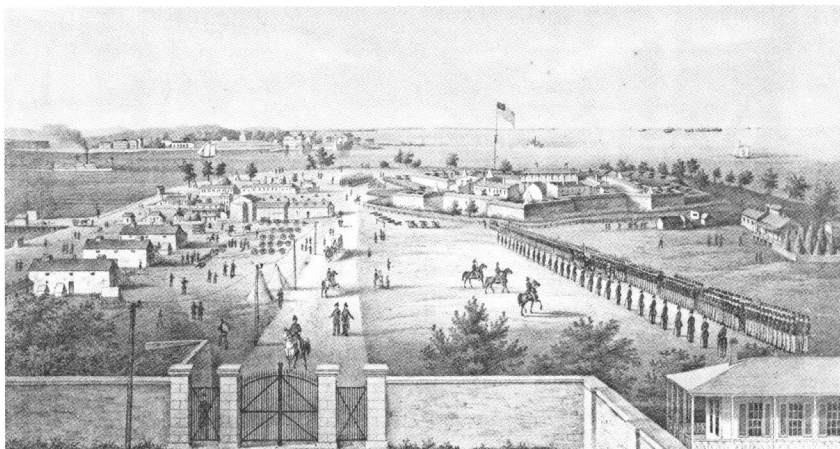

Fort McHenry, Baltimore, Maryland, lithograph, E. Sachse, 1862. Fort McHenry received nearly 7,000 prisoners after the battle of Gettysburg including the surgeons who were held there until November. Courtesy of Division of Home and Community Life, National Museum of American History, Smithsonian Institution

Another fight between a surgeon and a chaplain reported by Baruch may have been the fight recorded by Tinsley on September 2nd between Chaplain James M. Stokes, 48th Georgia, and Louis Giuseppe Contri. Contri was serving as assistant surgeon with the 34th Virginia Battalion of Stuart's Cavalry, when he was captured at Hagerstown on June 12, 1863. He never made it to Gettysburg but later joined the other surgeons as a prisoner at Fort McHenry. His sketchy history before and after 1863 is consistent with Tinsley's reference to a rumor that "one of our members had appropriated $75 given him for distribution. The report is traced to Dr. Contri who said he could not give his author."[51] On another occasion Tinsley reports that "an engagement takes place between Drs. Loyd & Contri. A disgraceful & disagreeable business. The former is said to have fought a Yankee Lieut in the forenoon."[52] Five days later Tinsley reports that Lloyd has been arrested on serious charges, probably related to fighting a Union officer. Another surgeon identified as Dr. H. was arrested stealing opium from the hospital stores. "It happened that one of the surgeons was an opium fiend, and to obtain the drug he had himself reported sick, and so managed to obtain small quantities of the drug. Very soon, however, the quantity became insufficient, and he would steal into the drug room at night to obtain a sufficient quantity to satisfy the increased craving. He was discovered one night, and two of our colleagues, who happened to be patients, witnessed the arrest of Dr. H."[53]

Some of the prisoners at Fort McHenry, unwilling to wait for exchange, took advantage of their relative freedom to escape. Seven surgeons and three chaplains were reported missing on October 10th. Simon Baruch remembered that some prisoners were able to bribe guards who allowed them to visit Southern sympathizers and then simply never returned. Surgeon William Riddick Whitehead described his escape with two chaplains on a Sunday evening (probably September 27) after obtaining civilian clothing and bribing a guard to delay going on duty so that they could go over the wall undetected. Whitehead made his way to Montreal, then to Halifax, Nova Scotia, and back to Richmond by way of Bermuda. The two chaplains with him were William B. Carson, 14th South Carolina, and Henry E. Brooks, 2nd North Carolina. The third chaplain, Paul Carrington Morton, 23rd Virginia, reportedly swam the river to make his escape.[54] Tinsley recorded the quandary of the remaining prisoners when it was announced that the Union and Confederate chaplains were to be exchanged on October 5th. It was proposed that surgeons Waters, Gregory, and Purefoy would impersonate escaped chaplains Morton, Carson, and Brooks. Several days after the exchanged chaplains left, the escapees were finally discovered when Dr. Guild, one of the escaped surgeons, was called as a witness to the theft of opium but was nowhere to be found.[55]

RELEASE OF SURGEONS

Negotiations for the release of surgeons continued after the Union and Confederate chaplains were exchanged in early October. On November 6th, Surgeon George Suckley, U.S. Volunteers, formerly medical director of the Eleventh Corps at Gettysburg and now acting medical director in the Middle Department at Baltimore, wrote to Gen. William Hoffman, Commissary-General of Prisons, complaining about the imprisonment of Confederate medical officers.

The effect of this cannot help but be detrimental to the service. The rebel surgeons state freely that they will not voluntarily again submit themselves to a long and tedious confinement, and I can add that the temper of our own surgeons is averse to a similar imprisonment in a filthy rebel prison. I must confess that in my own case, as things now stand, I should rather avoid than court captivity, whereas, to the contrary, if the terms of the cartel were adhered to, I would willingly submit to privations only temporary in character in order to minister to our wounded, and would, if on the field at any time, volunteer for the purpose.[56]

Hoffman's response coyly hinted that the hostage situation might be drawing to an end.

You need not doubt, however, that the more humane practice under the usage of war will be returned to at the earliest moment when it can be done without sacrificing the rights and interests of our medical officers. From recent occurrences I am under the impression this desired change will not be delayed much longer.[57]

In fact, Dr. Rucker had already escaped from his jail cell in Danville, Virginia, on October 18, 1863, assisted by friends. The surgeons at Libby learned on November 10th that Rucker had made good his escape and was now within Union lines. On November 23rd the Richmond newspapers announced, "An Exchange of Surgeons Effected."[58]

Col. Peter Porter, commanding Fort McHenry, reported to General Hoffman on the departure of 120 Confederate surgeons who "were allowed to take everything they possessed when captured, and a full suit, composed either of what they owned originally or had replaced by gift or purchase. Even thus restricted, they were richer in the aggregate by far than when they entered the lines."[59] Simon Baruch, for example, was able to retain a case of medical instruments that he had received as a gift from a Baltimore surgeon while at Gettysburg. The Confederate surgeons went to Fort Monroe and from there were taken by the Union truce boat, *New York*, to City Point for exchange.

Meanwhile, on November 24, 1863, the surgeons at Libby received the order, "Surgeons pack up to go north!!!!" William Spencer described how he and his ninety-two colleagues had lost money, now "in the hands of these thieves, and by a rough calculation we find the crowd is robbed in the aggregate, to the nice little sum of $5,000 to $6,000."[60] The process of exchange had begun. The Union surgeons boarded the Confederate truce boat, the steamer *Schultz*, in Richmond and arrived at City Point where they transferred to the *New York*. The Confederate surgeons boarded the *Schultz* to return to Richmond. The next day, the Union surgeons arrived at Fortress Monroe and boarded the steamer *Adelaide* bound for Baltimore. Aboard the *Adelaide*, on November 26th, they appointed a committee to prepare a report on the conditions and treatment of the Federal prisoners in Richmond, which they unanimously adopted and eventually published.[61] The testimony of formerly imprisoned surgeons carried considerable weight since they could describe their observations of nutritional and health conditions in professional terms based on scientific and medical knowledge.

The release of surgeons did not address the larger problem of overcrowded prisons that resulted from discontinuing all general exchanges, except for those held longest or in poor health. Many prisoners of both sides suffered under terrible conditions during the last two years of the war. The debate about who was responsible continued long after the war ended. Each side blamed the other for the failure of the cartel and the overcrowded prisons that resulted after 1863. *The Annals of the Civil War Written by Leading Participants North and South*, published by Alexander Kelly McClure in 1879, included both versions. Robert Ould, CSA Agent for Exchange throughout the war, blamed the Union, pointing to contradictory general orders issued by the Federal government and complaining that "The civilians of the War Department seem to have been under the belief that they could make and unmake the laws of war to suit emergencies." "The Union View of the Exchange of Prisoners" by Robert S. Northcott presented the perspective of a former prisoner at Libby Prison: "That the Confederate Government first violated the cartel, there can be no doubt," specifically citing the refusal to exchange Colonel Streight's and General Milroy's officers, and "holding of surgeons and chaplains as prisoners of war."[62] In his preface to the 1876 publication of *The Southern Side; or Andersonville Prison*, Dr. R. Randolph Stevenson, surgeon at the infamous Confederate prison at Andersonville, Georgia, acknowledged that the subject of prisoners was still too contentious.

> The future historian who shall undertake to write an unbiassed story of the War between the States, will be compelled to weigh in the scales of justice all its parts and features; and if the revolting crimes against prisoners which have formed the burden of recrimination between the South and the North have been indeed committed, the perpetrators must be held accountable. Be they of the South or of the North, they can not escape history.[63]

PART III
AFTER THE WAR

CHAPTER 10

Picking Up the Pieces

UNION VICTORY AT THE BATTLE OF GETTYSBURG DID NOT END THE Civil War. For nearly two more years Union and Confederate surgeons continued their grim work as casualties mounted, recuperating wounded filled the military hospitals of both North and South, and prisoners of both sides died of starvation and disease in overcrowded conditions. When the war finally ended in 1865, the transition from military service to life as a civilian physician required difficult adjustments for many surgeons. Some returned home to resume medical practices; others moved west or embarked on new careers in business and politics. Some became financially successful in medical or other fields, while others struggled to support themselves. For many surgeons the health problems they experienced during the war became long-term, chronic conditions.

SURRENDER AT APPOMATTOX

When Ulysses S. Grant took command of the Union armies in March 1864, he began an aggressive strategy that would eventually deplete Confederate resources and maneuver Lee's army into a decisive battle to end the war. Following the loss of Petersburg and the subsequent Union occupation of Richmond on April 3, 1865, Lee's Army of Northern Virginia had few options left. Assistant Surgeon William H. Taylor, 19th Virginia, provided a detailed account of the days leading up to the battle of Sailor's Creek on April 6, 1865, and the surrender at Appomattox.

Here my large and varied store of military experiences was enriched with the knowledge of how it feels to be part and parcel of a thorough-going panic . . . I felt no extraordinary apprehension. In fact, fear was driven out by despair, for all of us knew that this was our last stand, that overwhelming defeat was certain, and that escape would be well nigh impossible.[1]

Taylor avoided capture at Sailor's Creek and appears in the lists of Confederates who surrendered and received paroles at Appomattox Court House on April 9, 1865.[2] A number of the Gettysburg surgeons still serving with Confederate regiments at the end of the war do not appear on the official lists of parolees at Appomattox. Some, like Assistant Surgeon Joseph Sykes, 3rd Virginia, were among those captured before the surrender at Sailor's Creek on April 6, 1865. Sykes was held at the Old Capitol Prison in Washington, DC, until April 14 and then transferred to Johnson's Island prison before being paroled May 1, 1865. Eighteen surgeons assigned to duty in Virginia hospitals at Lynchburg, Richmond, Thomasville, Mount Jackson, Petersburg, and Winchester were taken prisoner and released on parole with their patients.

Approximately 40 percent of the Confederate surgeons present at the battle of Gettysburg still served with Lee's Army of Northern Virginia in 1865.[3] Records from the surrender at Appomattox include the names of at least 180 Confederate surgeons who served at Gettysburg. Others, not included in the lists of parolees, simply went home without surrendering. Hospital steward John Samuel Apperson, 4th Virginia, recorded the confusing final days of the Army of Northern Virginia in his diary. Traveling with the medical wagons of Gen. Bushrod Johnson's division, Apperson and other medical staff in the Stonewall Brigade evaded capture.[4] Apperson made his way to Lynchburg with Surgeon Samuel Sayers, 27th Virginia, where they learned on April 9th that the "Army had been surrendered."[5] Apperson and Sayers considered joining the Confederate army still fighting in North Carolina, but Apperson's mentor, Dr. Harvey Black, now paroled and at home, "gave me good advice which I shall take I think." Apperson ended his diary on April 23rd, "Returned home to Stay." Surgeon John D. Starry, 7th Virginia Cavalry, escaped capture at

Appomattox and returned home where he was paroled on April 28th in Charlestown, West Virginia.[6]

Several Gettysburg Confederate surgeons, no longer serving with the Army of Northern Virginia, were paroled in Greensboro, North Carolina, and other hospital locations after Generals William Sherman and Joseph Johnston reached agreement on surrender terms similar to Appomattox on April 26th. Two surgeons working in hospitals in Augusta, Georgia, were paroled between May and July under that agreement.[7]

The terms of surrender that Grant offered Lee were purposely generous.[8] As officers, Confederate surgeons were allowed to keep private horses and baggage, but records show that most had few remaining possessions to take with them. Assistant Surgeon James McCombs, 11th North Carolina, was paroled April 10th with one horse and two cases of instruments. Surgeon William Henry Daughtry, 14th Virginia, reported "2 horses and equipment, Haversack, 3 blankets, calf skin and bundle, sole leather and servant." Assistant Surgeon Francis Walker, 41st Virginia, reported clothing, blankets, and side arms at his parole on April 9th.[9]

A pass issued by the Union army supposedly provided safe passage and transportation for parolees, but the journey home presented challenges for many Confederate surgeons. Assistant Surgeon Carl Kleinschmidt, 3rd Arkansas, returning home to Washington, DC, after Appomattox "walked nearly all the way to Georgetown, arriving destitute."[10] Surgeon Henry Minor, 9th Alabama, among those who surrendered at Appomattox, later recounted,

> The next day we remained in the bull-pen awaiting our paroles. About night we (myself and my brother) got our paroles and our last order from General Lee, his farewell to his soldiers. Neither of us had a cent of money, no horse. It was between 800 and 900 miles to my home in Macon, Mississippi. We were weak from want of food. We had no baggage. We prayed for help and guidance to Him who is able to help and we started home.[11]

Surgeon Sylvester J. Farmer, 15th Georgia, "began life anew on twenty-five cents which he had managed to save from the general wreck. He soon built up a good practice in and around Crawfordsville, and still owning his plantation near town he gradually got that in shape again and resumed his planting interests along with the practice of his profession."[12]

Not all Confederate surgeons were able to achieve professional and financial success. Assistant Surgeon Henry Woodbury Moore, 2nd South Carolina Cavalry, provided an unusually detailed account of his struggles after the war for a biographical sketch published in a history of his 1853 graduating class from Dartmouth College. Following his graduation, he followed his father and uncle to settle in Gillisonville, South Carolina, and graduated from the Medical College of South Carolina in Charleston in 1856. He joined the Confederate army in 1861 and served until 1865.

> Before the abandonment of Bragg's forces, he was taken sick and after 3 weeks confinement, he and his nurse turned their horses homeward, thankful that they had seen the end . . . After the war, he followed hunting for several months, with his brothers, in the swamps of the Savannah River, marketing their game at the city of Savannah, Ga . . . During the reconstruction troubles in South Carolina, he was obliged to "refugee" with his family in Georgia, and he gives a racy description of his experiences as Principal of Morven Acad. for nine months, among the pine barrens of Brooks Co., Ga., in 1876–77.[13]

A classmate visiting him in 1884 reported that he supported himself by practicing medicine, teaching in the winter, and farming near Hendersonville, South Carolina.

While Confederate surgeons ended their military service abruptly and transitioned to civilian life with little or no support after the surrender, Union surgeons had options to continue military service or resume civilian lives. Some Union surgeons who served at Gettysburg had already mustered out with their regiments at the end of three years of service in 1864; others resigned after Gettysburg for health reasons. Assistant Surgeon Holt, 121st New York, was forced to resign October 17, 1864, with tuberculosis that left him an invalid until his death in 1868. Leaving military service, he described settling his accounts and receiving his final pay, "It does not seem possible that I am now a *civilian* in soldier's clothes."[14] As much as Union surgeons yearned for family and home, leaving the structure of military life could be complicated. Surgeon James Langstaff Dunn, 109th Pennsylvania, decided to resign in late March 1865 after Sherman's occupation of Greensboro, North Carolina, but found it difficult to muster out in the field. On April 15, 1865, he was finally able to end his term of service and close his affairs with the Surgeon General's Office in Washington, DC, writing, "I am once more a citizen."[15]

Assistant Surgeon William Child, 5th New Hampshire, writing to his wife in June 1865, was reluctant to resign before his regiment mustered out because his army pay was more than he could make at home, and he wanted to receive the additional three months pay promised to those who stayed to the end of the war. He was anxious to get home to his wife and children but also anticipated a difficult transition back to civilian life. "It will require great exertion on my part to content myself with living in Bath. After three years of such a life as I have had you must know that I can not at once be satisfied with the slow life in the dullest of country villages. But never mind, Dear Carrie, I shall after a time become accustomed to my old style of living and business."[16] At the end of the war, Surgeon William Watson, 105th Pennsylvania, wrote to his family describing the surrender at Appomattox, the assassination of President Lincoln, and the Grand Review of Union troops in Washington, DC. He too decided not to resign until he could collect the additional three-months' pay of $240, anticipating that the army would be disbanded immediately, "excepting the regulars." On May 15th he wrote home that you "must not expect too much from me when I return to Civil life for you know I was a pretty rough customer before leaving home and military life, I assure you, has not improved me."[17]

MILITARY CAREERS

Some Union surgeons chose not to return to civilian life and continued military careers with the regular army after the Civil War ended. In addition to assignments in army hospitals and various military posts, they served with the occupation forces in former Confederate states and in Indian Wars in the western territories. Of the sixty-one commissioned surgeons or assistant surgeons who served in Union regiments during the Gettysburg battle or in the hospitals at Gettysburg after the battle, seven remained in military service after the war. Of an additional twenty-four who sought regular army commissions between Gettysburg and the end of the war, at least seven decided to pursue long-term military careers.[18] Others returned to army life as contracted acting assistant surgeons or sought army commissions after the war. A few found opportunities to advance above the rank of assistant surgeon in a state regiment by seeking a commission as surgeon with newly formed regiments of U.S. Colored Troops during and after the war.[19] Some continued their government service as physicians in veterans' hospitals and soldiers' homes, or as pension examiners.

A few Confederate surgeons also sought military or government positions after Reconstruction. Confederate assistant surgeon Thomas Young Aby in Alexander's Artillery Reserve returned to Louisiana where he practiced medicine and was employed as a quarantine physician for the U.S. government in 1884. During the Spanish American War, he enlisted as a surgeon in the 20th U.S. Infantry and was at the 1898 battle of Santiago, Cuba. Surgeon William Spence, 47th Virginia, was appointed acting assistant surgeon in the Marine Hospital Service in Jacksonville, Florida, in 1889 at a salary of $360, after losing money he invested in growing oranges.[20] Surgeon James Dickie Galt, 19th Virginia, practiced medicine in Norfolk, Virginia, after the war, and in 1885 treated contagious cases for the U.S. Marine Hospital Services at the rate of $2.50 a day.[21]

Several Union surgeons who chose regular army careers achieved prominent positions. Assistant Surgeon John Shaw Billings, 7th U.S., remained in the army until 1896. During that time his accomplishments included developing the Army Medical Museum and Library, designing the Johns Hopkins hospital in Baltimore, and supervising vital statistics for the 1880 and 1890 censuses. After retirement from the army, he served as director of the New York Public Library.[22] Charles Smart served as assistant surgeon of the 63rd New York during the battle of Gettysburg and was commissioned an assistant surgeon in the U.S. Army in March 1864. Born in Scotland, with a medical degree from the University of Aberdeen, Smart had planned to enter medical service in the British army but sought an opportunity to gain battlefield experience in the American Civil War. He arrived in New York City in 1862, enlisted at Albany, and joined Meagher's Irish Brigade in the Army of the Potomac. Abandoning his plans for British service, in 1864 he took the examination for assistant surgeon in the U.S. Army, serving in San Francisco, Arizona, Virginia, Wyoming, and Utah. In 1879 he was transferred to Washington, DC, and served as an expert in sanitary chemistry with the National Board of Health. In 1883 he was assigned to the Office of the Surgeon General in charge of a division dealing with sanitation and statistics and was tasked with completing the third volume of the *Medical and Surgical History of the War of the Rebellion* in 1888. In 1889 he prepared and published the *Handbook for the Hospital Corps of the United States.* Following the Spanish American War, he was chief surgeon of the Division of the Philippines from 1902 to 1904.[23] William Henry Forwood, assistant surgeon of the 6th U.S. Cavalry at Gettysburg, went on to serve at various posts in the West and South, and accompanied exploratory expeditions to the Yellowstone region in 1880 and 1881 as both surgeon and naturalist. While serving as attending physician at the Soldiers' Home in Washington, DC, he taught on the faculty of the Army Medical School and briefly served as surgeon general just before his retirement in 1902.[24] Assistant Surgeon James Albert Hawke, 114th Pennsylvania, mustered out as surgeon of the 215th Pennsylvania Volunteers on July 31, 1865, but two years later joined the U.S. Navy as assistant surgeon. He was promoted to surgeon, medical inspector, and finally medical director of the U.S. Navy in 1899, retiring with the rank of rear admiral. During the Spanish American War, he commanded the medical corps at the New York Navy Shipyard.

FRESH STARTS

Not every surgeon who left military service returned home. Some Confederates could not bring themselves to rejoin the United States and accept the reality of a society without slavery. Reluctant to swear the oath of allegiance and live under military occupation during Reconstruction, they sought to distance themselves from the past and start over in a new place. For Surgeon Arthur R. Barry, 9th Virginia, who grew up in Washington, DC, and Prince George's County, Maryland, the difficult trip home prompted him to follow a different path. After walking from Appomattox to City Point, he took a steamboat to Fortress Munroe. Unable to get passage home to Baltimore because of travel restrictions following the assassination of President Lincoln, he instead sought passage to Mexico with other former Confederates who planned to support French efforts to establish Maximilian as emperor of Mexico and help reinstate slavery there. When Barry arrived in New Orleans with the other Confederates, mostly from Louisiana and Texas, they were received with great honor as the first Confederate soldiers to arrive. He never made it to Mexico. At first, he supported himself by lecturing about the Army of Northern Virginia and teaching school, but he eventually restarted his medical career in Texas.[25] Some Confederates chose to live abroad. William McClung Piggott, with Wofford's Brigade during the battle of Gettysburg, did not return home to James City, Virginia. Instead, he traveled first to Turkey and then settled in Sonora, Mexico, where William M. Edwards, a U.S. Army scout during the Apache wars, spent an afternoon with him.[26] Thousands of former Confederates chose Brazil as a place to start over, where slavery was still legal. Among them, James Gaston, chief surgeon of Gen. Robert Anderson's division at Gettysburg, emigrated to Sao Paolo Province in 1865 but later returned to Atlanta, Georgia, in 1883, where he practiced medicine until his death in 1903.[27]

Like other Civil War veterans, both Confederate and Union surgeons sought financial and professional opportunities in newly opened western territories. Many became leading citizens in their new communities and helped establish businesses and institutions. Surgeon William Riddick Whitehead, 44th Virginia, came from a wealthy family with financial holdings in both North and South. In 1865 he established himself in New York City where he was "employed by a few families of means as their family physician," living in a house on 42nd Street near Madison Avenue which he "leased and furnished sumptuously."[28] After his wife and child became ill with cholera, they moved to Denver, Colorado, for a healthier environment. In 1877 Whitehead visited Paris where he planned to practice medicine with his French diploma, but he instead returned to Denver during the Depression of 1877 and the subsequent discovery of silver and lead in Colorado. Assistant Surgeon William Maberry Strickler, 5th Louisiana, resigned from the Confederate army in 1864, completed his medical education at the Medical College of Virginia in 1869, and left Virginia to practice medicine in Colorado. Settling permanently in Colorado Springs in 1874, he eventually served on the City Council and as mayor.[29] Union surgeons also moved west. Assistant Surgeon George Stitzwell, 56th Pennsylvania, resigned in August 1863, after the battle of Gettysburg. By October 1863, he had moved his family from Pennsylvania to Nevada, Iowa, where he became prominent as a physician, an examining surgeon for U.S. pensions, and a member of the Grand Army of the Republic.[30]

CHANGED MEN

Whether they moved west or returned home, Civil War surgeons had to pick up the pieces of their former lives and careers and face an uncertain future. William Child wrote home to his wife a few days before he mustered out with his regiment: "It seems as though I had lived an hundred years in the last three . . . I feel that I am somewhat a changed man . . ."[31] Changed by their military experiences, Civil War surgeons returned to civilian life as a distinct group within a changing medical profession. Whether they moved on to new pursuits or returned home to practice medicine, they were not the same medical students or country doctors who had left home with limited medical experience. Silas Weir Mitchell later noted, "The war so trained vast numbers of country doctors that for a long time the cases for grave operations ceased to be sent to the cities as had been usual. The constant mingling of men of high medical culture with the less educated had also value, and the general influence of the war on our art was, in this and other ways, of great service."[32]

They had encountered physicians from varying backgrounds and training, shared expertise, and learned from each other. The endless medical reports they had to submit trained them to value and use data and statistics. Responsibility for the health of an entire regiment, brigade, or corps taught them to think about medicine not just as a response to an individual's illness but as a community-wide endeavor. They had seen firsthand the importance of clean water, proper nutrition, and sanitation. They endorsed medical care based on science, clinical observations, and results, rather than unsubstantiated medical theories. They learned how to organize and operate large-scale hospitals. Whether they practiced in large cities, small towns, or rural areas, their postwar careers reflect changes in their personal and professional lives resulting from their military service, as well as dynamic changes in medical practice and American society during the second half of the nineteenth century.

Surgeon Henry Janes, U.S. Sixth Corps, spent much of his military service during the Civil War as a hospital administrator, including responsibility for the hospitals at Gettysburg following the battle in 1863. He was later in charge of Sloan Hospital in Vermont until he resigned in 1866, continued his studies in Europe, and might have been expected to pursue a prestigious hospital career. Instead, he chose to practice medicine in his hometown of Waterbury, Vermont.

> Returning to his home in Waterbury in 1867, that he might be with his parents in their declining years, Dr. Janes resumed the practice of medicine and surgery there and soon became known throughout the State as one of its best and most highly esteemed physicians and surgeons. He published numerous important papers, notably on G. S. [Gun Shot] fractures and amputations. He was president of the Vermont State Medical Society in 1870; was consulting surgeon at Mary Fletcher Hospital, Burlington, and Heaton Hospital, Montpelier; surgeon general, Vermont National Guard; chairman Vermont Board Medical Censors; president, Vermont Board Medical Registration; trustee, University of Vermont, and President Waterbury Village trustees. He served as a member of the Vermont State Legislature in 1890, was a member of Bellevue Hospital Alumni Association, of the G. A. R. the M. O. L. L. U. S. [Military Order of the Loyal Legion of the United States] and of the Sons of the American Revolution.[33]

Dr. Janes's long list of accomplishments after the war echoes the obituaries and biographical sketches of many regimental surgeons who returned to private local practices but became active contributors in medical and civic affairs.

PUBLIC HEALTH

Assistant Surgeon William Henry Taylor, 19th Virginia, described the public aspects of medicine to his students at the Medical College of Virginia by explaining that a doctor was obliged to contribute to the general well-being of his community.

> Whatever promotes the public health is specifically his province, and his services are particularly valuable as a sanitary officer and as a member of the school board . . . In this State it is the custom to bestow the office of coroner upon a physician . . . Among other public stations reserved for the doctor are those of medical officer of almshouses and prisons, of some municipal departments, police and fire, for instance, and of superintendent of asylums for the insane.[34]

Doctors, he reminded them, were the first line of defense during epidemics like cholera and yellow fever that continued to plague American cities with outbreaks in the 1870s and into the first decade of the twentieth century. Taylor, himself, served as coroner of Richmond for thirty years, doing postmortem examinations for $25, testifying at murder trials, and drawing on his knowledge of chemistry to identify deaths by poison. His description of public service matches the postwar careers of many Gettysburg surgeons who went on to serve on boards of health, as coroners, and as superintendents and physicians of government-run insane asylums, prisons, soldiers' homes, and other institutional settings.

With wartime experience in setting up and managing military hospitals, many Civil War surgeons went on to play important roles in the development of sanitariums and insane asylums. Surgeon William H. Moore, 1st North Carolina Artillery, helped establish the Eastern Asylum for the Colored Insane in Goldsboro, North Carolina, in 1880, serving as superintendent until his death a year later.[35] Surgeon John F. Miller, 34th North Carolina, followed him as superintendent from 1887 to 1905. Miller's obituary describes how he expanded it from 200 patients to "more than

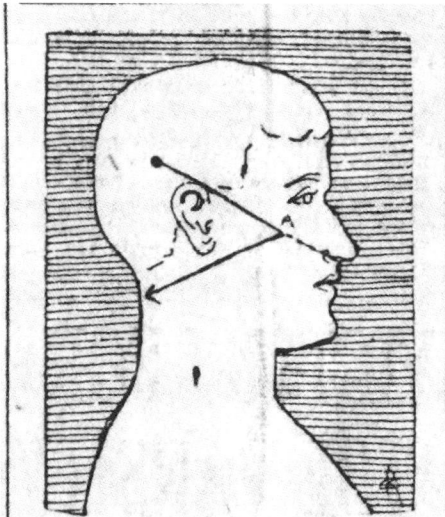

WOUND THAT KILLED J. A. SCOTT.

Dr. W. H. Taylor, City Coroner, made his post-mortem examination yesterday and remove the ball from J. A. Scott's head. He found it against the skull at the back of the head. The Coroner found that it had entered three inches behind the right ear and one inch above it and went forward in a line which would have given its exit below the left nostril, but was deflected at "a" by striking the bone, was sent backwards and lodged in the brain near the back of the skull.

Evidently Mr. Scott was stooping down when shot and was fired on at close range, the edges of the hole in the hat being apparently scorched by the flame. Dr. Taylor has the bullet. It is terribly battered. It is impossible to tell its calibre by comparing it with others. Its weight is 130 grains, and by comparing this figure with the weight of other pistol balls, the original size will be readily determined.

Coroner's Report, Richmond, Virginia, 1915. William H. Taylor served as coroner of Richmond for thirty years, testified at inquests and murder trials, and was often quoted in newspaper accounts. *Richmond Planet*, November 20, 1915

six hundred of the poor colored insane of North Carolina. His desire was to supply them with the best treatment and every comfort and need, and thereby restore as many of them as possible."[36] Surgeon Orpheus Everts, 20th Indiana, served as superintendent of the Indiana Hospital for the Insane, Central Hospital for the Insane in Indianapolis, and later a private sanitarium in Cincinnati, Ohio. We know something of his approach to mental illness from an article on psychiatric progress in Ohio that describes various forms of hydropathy, particularly Turkish baths and electricity, used to treat insanity.

> Orpheus Evarts urged active treatment for the insane "soon after impairment, even if the treatment be experimental." Evarts recommended discipline—to correct lack of control—rest, nutrition, and symptomatic medication. A particularly modern note is heard in his urging of baths, exercise, fresh air, sunlight, and occupation and amusement as accessory forms of therapy. He correctly warned against travel as a treatment for insanity, "since the patient would be preoccupied with himself and suicide is considered a constant danger."[37]

Everts had more than a purely clinical understanding of suicide. In 1891, his eighteen-year-old son, home on vacation from school, committed suicide with morphine, "laboring under depression of spirits" and "bad dreams and vision which harassed him beyond power of sleep."[38]

Although hydropathy had been considered a fringe sect advocated by eclectics before the Civil War, several Gettysburg surgeons trained in regular medical schools promoted medical uses of hydropathy after the war. Assistant Surgeon Simon Baruch, 3rd South Carolina Battalion, became an advocate of what he termed "hydrotherapy" to distinguish it from earlier forms of "hydropathy." Based on his own extensive clinical observations utilizing an eclectic, evidence-based approach to medicine, he claimed that hydrotherapy was "a valuable but an indispensable auxiliary to other treatments." He became an advocate of public baths in New York City for health and sanitary reasons.[39]

In addition to the health benefits of public baths in urban areas, mineral baths offered relief from various ailments. Samuel Brown Morrison, chief surgeon for Confederate general Jubal Early's division and a graduate of the University of Virginia, became proprietor of the Rockbridge Baths Sanitarium, Rockbridge County, Virginia, from 1874 to 1900. Located on the southern slopes of the Allegheny mountains, it offered baths in a natural thermal pool and mineral waters containing lithia and magnesium. The hotel promoted relief from rheumatism, rheumatic gout, bladder and kidney infections, nervous prostration, and liver problems.[40] Assistant Surgeon Isaac White, 62nd Virginia Cavalry, also a graduate of Virginia Medical College, served as resident physician at Montgomery White Sulphur Springs and Alleghany Springs resorts in Montgomery County, Virginia, and published a paper on the "Medical Virtues of the Alleghany Springs Water."[41] Montgomery White Sulphur Springs was used as a Confederate general hospital during the war and White served there as an acting assistant surgeon from September 3, 1862 to January 7, 1863. Assistant Surgeon Robert C. McEwen, 17th Connecticut, a graduate of the College of Physicians and Surgeons in New York City, moved to Saratoga Springs in 1866 where he served as consulting doctor for Hathorne Spring.[42] Surgeon George Frederick Adams, 67th New York, studied with Dr. Russell Thatcher Trall at the New York Hydropathic and Physiological School in 1853, and in 1860 practiced as a hydropathic physician in Brooklyn, New York. He later established Turkish baths in Boston from 1866 to 1869, moved to St. Louis, and returned to Medfield, Massachusetts in 1886.[43] In his preface to the *Turkish Bath Hand Book,* published in 1881, he expressed a commitment to the principles of clinical observation shared by both eclectics and allopaths:

> There is a pleasure in believing that among the rising generation of practitioners, there is a disposition to escape from the blind obedience hitherto exacted by established medical dogmas and medical elites. A spirit of free inquiry is at work to test all systems by their ascertained results, and the very changes that are perpetually occurring in medical practice is the best evidence of the fact that the old faith in assumed virtues, has been loudly shaken.[44]

In the field of public health, former military surgeons became leading advocates of vaccinations, clean water, and sanitary reforms to improve mortality rates in their communities. As coroners, they performed autopsies to record accurate causes of death and advocated for demographic statistics to monitor and track disease. The new emphasis on scientific methods and accurate statistics had tremendous impact on the development of public health efforts to eradicate childhood diseases, epidemics, and social ills in the second half of the nineteenth century. The endless reports that regimental surgeons complained about during their service established lifelong habits of record keeping and helped shape a medical field increasingly united in support of clinical observation and statistical analysis. The sharp distinctions between eclectics and allopaths faded after the war as most former Civil War surgeons practiced medicine as allopaths but also incorporated eclectic elements into their practice.

INDUSTRIAL MEDICINE

The regimentation and bureaucracy of their military experience prepared Civil War surgeons to work as company doctors for railroad, mining, and insurance companies in the growing field of industrial medicine. Railroad hospitals adopted the model of military hospitals to treat injured workers and passengers. Company medical systems ranged from highly organized hospital systems with salaried surgeons, to contract arrangements with local physicians or mutual benefit societies that functioned as insurance programs. By the turn of the century, it was estimated that as many as 14,000 physicians worked full- or part-time for a railroad medical organization.[45] Railroad medical services mirrored military medical departments by treating emergency trauma wounds after railway accidents and train wrecks but also advocating for preventive measures like vaccinations, regular medical examinations, and sanitary conditions. Just as military surgeons had to balance the medical requirements of individual men under their care with the regiment's need for soldiers in the ranks, company doctors had to negotiate conflicting obligations to workers and employers. Railroad surgeons worked for the many independent railroad companies throughout the country. Assistant Surgeon William Henry Harrison Cobb, 2nd North Carolina, served as a local surgeon for the Atlantic Coast Line Railroad and was also a medical examiner for insurance companies and fraternal organizations.[46] Surgeon William Samuel Love, 2nd Louisiana, was a surgeon for the Baltimore and Ohio Railway.[47] Surgeon Andrew Jackson Hobart, 1st Michigan, was surgeon for the Chicago and Northwestern Railway for sixteen years.[48]

Others found similar work as company doctors in the self-sufficient mining communities producing coal and iron. Suffering from lifelong chronic diarrhea after the war, Surgeon Curtis John Bellows, 7th Ohio, probably relocated to Michigan in hope that the climate of Lakes Superior and Michigan would benefit his health. He worked first as a physician for the Chicago-Northwestern Railroad in Escanaba, Michigan, from 1868 to 1870 until workers refused to pay $1 weekly fees for their medical care. He then served as the company doctor at the iron furnace of the Jackson Iron Company in Fayette, Michigan, from 1870 until his death in 1882. As Fayette's resident physician, Bellows treated industrial accidents, pregnancy, dental problems, and other health problems for about 500 residents. His two-story house on Main Street, not far from the superintendent's home, contained his office and infirmary on the first floor and living quarters on the second floor. Medical fees, along with store expenditures, rent, and other expenses were deducted from employee earnings each month.[49] Confederate surgeons also became company doctors. Surgeon Benjamin Mellichamp Cromwell, 1st North Carolina, moved from Albany, Georgia, in 1882 to become the resident physician of the Consolidated Coal Company at Eckhart Mines in Alleghany County, Maryland, a company town with a population of more than 700.[50] From 1885 to about 1890, Surgeon John Moore Hayes, 26th Alabama, worked as a physician at the Pratt Coal and Coke Company, located 6 miles outside of Birmingham, Alabama. The company employed prison labor provided by freed Blacks who were often sentenced to years of forced labor for petty crimes.[51] An 1887 description of the Pratt Mines provided a sanitized version of the conditions. It estimated 1,000 to 1,500 employees of which 500–600 were unpaid state convicts. "The convict miners are closely inspected by the state authorities and moderately worked, the mortality rate among them is very low."[52] As the state-employed physician, Hayes would have provided medical care and oversight for the convicts.

MEDICAL CONTRIBUTIONS

The sheer volume and severity of cases encountered in battlefield medicine helped prepare some Civil War surgeons for specialized medical careers after the war. Assistant Surgeon William Williams Keen and Acting Assistant Surgeon S. Weir Mitchell were among those dispatched to assist with the wounded after Gettysburg. Both had extensive experience in the Philadelphia hospitals where their work and research devoted to neurological disorders at Turner's Lane Hospital led to specializations in mental illness and brain surgery.[53] Morris Joseph Asch, medical director of the U.S. Artillery Reserve at Gettysburg, resigned from the army in 1873, practiced medicine in New York City, and specialized in diseases of the nose and throat. He is credited with developing a new operation for the cure of septal deviations, afterwards known as the Asch operation.[54] Several Confederate and Union surgeons went on to specialize in obstetrics and gynecology.[55] Among them, Assistant Surgeon William Shaw Stewart, 83rd Pennsylvania, helped found the Medico Chirurgical College of Philadelphia, served as professor of obstetrics and gynecology, and invented an obstetric forceps with detachable blades.[56]

Both the Confederate and Union medical departments encouraged surgeons to interact with colleagues from diverse backgrounds and medical experiences through formal and informal training, publishing case histories, and collecting specimens. After the war many surgeons continued to share information by remaining active in medical societies, submitting papers to medical journals, and working to improve medical practice. A few contributed technical advances. Assistant Surgeon Ai Waterhouse, 7th Maine, practiced medicine in Jamestown, New York, while he pursued his interest in scientific research as a member of the American Association for the Advancement of Science, the American Society of Microscopists, and as president of the Jamestown Microspical Society. Surgeon Augustus Clarke, 8th New York Cavalry, graduated from Harvard Medical School in 1862 and then studied in Leipzig and Paris for a year after the war. His obituary notes that "He was one of the earliest advocates of the adoption of antiseptic measures in carrying out successful surgical work . . . he was continually absorbed in research work, especially along gynecology and abdominal surgery lines and frequently contributed articles on both subjects to medical journals."[57] Assistant Surgeon Benjamin Howard, 6th U.S., designed the Howard Ambulance, later adopted by the French army and the metropolitan ambulance corps in London. Although his self-promoted method of hermetically sealing chest wounds initially showed little success, he is credited with the widely used Howard Method of artificial respiration to resuscitate drowning victims. Surgeon William Alexander Greene, 11th Georgia Battalion, advocated the use of the hypodermic syringe and invented a widely used syringe and improved needle.[58]

MEDICAL EDUCATION

Former military surgeons also became harsh critics of their own medical education and advocated for improved education and licensing standards. Many shared their military experience with a new generation of physicians by serving as faculty of medical colleges. More than forty of the Confederate and Union regimental surgeons at Gettysburg later held professorships in the fields of surgery, physiology, anatomy, *materia medica*, ophthalmology, obstetrics, and chemistry. They taught in established medical schools in New Orleans, Richmond, Philadelphia, Baltimore, Charleston, Albany, New York, Chicago, Cleveland, and Cincinnati, as well as newer schools like the University of Colorado, established in 1876, and Arkansas Industrial University founded in 1871. Hunter Holmes McGuire, medical director of Ewell's Second Corps, served as chair of surgery at the Medical College of Virginia and helped found several medical schools in Richmond, which later incorporated into the Medical College of Virginia. William Riddick Whitehead helped found medical schools at the University of Denver and University of Colorado. Like so many other Civil War surgeons who had acquired medical skills on the battlefield, he was a proponent of improved medical education and advocated for more consistent government licensing.

The general government should as a matter of public safety take away the licensing power of the medical diploma, from every college, and vest this power in medical examining boards, at least equal to those for the examination of surgeons to the United States Army and Navy. The government owes as much to its people as to its soldiers.[59]

MEN OF SCIENCE

As members of the medical profession in postwar America, former Civil War surgeons clearly identified themselves as men of science. William Henry Taylor counseled his chemistry class at the Medical College of Virginia that, as scientists, "All Nature is yours to roam over and explore. Our aim is the truth."[60] For some, interest in science was part of their medical practice. Others actively pursued lifelong interests in a variety of scientific fields, especially climate, ethnology, and natural history.

Surgeon John Geddings Hardy, 6th North Carolina, and William Henry Geddings, medical purveyor of the Army of Northern Virginia, both studied the value of climate on health. Since their fathers, who studied and taught at the Medical College of South Carolina in Charleston, remained lifelong friends, the sons probably knew each other. They shared a growing interest among medical professionals in the relationship between health and the environment, theorizing that patients suffering with consumption, in particular, could help restore their health by seeking warmer climates offering fresh outdoor air during the winter months. Hardy's meteorological observations in Asheville, North Carolina, became the basis for promoting the area for chronically ill tuberculosis patients. Geddings maintained a practice in Aiken, South Carolina, during the winter months and a summer practice in Bethlehem, New Hampshire. Convinced that Aiken offered an ideal climate for pulmonary diseases, he set about documenting the weather with "tri-daily observations with improved meteorological instruments and following rigidly the instructions furnished by the Smithsonian Institution and United States Signal Service."[61] Assistant Surgeon Greenly Vinton Woollen, 27th Indiana, was appointed superintendent of the City Hospital in Indianapolis in 1866 and three years later began recording weather observations there for the Smithsonian Institution.[62] Surgeon George MacIlvane Ramsey,

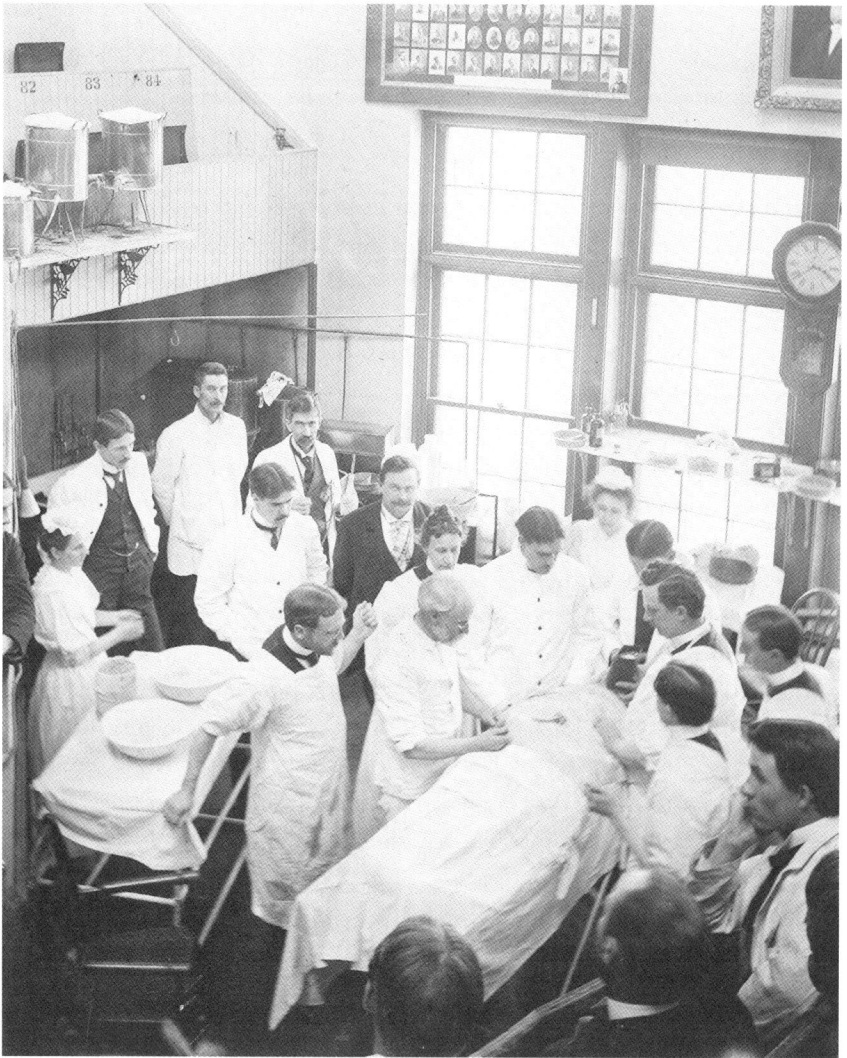

Dr. Breakey's Clinic, University of Michigan, c. 1897. William Fleming Breakey, 16th Michigan, returned to Ann Arbor to practice medicine and held professorships at the University of Michigan Medical School in surgery, dermatology, and syphilology. Courtesy of University of Michigan Bentley Historical Library

95th New York, grew up in Washington County, Pennsylvania. Due to failing health at the age of twenty-six, his physician advised him to go to the South for several winters. He spent time in Louisiana, Alabama, Missouri, and Arkansas before returning home to begin the study of medicine in 1849, graduating from Jefferson Medical College in 1852. A history of Washington County describes his fondness for scientific studies and in particular pursuing theories to explain the diurnal motion on earth and the eastward flow of winds.[63]

Some surgeons pursued their interests in natural sciences. Assistant Surgeon Hamilton Gamble, 25th Virginia, returned home to Moorefield, West Virginia, to practice medicine and surgery but is best known for his collection of more than 157 plant specimens gathered locally along the Potomac River, which he donated to the West Virginia University Herbarium.[64] Assistant Surgeon Isaiah Fawkes Everhart, 8th Pennsylvania Cavalry, studied natural science at Franklin and Marshall College in Lancaster, Pennsylvania, before earning a medical degree from the University of Pennsylvania in 1863. After the war he traveled through Europe and then returned to Scranton to practice medicine and oversee the family businesses in brass, coal, and iron. Everhart continued his interest in the natural sciences and assembled an extensive collection of birds, animals, woods, and seeds native to Pennsylvania. With family inheritance he was able to build and endow the Everhart Museum of Natural History, Science and Art that opened in 1908 as a gift to the city of Scranton.[65] Assistant Surgeon Jeremiah Bernard Brinton, medical purveyor for the Army of the Potomac, returned to Philadelphia to practice medicine briefly before pursuing other business interests that allowed him to devote more time to his lifelong interest in botany. An authority on the Pine Barrens of New Jersey, he was an active collector, known for the accuracy of his observations and scrupulous care in preserving specimens.[66]

Surgeon Daniel Garrison Brinton, medical director of the 2nd Division U.S. Eleventh Corps, became a distinguished ethnologist, serving as professor of ethnology and archaeology in the Academy of Natural Sciences and as professor of American archaeology and linguistics at the University of Pennsylvania.[67] Surgeon Edward Donnelly,

2nd Pennsylvania, was charged with "inhuman vandalism" for picking up bones on the Manassas battlefield but was acquitted due to his long history of biological collecting in Africa and Brazil before the war. Thomas Hewson Bache, medical inspector, U.S. First Corps, served as curator of the Mütter Museum of the College of Physicians from 1866 to 1883. During his tenure the museum acquired some of its most notable collections including the skull collection of Austrian anatomist Joseph Hurt and the anatomical models made by Louis Thomas Jerome Auzoux.[68]

BUSINESS AND POLITICS

Some former surgeons abandoned medical practice after the war for more lucrative fields in business and commerce. Some responded to the demand for manufactured pills and patent medicines by opening retail drug stores, sometimes temporarily after the war, or in combination with continued medical practices. Assistant Surgeon Charles M. Trask, 5th New Hampshire, practiced medicine until 1872, "when, on account of failing health, he entered the drug business" first in Boston and then White River Junction, Vermont, until his death in 1891 "from disease contracted in the United States service."[69] Assistant Surgeon Henry Washington Williams, 5th North Carolina, moved to Sherman, Texas, in 1873 where his drug business succeeded in "accumulating a snug little fortune." In 1883 he moved his growing business to Fort Worth where he became the largest wholesale drug business in the state, with annual sales of $500,000.[70] Assistant Surgeon Azro Melvin Plant, 14th Vermont, advertised in St. Albans, Vermont, as "physician and surgeon, dealer in drugs, manuf. and dealer in Red Star Bitters and Plant's Kidney Remedy."[71]

Former surgeons also pursued non-medical careers in banking, politics, and business. Surgeon Castanus Blake Park Jr., 16th Vermont, "came to Poweshiek County, Iowa, in 1867, and to Grand Junction two years later, hoping to quit his practice altogether; but his reputation followed him, almost compelling him to practice a portion of the time." In addition to practicing medicine, his successful business enterprises included the first lumber yard; sales of grain, implements, and coal; investments in real estate; and the first herd of short-horn cattle in the county. Thirteen years later, he "sold out all his other business except his farm and stock, and in 1879 built and started the banking house of C.B. Park, at Grand Junction."[72]

Many of the Gettysburg surgeons became active in politics, serving in local government as mayors and councilmen, in state legislatures, and in national politics. While Union surgeons identified as both Republicans and Democrats, former Confederates allied exclusively with the Democratic Party. Assistant Surgeon Whiteside Godfrey Hunter, 149th Pennsylvania, was elected as a Republican representing Kentucky's 3rd and 11th Districts in the U.S. House of Representatives and served as U.S. minister to Guatemala and Honduras in 1897. Assistant Surgeon William Hinson Cole, 8th Georgia, was elected as a Democrat to the 49th U.S. Congress in 1885. Surgeons William Allen Robertson, 6th Louisiana, and Sampson Pope, 22nd Georgia, both took part in contesting electoral votes from Louisiana and South Carolina in the disputed Hayes-Tilden election of 1876. Testimony in a U.S. Senate investigation accused Robertson, then president of the Louisiana State Senate, of offering $200,000 to an elector to vote for the Democratic candidate, Samuel J. Tilden.[73] Pope's obituary reports that he took part in the so-called redemption of South Carolina in 1876, a sometimes-violent effort to disrupt and intimidate voters, and served for a number of years in the state legislature.[74]

DISABILITIES

Many surgeons suffered from the long-term consequences of their military service. Surgeons were vulnerable to all the injuries and camp illnesses that they treated, and many returned with debilitating physical and mental conditions resulting from their wartime experiences. Ill health forced Surgeon Thomas Whitaker Salmond, 2nd South Carolina, to return home at the beginning of 1864. The examining doctor, Dr. John J. Chisolm, reported that he was "suffering from involuntary discharges of urine which are excessively annoying to him. He has been under treatment for sixty days without benefit. The disease is of twelve months duration and for its persistence renders him unfit to perform the duties required of him in the Brigade."[75] In April 1869 the South Carolina House of Representatives adopted a resolution, to pay Dr. Salmond $20 for postmortem examinations and $65 to care for prisoners in jail, but only a few months later he died after what was described as "a long and painful illness."[76] Surgeon James W. Anawalt, 11th Pennsylvania, suffered from multiple chronic illnesses during his military service and never fully recovered. In February 1862 he contracted chronic diarrhea with intermittent constipation, the next winter he contracted malarial fever, and in March 1863 he "experienced sciatica which caused recurrent hemiplegia of his left leg." He still managed to serve to the end of the war and was discharged in July 1865. After the war he practiced medicine in Greensburg, Westmoreland, Pennsylvania. Pension records describe Anawalt's "severe rheumatism along with chronic diarrhea which required him to wear a 'rectal pad.'" He began receiving a pension of $25 per month in 1888 for chronic diarrhea and rheumatism, requiring constant care of an attendant who assisted him with dressing and undressing. In 1892 he was admitted to the Military Soldiers Home in Dayton, Ohio, and died four years later from "chronic Meningitis."[77]

In some cases, physical disabilities made it difficult or impossible to continue a medical career. Assistant Surgeon Louis Evans Atkinson, 1st Pennsylvania Cavalry, was discharged in December 1865 as surgeon of 188th Pennsylvania at twenty-four years of age with joint disease of his legs that required crutches. Unable to practice medicine, he studied law, was admitted to the bar in 1870, practiced law in Mifflintown, Pennsylvania, and served as a Republican congressman from 1883 to 1893.[78] Assistant Surgeon Edgar Parker, 13th Massachusetts, was wounded in the head on July 1st on the steps of Christ Church in Gettysburg. He later abandoned medicine to pursue a career as a portrait painter and became a successful artist in Boston, specializing in portraits and historical subjects.[79]

Not all disabilities were as visible as amputated limbs or scarred bodies. Gettysburg surgeons, like other Civil War veterans, suffered from alcoholism, drug addiction, and mental illnesses during and after the war. Assistant Surgeon Thomas Upshur, 2nd North Carolina Cavalry, struggled with alcoholism during the war. In August 1862 he was court-martialed for drunkenness, reprimanded, and given a one-month suspension. His military records provide a detailed description of his erratic behavior and habitual abuse of alcohol.[80] In 1914, when Ewing Jordan was assembling information for his publication, *University of Pennsylvania Men Who Served in the Civil War*, he contacted Upshur's children who provided what little they knew about their father's postwar life. Their letters to Dr. Jordan describe his return to his family, "broken in health and spirit, with fortune gone, having lost all by the war he tried to establish himself in his profession again." He was not successful, and after 1869, abandoned his wife and children to live with a brother in Mississippi and later reportedly "lived in the mountains."[81] Upshur was not the only veteran surgeon with wartime alcohol problems that carried over into civilian life. Surgeon Tazewell Tyler, 13th South Carolina, was the youngest son of President John Tyler. After the war. Tazewell Tyler moved to San Francisco, divorced his wife, and died in 1874, "after turning to alcohol." One account suggests that he suffered from what we today call post-traumatic stress disorder, but a fellow surgeon complained during the war that "Dr. Tyler is too fond of drink and gambling."[82] Suffering from mental illness, Surgeon Melson Rowland, 118th Pennsylvania, is listed as an inmate in the Philadelphia Hospital for the Insane in the 1870 census and later the Norristown Hospital for the Insane, where he remained until his death from influenza in 1901. When Surgeon James Lorenzo Farley, 84th New York, died in 1886, a medical journal reported it as "Another case of the bad effects of cocaine." Dr. Farley had been treating himself for nervousness with hypodermic injections of cocaine, became insane, and died at the Flatbush Asylum.[83]

Despite his misgivings about leaving army life, Dr. William Child was among those who successfully weathered the transition from military service to civilian life as a physician in his community. A biographical sketch in 1908 described how he "resumed his practice at Bath and entered upon the quiet duties of citizenship . . . His professional life has been in the main the quiet uneventful one of the country practitioner."[84] He remained connected to his military service by participating in the Grand Army of the Republic and authoring the history of his regiment. As an active member in the New Hampshire Medical Society, he regularly presented papers.

> These published papers show that he held advanced views on sanitary matters, had little faith in drugs, no faith in so-called disinfectants, claiming that to be "clean" was the essence of modern sanitation and surgery. He does not claim to have made discoveries or advancements; does not suppose that the profession has arrived at perfection; expects that there will be much greater progress, that much useless medical and surgical lumber will be abandoned and that we shall finally have a practice based upon knowledge of the human body and mind and common sense, and that all "shades and shadows" will be eliminated from the profession.[85]

In 1895, due to disabilities contracted during the war, he retired from active practice to a farm where it was reported that "he hopes to live his appointed days."[86]

Chapter 11

"Death Makes No Distinction"

The Good Death

Andrew B. Cross somberly observed in his account of the Christian Commission's work at Gettysburg, that "Death makes no distinction. There is no discharge in the war with death and the grave."[1] Death may have been the common enemy of the surgeons, but it was also a constant presence for the many caregivers who struggled to make sense out of the suffering and loss that followed the battle of Gettysburg. Christian Commission delegates, chaplains, and volunteer nurses all described emotional deathbed scenes in the hospitals and wrote letters home to grieving families that incorporated the required elements of what was widely considered a "Good Death." The deceased understood and accepted his fate, expressed a belief in God and his salvation, and sent messages to loved ones at home.[2] For patients facing death far from home without family and friends at their bedside, nurses and chaplains filled in as surrogates for absent loved ones, oversaw burials in hospital cemeteries, and conducted simple religious services. Graves were marked whenever possible according to army regulations, in hopes that bodies could be identified and returned home or reburied in the newly established National Cemetery at Gettysburg. Focusing on individual stories of faith and heroism, civilian volunteers attempted to understand the massive loss of life in religious and patriotic terms of spiritual redemption and national renewal. Anna Holstein, serving as matron at Camp Letterman, described one young man from Montgomery County, Pennsylvania, who lay from July until October, calmly bearing untold agony from a wound which he certainly knew must result in death; yet his one anxious thought, constantly expressed, was: "Mother, do not grieve; it is best and right; bury me with my comrades in the field." So, at sunrise one bright autumn morning, his soul went up to God, and the casket which had held it, we laid to rest among the nation's honored dead in Gettysburg Cemetery.[3]

If his soul belonged to God, Holstein found solace in the fact that his body remained to consecrate the ground that Lincoln described as "a final resting place for those who here gave their lives so that the nation might live."

Scientific Naturalism

Death was no stranger to the surgeons who provided medical care during and after the battle. During their medical training they had stolen bodies from graveyards and spent long hours examining corpses in dissection rooms. They had witnessed the deadly cholera and yellow fever epidemics that devastated their communities. In their personal lives, some had already lost wives and children to childbirth and disease. But nothing they had experienced in civilian life matched the sheer numbers of dead they encountered at Gettysburg. Samuel Brown Morrison, chief surgeon of Confederate general Jubal Early's Division, wrote home to his wife after Gettysburg in a rare personal description of the dead:

> I saw the dead scattered over the field & many have seen the dead body of this poor woman's husband, or his desolate corps. No wife looked, no child shed a tear. The thought of being killed in battle and been buried as I have seen many a soldier buried, in a heap on the battle field (he may sleep with his "Marshales Cloak around him"-but) I have no fancy for such a death & burial—When I die I would wish to be buried where my dust might mingle with yours and be near to those who were dear to me on earth.—I saw fifty soldiers buried in one hole at Gettysburg, carelessly covered with earth, many more left unburied upon this field.[4]

Morrison's account is unusual because, unlike many civilian accounts, surgeons rarely described battle and hospital scenes so emotionally, more often describing death in a medical context, using anatomical and clinical terms. They described and quantified death in patient reports and case histories, many of which were later published in the *Medical and Surgical History of the War of the Rebellion.*[5] In a volume of patient notes, later compiled by Dr. Henry Janes, Dr. Henry C. May reported the treatment and death of Isaac Johnson, aged twenty-one, wounded in the thigh on July 2nd in the standard medical format:

> Compound fracture of left thigh amputated July 3rd. August 20 improving. August 25–31 severe diarrhea and hectic fever. Sept. 5 admitted. Health very poor. Discharge from Stump free and unhealthy. Diarrhea continued, Oct. 10 secondary hemorrhage with loss of four ounces of blood. Large abcess in gluteal region. Discharging through face of stump. Oct. 19 died.[6]

Compared to civilian caregivers who provided emotional and spiritual support, surgeons were often criticized for being cold and uncaring. Some surgeons were deeply religious, including a few who later became ministers; some were closely affiliated with a religious denomination; others self-identified more generically as "Christian"; and still others espoused more secular and scientific philosophies. Whatever their personal beliefs, surgeons during the Civil War moved away from the religious symbolism and sacredness of the body after death to adopt a more pragmatic scientific naturalism based in materialism and scientific knowledge. Two Confederate surgeons, who later in life wrote about both religion and death, provide important insights into how surgeons came to view their work differently from civilians and non-medical caregivers. William Henry Taylor did not espouse what he called "ecclesiastical religion" and presented his materialist views in a lecture on "Science and the Soul," explaining:

> Of those who see many dead bodies, as your teachers now do and as you, too, will when you are in practice, the impression is irresistibly made that, in the matter of the soul, there is no apparent difference

between a dead man and a dead dog. On occasion we doctors cut up our subjects as the butcher cuts up his; the materiality of all we are dealing with is fixed upon our minds as it is upon his, and the idea of an associated spirit is no more imposed upon our conceptions than upon his . . .[7]

Taylor received criticism for this lecture but defended his remarks by explaining that for the man of science, "His religion, if it be not in subjection to conventional formulas, yet it is as pure and practical as any that is set forth in creeds, and his system of morals is as exalted and as faithfully observed as that of any other man . . . he, too, weeps bitter tears where he sees his loved ones sink into the grave. Nor is he, in that dark hour, without hope . . . "[8] William Maberry Strickler, who came from a religious background in the Methodist Episcopal Church and served as the chaplain for his regiment during the Civil War, nonetheless quoted George Herbert Palmer, Harvard professor of natural religion, moral philosophy, and civil polity, describing a surgeon at work:

> I suspect his thoughts can hardly travel so far from his knife as to consider even the poor sufferer before him. I doubt if he greatly pities the patient before him on whom he is engaged or takes much satisfaction in restoring him to health . . . as he cuts, he may wisely exclude all thought of God and his neighbor, being a surgeon and nothing more. He requires a certain narrowing of his vision, a certain exclusion of the infinite aspects of his task, in order to perform that task well.[9]

POSTMORTEM EXAMINATIONS

Cornelia Hancock, who began her nursing career at Gettysburg, chronicled her own changing attitude toward death and the work of the surgeons in her letters home from Civil War hospitals. Writing from Gettysburg in August 1863, she admits that "it does not seem to me as if I should ever make any account of death again. I have seen it disposed of in such a summary manner out here." Seven months later at the Second Corps Hospital at Brandy Station, Virginia, she described how surgeons made use of amputated limbs and dead bodies. An hour after a man's leg was amputated, "I saw one of the Drs. cut it up into three pieces for the sake of practice. One can get used to anything. One of my favorite resorts is our dead house, some such fine looking men die. Sometimes Dr. Dudley embalms them and keeps them quite a while just to look at."[10] While the dead house as a favorite resort might seem macabre, postmortem autopsies and dissections performed during the Civil War became routine functions for the medical staff. The seemingly limitless supply of bodies available to military staff was recognized as an opportunity for medical study by both armies. U.S. Surgeon General William Hammond's special order No. 2, dated May 21, 1862, directed surgeons to prepare reports of postmortem examinations and "to collect and forward to the office of the Surgeon General all specimens of morbid anatomy surgical or medical which may be regarded as valuable."[11] The program was well underway by the battle of Gettysburg under the direction of U.S. Surgeon John H. Brinton who visited Gettysburg and other battlefields to collect specimens and encouraged surgeons in the field to contribute to the newly established Medical Museum in Washington, DC. Brinton described his collecting efforts during visits to battlefields.

> Many and many a putrid heap have I had dug out of trenches where they had been buried, in the supposition of an everlasting rest, and ghoul-like work have I done, amid surrounding gatherings of wondering surgeons, and scarcely less wondering doctors.[12]

Acting Assistant Surgeon Henry K. Neff wrote to Brinton from Camp Letterman, "I have numerous specimens for you and have packed them in ale with some whiskey and chlorismatia Inda—we have more in the ground and will have more everyday for a month to come."[13]

Autopsies reported in the *Medical and Surgical History of the War of the Rebellion* most often took place in hospital settings, but the U.S. Army prepared a printed checklist to assist regimental surgeons in the field in preparing postmortem reports. While families or comrades might object to postmortem examinations of deceased soldiers, surgeons had undisputed custody of the dead bodies of prisoners. Acting Assistant Surgeon John T. Lanning reported on an autopsy of W. D. Shivers, twenty-one, of the 1st South Carolina Cavalry, who died on August 14th:

Wounded July 1 by a minnie ball causing fracture and comminution of the Right Elbow joint Amputation of arm at its middle third performed July 6. July 31 Stump is very sensitive. Patient has symptoms of Pyaemia. Aug 4 Delirium attended the fever today. Aug. 8 The stump is swollen and hot. The discharge very small granulations are unhealthy. The delirum attended the fever today. Aug 14 The Patient has profuse prespiration—is rational—Died. Autopsy-there was effusion of Serum in the Plura and pericardium. The left Lung contained numerous abcesses filled with pus.[14]

Fewer medical records of the Confederate Medical Department survived the war, but articles submitted to the *Confederate Medical Journal* document numerous autopsies conducted by Confederate surgeons. Surgeon J. L. Cabbell, in charge of the Charlottesville Hospital, submitted reports of various head wounds, including one autopsy in December 1862:

Autopsy showed the external table slightly fractured, and the internal, also, for about an inch, but nearer to the middle line of the skull. About one ounce of extravasated blood was found between the skull and dura-mater, and a like quantity between the latter and the brain. The brain itself was disorganized to the depth of three-fourths of an inch and to the extent of about two square inches.[15]

Later in the war, Confederate surgeon Joseph Jones used the bodies of deceased Union prisoners to conduct autopsies as part of his study of mortality at Andersonville Prison. The order issued by Confederate surgeon general Samuel P. Moore, dated August 6, 1864, echoes U.S. Surgeon General Hammond's commitment to the value of postmortem investigations in furthering medical science. Moore wrote to Surgeon Isaiah H. White in charge of the hospital at Andersonville:

The field of pathological investigation afforded by the large collection of Federal prisoners in Georgia is of great extent and importance, and it is believed that results of value to the profession may be obtained by a careful investigation of the effects of disease upon a large body of men subjected to a decided change of climate and the circumstances peculiar to prison life. . . . The medical officers will assist in the performance of such post mortems as Surgeon Jones may indicate, in order that this great field of pathological investigation may be explored for the benefit of the medical department of the Confederate army.[16]

EMBALMING

Obtaining medical knowledge from the dead through autopsies and specimens often conflicted with the desire of grieving families to fulfill the rituals of the good death by reclaiming the bodies of departed loved ones so that they could be reburied at home. Several embalming firms offered their services at Gettysburg to help families locate bodies for exhumation and then disinfect or embalm them for transport home for burial. After Pennsylvania governor Andrew Curtin personally visited the battlefield, he appointed local Gettysburg lawyer David Wills as his state agent to take charge of helping Pennsylvania families identify graves and ship bodies home. As early as July 11th, William Bunnell had set up an embalming tent on East Cemetery Hill, and by the end of July the embalming firms of Dr. Richard Burr, Chamberlain & Lyford, and Brown & Alexander had also established offices in Gettysburg.

Most of the embalmers had some medical training. William J. Bunnell was not a trained physician but had been taught embalming by his brother-in-law, Dr. Thomas Holmes. Dr. Richard Burr, an 1847 graduate of the Philadelphia College of Medicine, served briefly as surgeon of the 72nd Pennsylvania from November 1861 to February 1862 before establishing himself as an embalmer. C. B. Chamberlain, a graduate of the Homeopathic Medical College of Philadelphia, and Benjamin F. Lyford, graduate of the Philadelphia Medical College, were partners in an embalming business at Gettysburg and appear in photographs taken at Camp Letterman. Charles De Costa Brown, who attended the University of Pennsylvania, and Joseph Bell Alexander advertised in the *Philadelphia Inquirer* July 25, 1863, for "Embalming of the dead. Drs. Brown and Alexander opened branch office in Gettysburg—exhume, disinfect and embalm when practicable bodies of the dead."[17] The work was lucrative. At least one Union surgeon, Assistant Surgeon Perrin

Gardner, 1st West Virginia Cavalry, admitted under investigation that he made $1,000 after the battle by embalming bodies.[18] Reverend Hiram O. Nash of Ridgefield, Connecticut, kept a detailed record of his journey to Gettysburg to retrieve the remains of his nephew, Pvt. Rufus Warren of the 17th Connecticut. Nash found his way to the 11th Corps Hospital where he learned that Warren had died July 17th, and, with the help of a member of his unit, was directed to his marked grave. Nash paid $1.00 to have the body exhumed and then had it taken to the office of Dr. Bunnell "where it was disinfected, then covered with charcoal and chloride of lime, then put into an airtight coffin with gutta percha edges and packed for shipping. Disinfection cost $15 and the coffin $23."[19] Embalmers remained unregulated until General Order #39, issued by Gen. Ulysses Grant on March 15, 1865, established the need for standard fees and required embalmers to be licensed by provost marshals based on their skill and the process used.

CASUALTIES OF WAR

As noncombatants, surgeons were less likely to be wounded, but they too became casualties of the war. At the battle of Gettysburg twelve Union medical officers and at least three Confederate surgeons were wounded in the course of their duties.[20] Most were assistant surgeons at field stations close to the action. Two died: Assistant Surgeon William S. Moore, 61st Ohio, struck by an artillery shell on July 3rd that shattered his thigh, died on July 6th; Assistant Surgeon James Alston Groves, 16th Mississippi, died from his wounds on July 2nd. Thirty-nine (3 percent) of the Union and Confederate surgeons who served at Gettysburg died during the remaining two years of the war following the battle. Eleven were killed during combat or by snipers. Two died in accidents, but the largest number died of camp diseases that included tuberculosis, pneumonia, typhoid, and cholera. For those who remained in the U.S. Army following the war, service on military posts in the West and South proved deadly during outbreaks of cholera, typhoid, and yellow fever. An outbreak of cholera at Hart's Island in New York City in 1866–67 claimed the lives of at least two U.S. surgeons, James T. Calhoun and George McCulloch McGill. The long-term effects of wartime service continued to cause early deaths

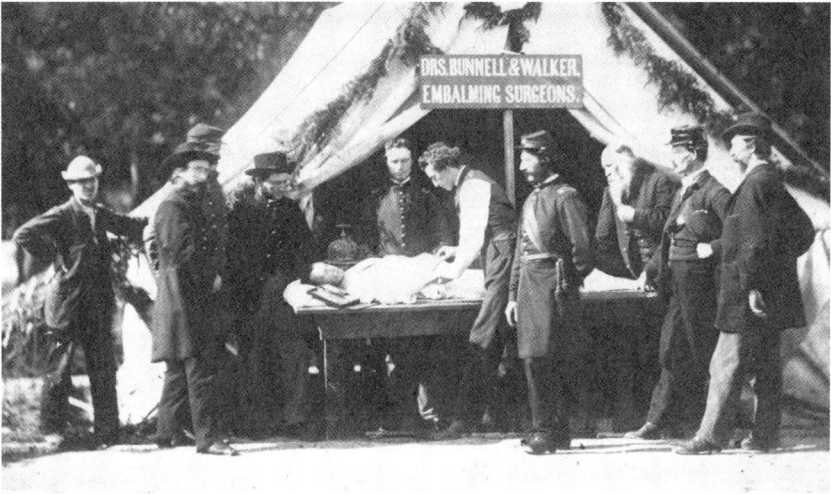

Drs. Bunnell & Walker, Embalming Surgeons. Peter S. Weaver, photographer, September 1863. Courtesy of the collection of Fred Sherfy

among surgeons from chronic dysentery, tuberculosis, liver diseases, nephritis (known as Bright's disease), and other disabilities. During the ten years following the war, 136 (11 percent) of the Union, Confederate, and contract surgeons who were at Gettysburg died. Even years later, deaths were attributed to diseases that began during military service. Surgeon Curtis J. Bellows, 7th Ohio, died from chronic dysentery at the age of sixty-two, resulting from the long-term effects of his military service. Some surgeons died from train and carriage accidents; some met violent deaths from murder and suicide; others lived long lives and died peacefully from old age.

Facing Death

Gettysburg surgeons often approached their own deaths with the same clinical distance that they applied to their medical practice. William Strickler's essay on "The Fear of Death," written a few years before he died, describes the natural process of dying:

> The heart in course of years, will lose its irritability; the glands of the stomach will shrink and lose their efficiency; all the tissues will become

inflexible and stiff; the eye by reason of changes in the shape of its lense, will become dim; the cells of the brain will dwindle and finally disappear, and that organ will lose the power of thought or reacting at all. In fact, the whole body will become a worn-out machine, and death is desirable to remove it. And we find that the aged pass out of life as naturally and easily as they came into it. Whatever hope religion affords is that much positive consolation.[21]

Strickler had already suffered temporary paralysis from a stroke in 1890 and goes on to argue that in cases of paralysis and dementia death is a welcome relief: "If death be beneficent in any class of cases, why not in all the aged."[22] In the end, he took his own advice. *The Medical Record* reported in 1908 that he died at his brother's home in Denver, Colorado, from "the effects of an accidental overdose of morphine."[23] William Henry Taylor also wrote about suicide as an acceptable end, and newspaper accounts of his death hint that the longtime coroner and chemist who specialized in poison may have chosen death. Recovering from a severe cold, he "told his butler to bring him a large dinner. An hour later his breathing became hard and short and in less than ten minutes he had passed away. His death came quickly and without suffering, as he had often expressed the wish that he might die."[24] One newspaper reported the cause of his death as "a form of poisoning resulting from an attack of grippe." Dr. W. J. Underwood reportedly approached his own death from Bright's disease at the age of fifty in stark clinical terms.[25] "He traced the progress of his illness to the last with a perfect realization of his condition at all times and bore himself with the greatest fortitude. He predicted the final symptoms of his disease and passed away, as he had expected, with little struggle."[26]

Final Resting Places

Samuel Brown Morrison got his wish to be buried at home next to his wife. After a long career as the proprietor of the Rockbridge Baths, Rockbridge, Virginia, he died in 1901 "of a complication of diseases [including Bright's disease], the chief malady being the effects of paralysis with which he was attacked nearly two years ago." Others died far from home. Surgeon Nahum Alvah Hersom, 17th Maine, suffered from effects of malarial fever after the war and died in Dublin while traveling alone for his health in 1881. His body was embalmed and returned home for burial twenty-five days later. His funeral was attended by veterans of the 17th Maine, the local GAR veterans post, and other physicians in Portland, Maine, where he had established a successful practice.

Two surgeons from Ireland, both buried at Philadelphia's Mount Moriah Cemetery, illustrate how postwar surgeons, despite similar military careers, could end their lives under very different circumstances. Assistant Surgeon William Craig, 26th Pennsylvania, was born in Ireland in 1832. Before he graduated from Penn Medical College and the Philadelphia University of Medicine and Surgery in 1862 at the age of thirty as an eclectic practitioner, he worked as a clerk for his brother-in-law's bottling and mineral water business. He passed the Pennsylvania examination for assistant surgeon with a score of five and was appointed assistant surgeon of the 26th Pennsylvania from March 1863 until it mustered out in June 1864. A year later he was appointed assistant surgeon in the 37th U.S. Colored Troops on duty in North Carolina where he was stricken with malarial fever. Craig never married, practiced medicine in Philadelphia, and lived with his older sister and brother-in-law until 1890. He is later listed as a nurse at the Alameda County Infirmary where his medical school classmate, Dr. Adam Shirk, had recently taken charge. From 1896 until his death in 1912, Craig was a patient at various Homes for Disabled Veterans in Los Angeles, Virginia, Tennessee, and finally Danville, Illinois. He died there from chronic nephritis with personal effects of 26 cents in money, and belongings worth $8.95. His next of kin, a sister in Philadelphia, arranged for his simple burial at Mount Moriah Cemetery.[27] Hugh Douglas McLean was born in Coleraine, County Londonderry, Northern Ireland, in the 1830s, attended Lafayette College, and graduated from Jefferson Medical College in 1854 in his twenties. He too passed the Pennsylvania examination with a score of five and was appointed assistant surgeon in the 106th Pennsylvania from November 1862 until his discharge in December 1863. He returned to Philadelphia where he practiced medicine and invested in real estate. His will, dated January 24, 1906, lists real estate holdings valued at almost

$85,000. He made generous bequests: $1,000 to Mount Moriah Cemetery for care of his lot, $5,000 to the Masonic Home of Philadelphia, and $5,000 to the Home for Aged Couples and Men. His funeral expenses were $428.25, and the cost of marble and cemetery work for his plot totaled $2,200.[28]

Familiarity with the process of death sometimes prompted former military surgeons to leave unusually specific instructions about the disposal of their bodies. Surgeon Morris W. Townsend, 44th New York, specified in his will that "I leave my body to my wife and daughter to dispose of as they wish, preferring that it shall not be subjected to the so-called process of embalming; that after my death is certain and decay evidently commenced it be burned and that no expense be incurred thereafter exceeding $15."[29] John McNulty, medical director of the U.S. Twelfth Corps, left even more specific directions. McNulty was the only medical director in the Army of the Potomac at Gettysburg who disregarded Gen. George Meade's order to leave medical supply trains in Maryland. During the battle, the Twelfth Corps hospital was fully equipped with tents and bedding, while other Corps hospitals had to wait for the hospital supply trains to arrive days after the battle. The specificity in McNulty's will suggest that his disregard of Meade's orders was no oversight, but the choice of someone with strong opinions who valued order and control. He left detailed instructions about his death and burial.

> First-I have a horror of being buried alive, the body shall not be prepared for burial until injected, so until decomposition sets in, my body shall be unburied for twenty four hours, after apparent death . . . there shall be injected into the aorta near the heart a very strong (underlined) solution of corrosive sublimate and alcohol with sufficient force to fill the remote small muscles. My body shall be dressed in full uniform placed in a plain hard-wood box without lining, paint or putty plain iron handles. Such a box is now in the keeping of Dr. H.G. Riskin. My body in such box is to be carried to the Episcopal Church. Should such church be closed the Methodist Church shall be selected. All the religious services shall be performed in the church, the clergyman performing such services shall receive five dollars from my executors. The

burial service alone shall be said, no sermon or remarks. The box shall be carried to the grave on the caisson of the cannon or if that is not practicable in a common vehicle. Under no circumstances is a hearse to be used. The grave shall be north and south with the head to the boulder. The box must be entirely surrounded four inches thick with the cement mixed at the time of burial. No organized body of men except military will participate. Ten dollars shall be paid by my executors to the artillery for its service.[30]

A further codicil in January 1897 reiterated that "I further direct that attending the services of my death and burial no crepe or other badge of mourning shall be used. Further in my will heretofore made as a part and parcel of the same I have added in the line the following words 'Faradization shall be used.'"[31] Faradization refers to stimulating muscles or nerves with electric current. McNulty was not alone in his fear of being buried alive. Nineteenth-century accounts of premature burial appeared in both fiction and newspaper reports and confirming putrefaction before burial was a common practice.[32]

Civil War surgeons clearly understood the real possibility of premature burials. In the chaotic aftermath of battle, the removal and burial of the dead was often left to regimental comrades and stretcher bearers. Anna Holstein recounted one such premature burial at Gettysburg. Luther [*sic*] White, Co. K 20th Massachusetts, was seriously wounded in the head and appeared to sink away and die.

> One sultry afternoon in July the stretcher bearers came tramping wearily, bearing three bodies of those who had given their lives for freedom; as the last reached the place, the men dropped with a rough jolting motion the army couch whereon he rested. The impatient effort to be rid of their burden was probably the means of saving a precious life; for the man—dead, as they supposed—raising his head, called in a clear voice: "Boys, what are you doing?" The response was prompt: "We came to bury you, Whitey." His calm reply was: "I don't see it boys; give me a drink of water and carry me back."[33]

This account is verified in the patient record for Lishur White, Corporal of Company K, 20th Massachusetts, who suffered a scalp wound and was later admitted to Camp Letterman General Hospital at Gettysburg on August 4th. Acting Assistant Surgeon A. B. Stonelake wrote that "it is a well authenticated fact in regard to this patient that immediately after the battle, and there in a comatose condition, he was laid by the grave for interment, but the patient, recovering for the moment, requested his considerate friends to 'delay the ceremony a short time longer.'"[34]

REMEMBERING THE SURGEONS

Despite lingering diseases and disability, more than 500 of the Union, Confederate, contract, and volunteer surgeons who served as caregivers at Gettysburg survived into the twentieth century.[35] William Williams Keen Jr., Assistant Surgeon, USA Volunteers, was the last surviving member of the group when he died June 7, 1932. Their experiences and the medical skills they acquired during the Civil War helped change the medical profession through medical education and medical practice. Some taught, conducted research, and helped establish new specialties, but others simply provided better medical and surgical care in their local practices. While former surgeons continued successful professional lives and contributed to the medical and civic health of their communities, many regretted that their service during the Civil War had been overlooked and generally forgotten.

Forty years after the battle, Dr. Henry Janes was asked to talk to his colleagues at the Vermont Medical Society about his Civil War experiences. He addressed the lack of recognition for the medical corps in a brutally honest account that asked, "Why Is the Profession of Killing More Generally Honored Than That of Saving Life?" Rather than the pageant of an army in full array with bands playing and colors floating, Janes invited his listeners to come with him "over the field, after a hotly contested battle," and described the conditions of mangled wounded and their suffering in chilling detail. "The army surgeon sees little glory in war . . . he may for a few minutes participate in the excitement of the fight; but the wounded, picked up mangled and helpless, covered with blood and filth, must soon absorb all his attention to the exclusion of any thought for the details of the battle." Arguing that physicians were better trained for their work than other officers and bravely risked their lives during battles and epidemics, he noted, "In all the army reunions which I have attended since the close of the war, I never but once have heard any sentiment expressed that the army had any medical department."[36]

No one did more to advocate for the memory of Civil War surgeons than Silas Weir Mitchell, who served as a contract surgeon in Philadelphia hospitals and was among the surgeons sent to assist the wounded after the battle of Gettysburg. Although it was his only battlefield experience, and he mentions it only in passing, his Gettysburg experience remained an indelible memory. In personal recollections he regretted that the part played by Civil War surgeons remained largely untold, except for the technical work they had done.

> I know of no book which tells the personal life of a war surgeon, what he did day by day on the field or in the hospital . . . We had served faithfully as great a cause as earth has known. We built novel hospitals, organized such an ambulance service as had never before been seen, contributed numberless essays on diseases and wounds, and then passed again in to private life, unremembered, unrewarded servants of duty.[37]

After the 50th Gettysburg Reunion in 1913, Mitchell worked with the Gettysburg Park Commission and the Surgeon General's Office to assemble information for markers identifying the major Union Corps hospital sites at Gettysburg. For the surgeons of Gettysburg who faced a common enemy in the war with death and the grave, Mitchell's efforts resulted in the first national memorial honoring their service installed in 1914, just before his death. The bronze shields marking Union hospital sites include the names of the surgeons in charge that Mitchell helped identify. Mitchell has left us with a fitting epitaph for them all: "He fired no shot but was often forced to operate under fire."[38]

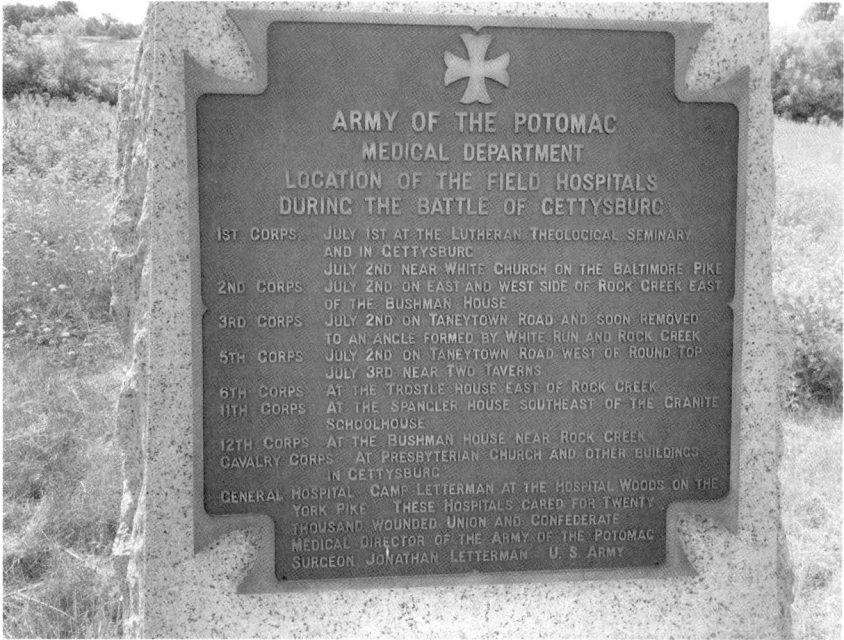

Hospital Marker, Route 30, Gettysburg. Author's photograph

ACKNOWLEDGMENTS

A ten-year project involving multiple aspects of the surgeons' lives required the help and support of many organizations and individuals. My thanks to the Seminary Ridge Museum for starting me on this journey and to Mark Simpson-Vos of the University of North Carolina Press for introducing me to the methodology of prosopography. Indiana University's Lilly Medical Library Database of Civil War Surgeons and F. Terry Hambrecht's unpublished database of Confederate surgeons provided examples that helped shape the content and structure of the Gettysburg Surgeons database. David Hacker from the University of Minnesota Population Center generously shared advice about the pitfalls of misusing statistics, and Lorien Foote, author of *Rites of Retaliation*, reviewed the chapter on the imprisonment of surgeons. Andrew Dalton and Tim Smith of the Adams County Historical Society read the sections describing the three days of battle for accuracy.

A wealth of information has come from repositories and collections of all sizes from the vast storehouse of the National Archives to a single diary in a small local historical society. It is a reminder that historical organizations of all sizes play an essential role in preserving our history, including local volunteer organizations, and deserve support for the important work they do. Research and writing can be solitary pursuits, so I am very grateful to colleagues like Doug Arbittier, Brad Hoch, Carolyn Ivanoff, Pete Miele, Peter D'Onofrio, John Seitter, and others who provided advice, feedback, and support throughout this project. In particular, I want to thank Robert Hicks and Peter Stanley, who provided the brutal critique I requested from them. Samantha Mayer helped edit the final versions.

Thanks to author Charles Fergus for his encouragement and for introducing me to Stackpole Books. Editor Dave Reisch has overseen the transformation of a manuscript into a book. I am grateful for the indulgence of family, friends, neighbors, and colleagues who endured my enthusiastic accounts of new discoveries and read early versions of chapters. Finally, I would like to thank my late husband, Jack Mayer, who listened patiently and was willing to share our home with 1,200 "dead doctors."

Appendix

Selected Profiles of Union and Confederate Surgeons

Morris Joseph Asch
Medical Director, Artillery Reserve, U.S. Army of the Potomac
7/4/1833–10/5/1902
Jefferson Medical College, 1855
Born in Philadelphia into a Jewish family of successful furriers from
Poland, Asch graduated from the University of Pennsylvania in 1852 before
attending medical school. He studied surgery with Dr. Joseph Pancoast
and later worked as clinical assistant to Dr. Samuel Gross. At the outbreak of the war he joined the U.S. Army as assistant surgeon, first in
the Surgeon General's Office, and then in the field with the Army of the
Potomac. At Gettysburg he was medical director of Artillery Reserve,
and later served as staff surgeon for Gen. Philip Sheridan from 1865 to
1873. He resigned from the army to practice medicine in New York City,
specializing in diseases of the nose and throat. He was a founder of the
American Laryngological Association and a member of the New York
Academy of Medicine. His operation to cure septal deviations became
widely known as the "Asch operation." He was active in social clubs,
including the Military Order of the Loyal Legion, as well as University,
Century, and New York Yacht clubs. He died in New York and is buried
in Salem Fields Cemetery in Brooklyn, New York.

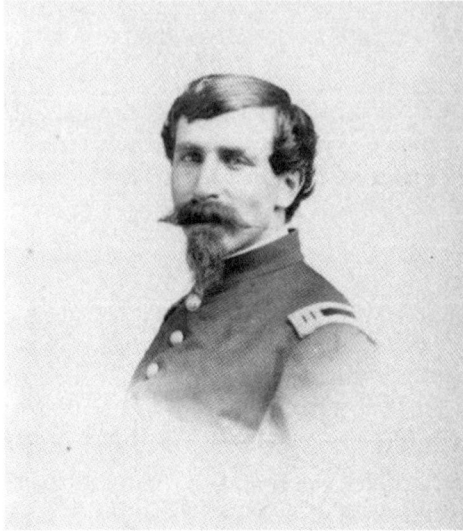

Morris Joseph Asch, Medical Director, Artillery Reserve, U.S. Army of the Potomac.
Douglas Arbittier, MD, MBA, www.medicalantiques.com

SMITH BUTTERMORE
Assistant Surgeon, 31st Virginia
2/29/1830–12/28/1897
Cleveland Medical College, 1854
Buttermore was born in Connellsville, Pennsylvania, where he studied medicine with a local doctor before graduating from medical school in Ohio. He practiced medicine in California for five years and then moved to Clarksburg, Virginia, where he enlisted in the Confederate army when the war broke out. His biography in the *History of Fayette County* described how he accepted a commission because the conflict and confusion along the border made practicing medicine too difficult. He served throughout the war and surrendered at Appomattox. He returned to Connellsville after the death of his father in 1868 and became a leading citizen in his hometown, eventually representing Fayette County in the Pennsylvania legislature as a Democrat in 1881. He was a strong supporter of education and the public schools. His daughter, Virginia Buttermore Donahoo, a graduate of the Women's Medical College of Philadelphia, was also a physician.

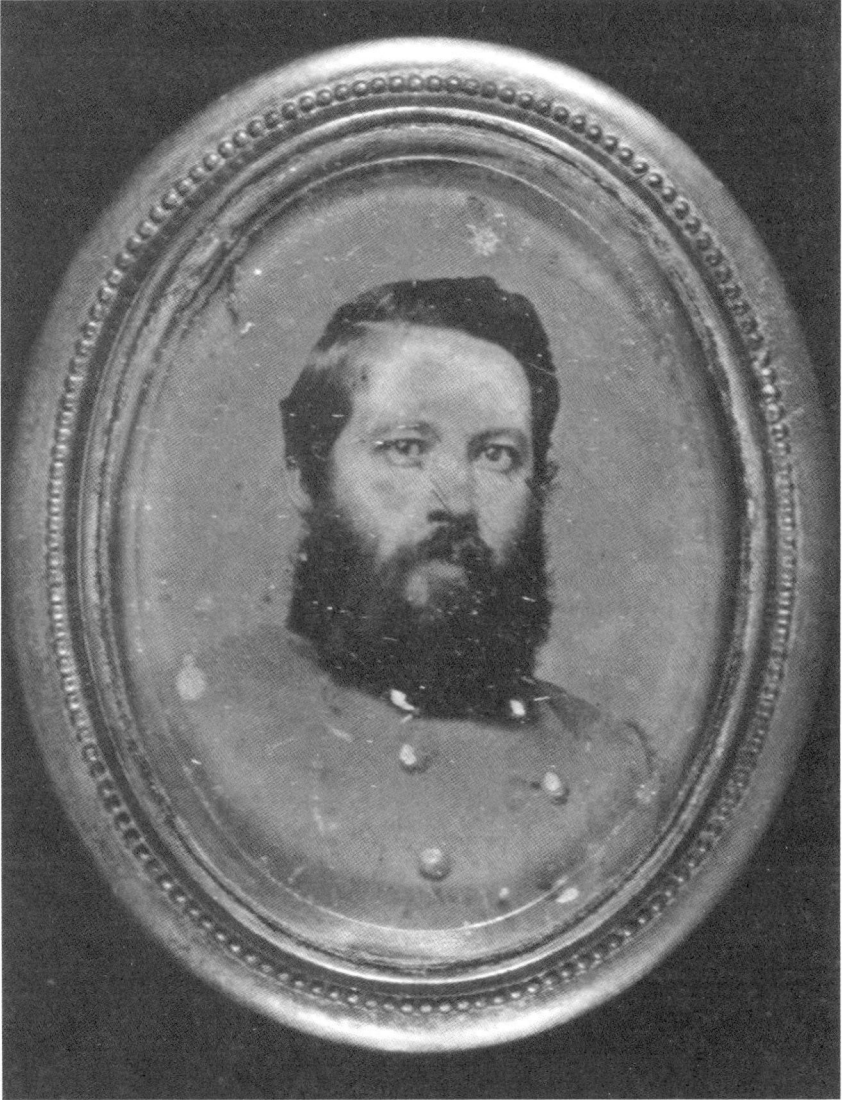

Smith Buttermore, Assistant Surgeon, 31st Virginia. Copy of family photograph.
Courtesy of Appomattox Court House National Historical Park.

James Lorenzo Farley
Surgeon, 84th New York
3/4/1836–3/9/1886

Columbia College of Physicians and Surgeons, 1857

Although Farley's military records indicate he resigned for disability in June 1863, he was still with his regiment at Gettysburg in July. From February 25 to early June, he was in Washington, DC, for either disability or hospital duty. On May 25, 1863, John Letterman requested that Farley rejoin his regiment to which Dr. Meredith Clymer, assistant surgeon general, responded, "I have no use for him." An article in the *New York Herald,* July 24, 1863, reported Farley at the Washington Hotel in Gettysburg, where the patients spoke in "highest terms of affection about him," but Dr. Theodore Dimon, a volunteer physician from New York, described how the surgeon there, undoubtedly Farley, spent his time "concocting iced drinks for himself and visiting friends." After the war, Farley became a popular elocutionist and gave presentations in New York and Boston accompanied by composer George F. Bristow. The *Eastern Medical Journal* for February 15, 1886, reported his death as "Another Case of the Bad Effects of Cocaine" and described how Farley "had been treating himself for nervousness with hypodermic injections of cocaine, but the drug soon ceased to relieve his sufferings."

JAMES MCFADDEN GASTON
Chief Surgeon, Confederate Third Corps
12/27/1824–11/15/1903
Medical College of South Carolina, Charleston, 1846
The son of Dr. John Brown Gaston Sr., James graduated from South Carolina College before attending his first course at the University of Pennsylvania and then graduating from the Medical College of South Carolina. After practicing with his father in Chester, South Carolina, for several years, he married and set up a medical practice in Columbia. He enlisted in the Confederate army in April 1861 and served in various hospital and staff positions throughout the war. Among his first assignments was setting up a hospital at Fort Sumter, Charleston Harbor, in April 1861. At Gettysburg he served as chief surgeon of Anderson's Division in General A. P. Hill's Corps and was stationed at the division hospital at the Adam Butt Farm. In 1865 he emigrated to Campinas, Sao Paulo Province, Brazil, where he practiced medicine for nearly two

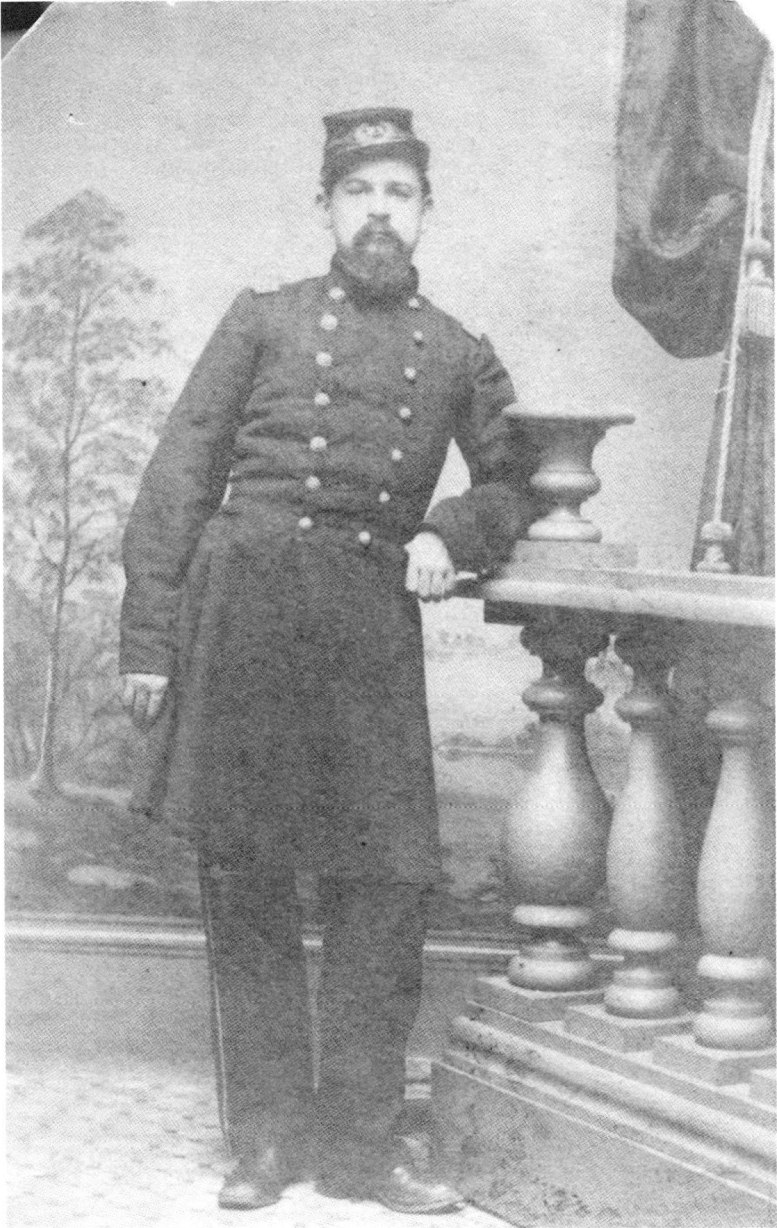

James Lorenzo Farley, Surgeon, 84th New York. Courtesy of New York State Military Museum

decades. He joined an estimated 10,000 or more former Confederates, lured by promises of cheap land, transportation, and inexpensive slaves in a country where slavery would remain legal until 1888. In 1883 he returned to Georgia where he practiced medicine and later taught surgery at the Southern Medical College, Atlanta, Georgia.

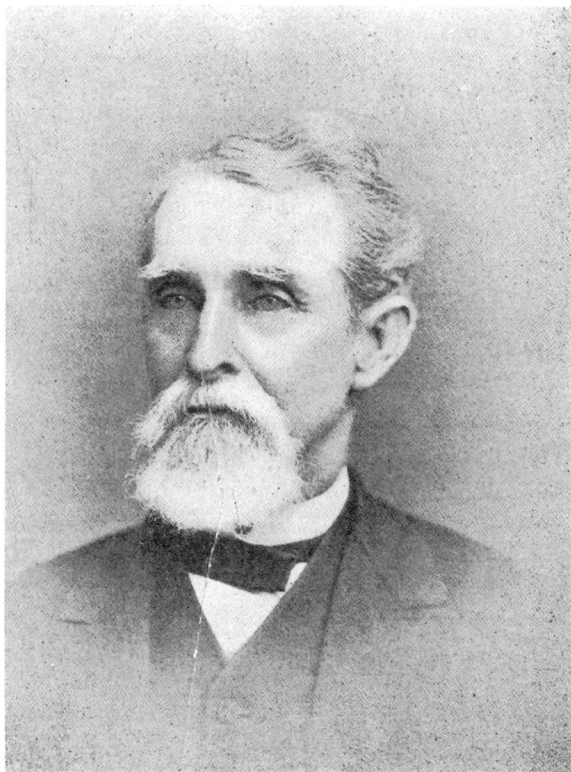

Robert Gibbon, Surgeon, 28th North Carolina. J.B. Alexander, *History of Mecklenburg County* (1902), 190. Courtesy of Robinson-Spangler Carolina Room, Charlotte Mecklenburg Library.

ROBERT GIBBON
Surgeon, 28th North Carolina
12/31/1822–5/14/1898
Jefferson Medical College, 1848

Robert Gibbon and his brother John Gibbon were both on the field during the battle of Gettysburg, but on opposing sides. Gen. John Gibbon commanded the U.S. Second Corps 2nd Division against the Confederate charge on July 3rd until he was wounded. Surgeon Robert Gibbon, 28th North Carolina, worked in the hospital at the Heintzelman Farm caring for the Confederate wounded of Pender's division. Both men were born in Pennsylvania. Their father, John Heysham Gibbon, graduated from the Medical Department of the University of Pennsylvania but later took up the study of minerology and relocated the family to North Carolina around 1838 where he took a position as chief assayer at the U.S. Mint in Charlotte. John Gibbon, a graduate of West Point and a career military officer, remained loyal to the United States, while his brothers joined the Confederate cause as North Carolinians. Dr. Robert Gibbon returned to Charlotte after the war where he practiced medicine and helped found the Presbyterian hospital there.

JOHN MOORE HAYES
Surgeon, 26th Alabama
8/7/1836–4/25/1905
Nashville Medical College, 1858
Born in Athens, Alabama, Hayes practiced medicine in Florence, Alabama, until he enlisted in the Confederate army in June 1861. He served as assistant surgeon in the 9th Alabama before promotion to surgeon of the 26th Alabama in March 1862 when his friend Edward O'Neal was appointed colonel. At Gettysburg, Hayes was taken prisoner while caring for wounded at the Schriver Farm, remained at the Seminary Hospital until August 6, and then transferred to Letterman Hospital until October 22. During his stay at Gettysburg, he had his photograph taken at Tyson Brothers Studio. He was transferred with other Confederate surgeons to Fort McHenry and held prisoner there until the surgeons were exchanged November 21, 1863. From February to May 1864, he was detailed to transport prisoners to Andersonville Prison. When the 26th Alabama surrendered at Greenville, North Carolina, Dr. Hayes's slave concealed the regimental flag and returned it to Florence. After the war, Hayes married the daughter of Col. James Saunders of Rocky Hill,

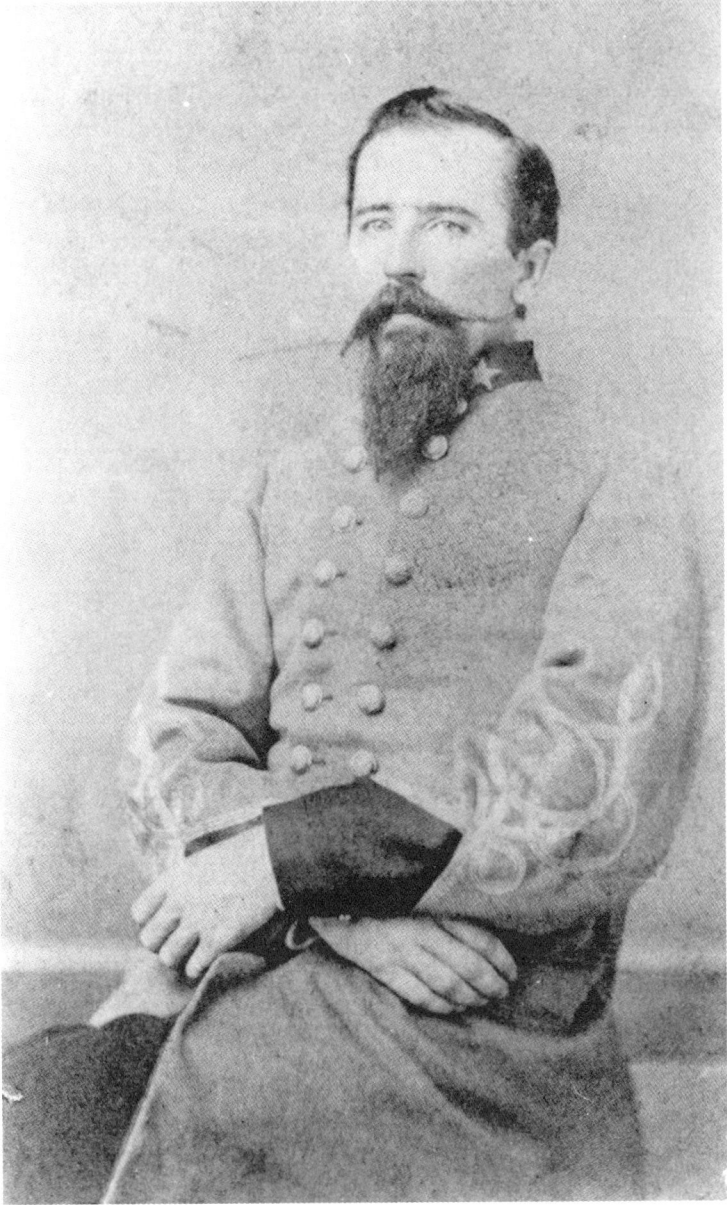

John Moore Hayes, Surgeon, 26th Alabama. Tyson Brothers Photographic Studio, Gettysburg, Pennsylvania, 1863. Courtesy of U.S. Army Heritage and Education Center, Carlisle, Pennsylvania.

Courtland, Alabama. From 1885 to 1890 he worked as a state physician at the Pratt Mines, overseeing care of the prison laborers employed there. Before his death, he presented the regimental flag to the widow of his friend Colonel O'Neal, and it was later donated to the Alabama Archives in Montgomery.

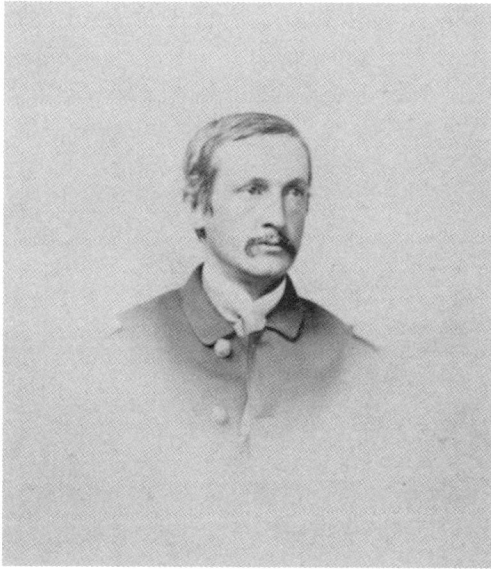

Nathan Hayward, Surgeon, 20th Massachusetts. F.L. Lay's Photographic Atelier, Boston, Massachusetts. Courtesy of Medford Historical Society and Museum.

NATHAN HAYWARD

Surgeon, 20th Massachusetts
1/8/1830–8/17/1866
Harvard Medical School, 1855
Nathan Hayward's prominent Boston family included his father, James T. Hayward, treasurer of the Boston Sugar Refinery, his maternal grandfather, Judge Thomas Dawes, and his great grandfather William Greenleaf, the sheriff of Suffolk County who read the Declaration of Independence from the Old State House in Boston in 1776. Hayward's education was the best available: Boston Latin School; Harvard University, 1850; medical studies at Berlin and Göttingen Universities

in Germany, 1852–1854; and graduation from the Tremont Medical School of Harvard. An accomplished sketch artist, he published a compilation of *College Scenes* depicting student life at Harvard in 1850. He was first commissioned assistant surgeon in the 20th Massachusetts in July and promoted to surgeon in September 1861. During the battle of Gettysburg, he was an operator in the Second Corps hospital until it closed and then moved with his patients to Camp Letterman. After the war, he relocated to St. Louis, Missouri, to practice medicine and died there a year later in 1866 during a cholera epidemic.

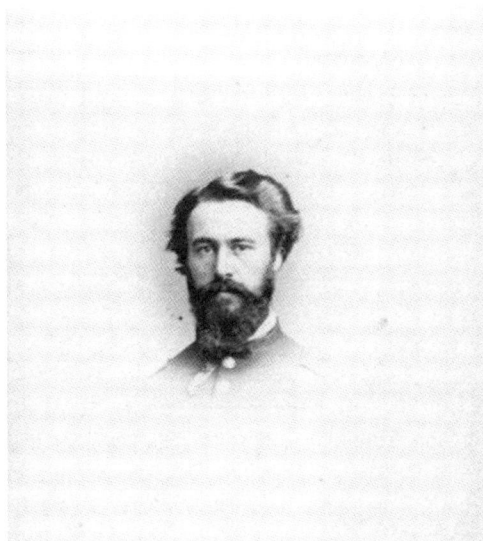

Benjamin Howard, Assistant Surgeon, U.S. Army. Charles D. Fredricks & Co., New York. Courtesy of Douglas Arbittier, MD, MBA, www.medicalantiques.com.

BENJAMIN HOWARD
Assistant Surgeon, U.S. Army
3/21/1836–6/17/1900
College of Physicians and Surgeons, New York, 1858
Born in England, Benjamin Douglas Howard emigrated to the United States to pursue his education. In 1861, while assistant surgeon in the 19th New York, the regimental surgeon, Theodore Dimon, described how

Howard routinely stole hospital supplies. Dimon found him well educated and competent as a physician, but "utterly selfish and unscrupulous and assuming a pious outside to cover his rascally conduct." Dimon was happy to see Howard leave when he received a commission in the regular army in August 1861. Howard served on General McClellan's staff at Antietam and later at Gettysburg. At one time he was medical purveyor and acting medical director of the Department of the Ohio. Following the war, he practiced medicine in New York until 1875, and then traveled widely in Europe, Asia, and Africa. He continued to promote his medical methods of hermetic sealing of chest wounds and artificial respiration, as well as ambulance designs that were later adopted in France and England. He authored several popular travel books based on his study of Russian prisons, but critics questioned the credibility of his accounts.

John Jefferson Milhau
Medical Director, U.S. Fifth Corps
12/28/1828–5/8/1881
College of Physicians and Surgeons, New York, 1850
After graduating from medical school, Milhau joined the U.S. Army as assistant surgeon in 1851. His service before the Civil War included an expedition to Utah and later against the Snake Indians in 1855. While stationed in Oregon he was the first to record the Coos and Lower Umpqua Indian language. With the outbreak of the Civil War, he was named medical director of the Army of the Potomac, and in 1862 served as medical director of the hospitals in Frederick, Maryland, and then medical director of the Third and Fifth Corps, before being transferred to New York City. After the assassination of President Lincoln, he was chosen as a guard of honor to protect the president's body. At Hart's Island during the cholera epidemic of 1866, he was the only surgeon who remained well enough to treat the prisoners. From 1867 to 1869 he was medical director of the Military District of the South. He resigned his commission in 1876 but remained active as a member of the Military Order of the Loyal Legion and represented the organization at the funeral of Gen. Ulysses Grant.

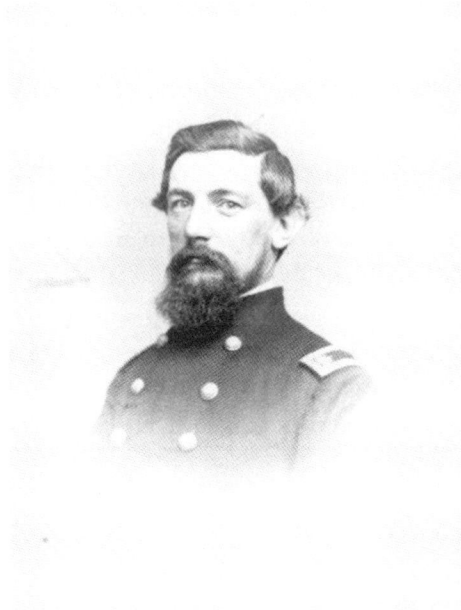

John Jefferson Milhau, Medical Director, U.S. Fifth Corps. Courtesy of Douglas Arbittier, MD, MBA, www.medicalantiques.com

SAMUEL BROWN MORRISON
Chief Surgeon, Jubal Early's Division, Confederate Second Corps
9/13/1828–2/4/1901
University of Virginia Medical College, 1853
Seeing the dead lying on the battlefield at Gettysburg, Samuel Brown Morrison expressed his desire to be buried at home next to his wife and those he loved. Except for medical school and the years of the Civil War, Morrison spent most of his life in and around Rockbridge County, Virginia. Born near Brownsburg, he attended Washington College in Lexington, the county seat, and then graduated from the University of Virginia Medical College in nearby Charlottesville, Albemarle County. Before the war, he practiced medicine in Lexington. During the Civil War, Morrison served as surgeon of the 58th Virginia Infantry before being appointed chief surgeon of Gen. Richard Ewell's division on August 16, 1862; two weeks later he amputated Ewell's leg after the battle of Groveton. He continued as division surgeon under Gen. Jubal

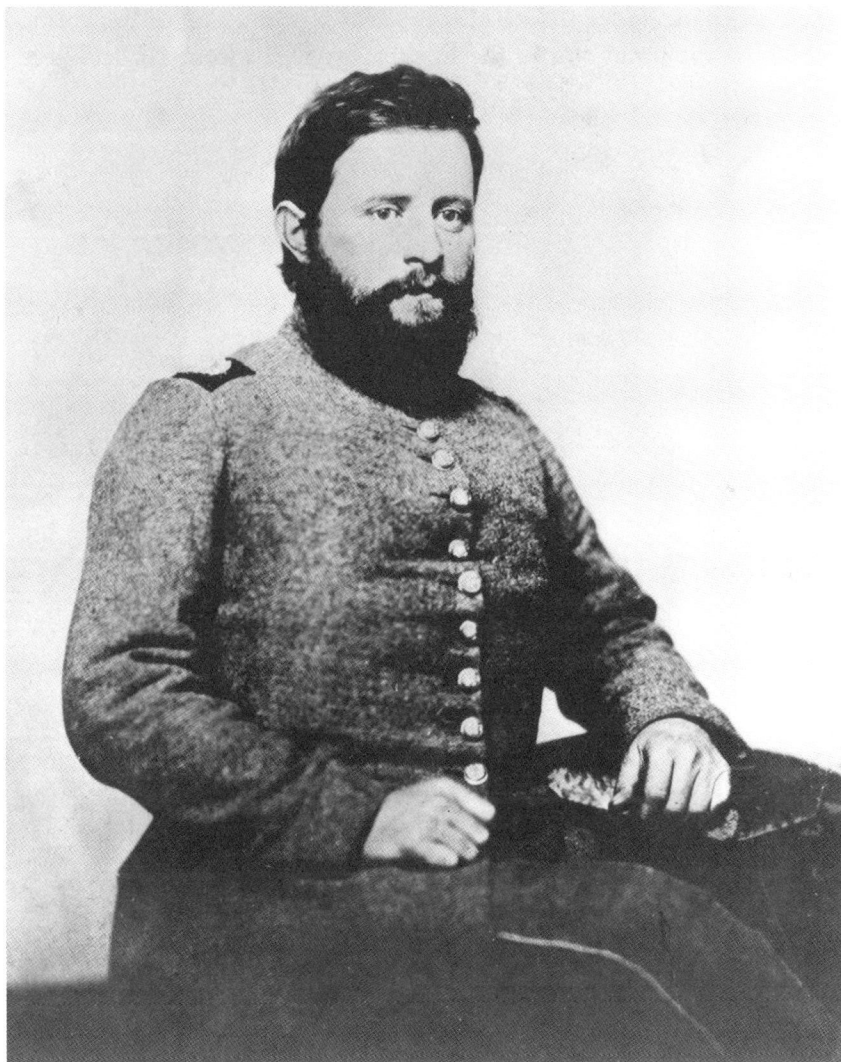

Samuel Brown Morrison, Chief Surgeon, Jubal Early's Division. Courtesy of Virginia Military Institute Archives

Early. In May 1863 Morrison was called to the bedside of the mortally wounded Gen. "Stonewall" Jackson. On seeing Morrison, Jackson said, "That's an old familiar face." Morrison knew him well and was related to Jackson's second wife, Mary Anna Morrison. After the war Morrison served in the state legislature (1871–1872) but returned to Rockbridge to become the proprietor of the Rockbridge Baths from 1874 until his death in 1901.

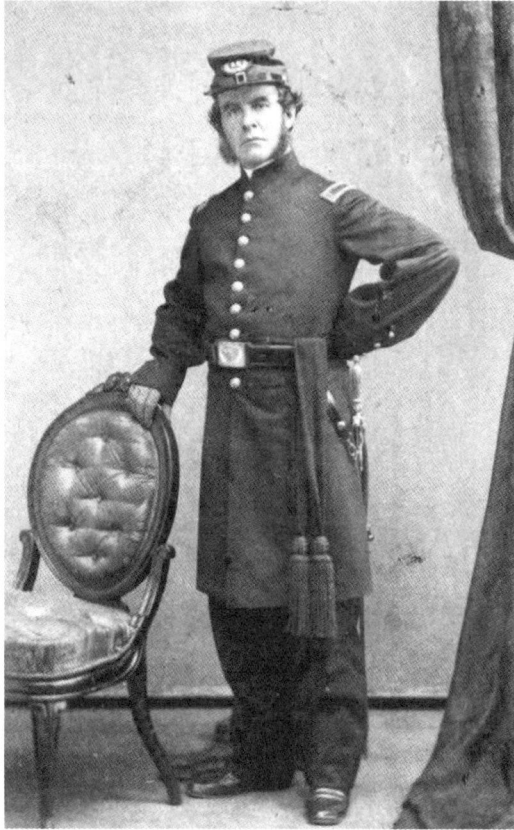

Thomas Fletcher Oakes, Assistant Surgeon, 1st Massachusetts. Courtesy of U.S. Army Heritage and Education Center, Carlisle, Pennsylvania

THOMAS FLETCHER OAKES
Assistant Surgeon, 1st Massachusetts
c. 1820–2/9/1876
Harvard Medical School, 1852

Oakes started his medical career as an apothecary in Boston, Massachusetts, and began practicing medicine after he graduated from the Harvard Tremont Medical School in 1852. In 1858 he married Elizabeth Howland Sherman; their son, Frank was born in 1861. Oakes was commissioned assistant surgeon in the 1st Massachusetts in July 1862 and served in that capacity at the battle of Gettysburg. In August 1863 he joined the 56th Massachusetts as surgeon and served until he mustered out in July 1865. There is no record that he returned to Massachusetts, and it appears that he abandoned his wife and son. By 1866 he was practicing medicine in Titusville, Pennsylvania, a booming oil town, and was active in the Crawford County Medical Society. Three other Gettysburg surgeons also saw opportunities in Titusville. Two practiced medicine and one became an oil producer. The 1870 census shows Oakes listed among the single men boarding at the Bush House. A family history reported that he married again in 1871 to Kate Bevins. His first wife remarried in 1874 and again in 1894. He died in 1876 from pneumonia after a short illness.

Daniel Parker
Assistant Surgeon, 8th Alabama
9/13/1835–6/18/1918
University of Louisiana Medical School (Tulane), 1860
Daniel Parker grew up in Brookfield, Vermont, where his father, the Reverend Daniel Parker, was a Congregational minister until his death in 1849. Daniel left Vermont in 1856 after his mother died and relocated to Marion, Alabama, to teach school. He was able to make enough money teaching to pay for his medical education in New Orleans. At the outbreak of the Civil War, he was single, twenty-five years old, and practicing medicine in Perry County, Alabama. He was appointed assistant surgeon of the 8th Alabama on July 3, 1861. At Gettysburg he was left with the wounded of Anderson's division at Butt's Farm, taken prisoner on July 5th, and was among the last Confederate surgeons to leave Camp Letterman on October 22nd. He remained a prisoner at Fort McHenry in Baltimore, Maryland, until the surgeons were exchanged November 21, 1863. On November 26th he was admitted to the hospital in Richmond with a case of scabies acquired during his imprisonment. After the war,

he married and practiced medicine in Perryville, Alabama. He relocated to Calvert, Texas, in 1875 where he practiced medicine and became involved in politics as mayor of Calvert, justice, and representative to the state legislature.

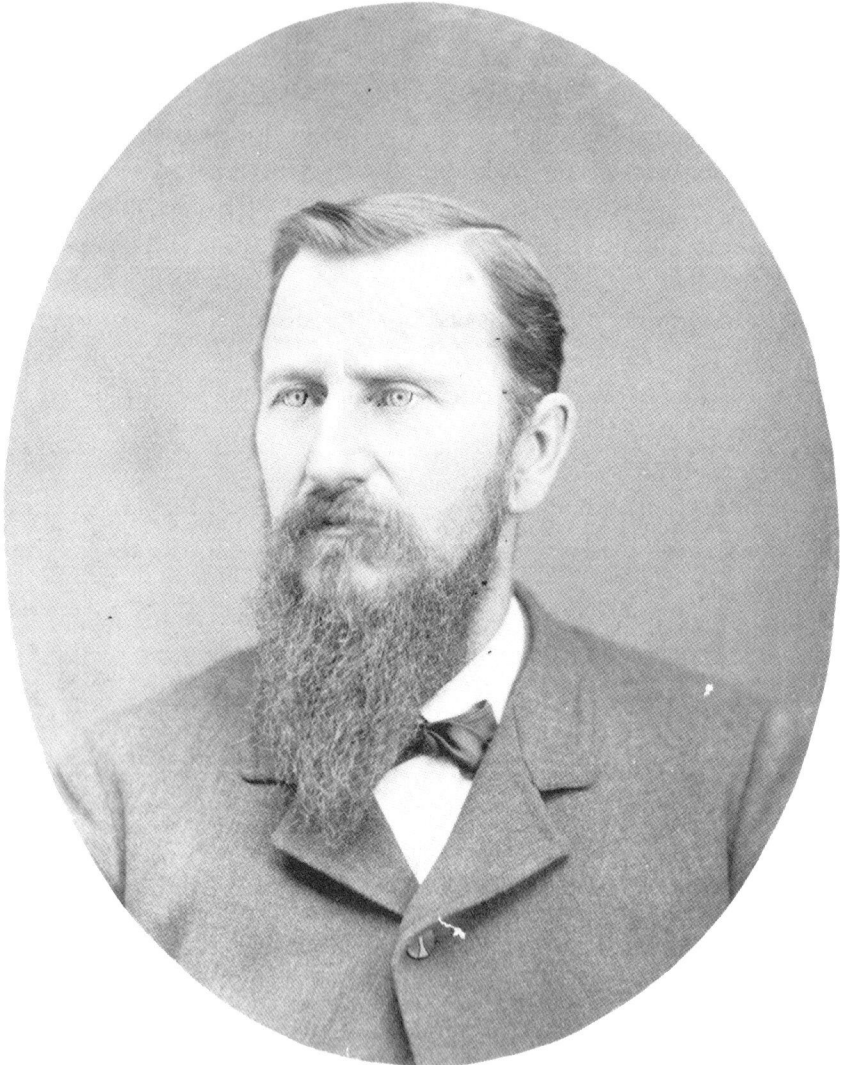

Daniel Parker, Assistant Surgeon, 8th Alabama. Courtesy of Thomas Parker

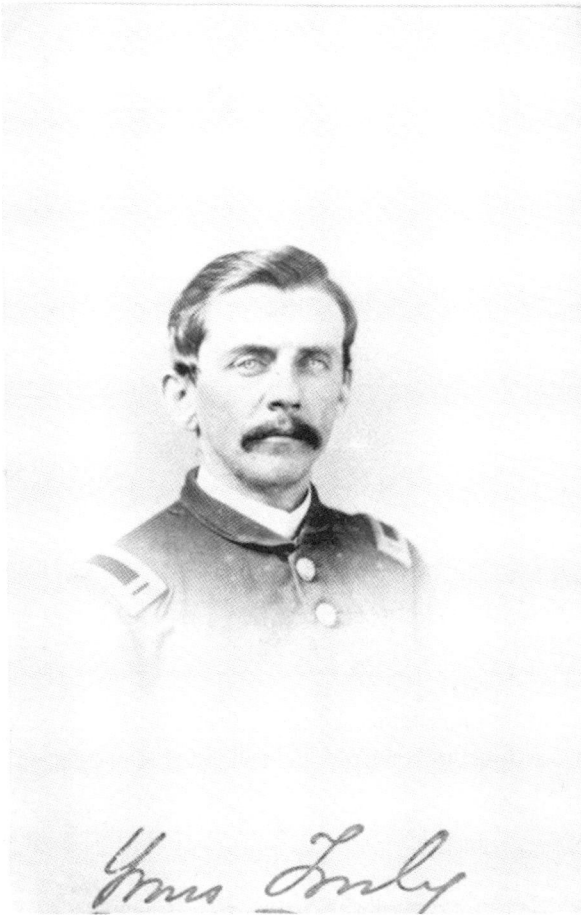

Dewitt Clinton Peters, Assistant Surgeon, U.S. Army. Courtesy of Douglas Arbittier, MD, MBA, www.medicalantiques.com

DEWITT CLINTON PETERS
Assistant Surgeon, U.S. Army
7/30/1829–4/23/1876
University of the City of New York Medical College, 1853
Dewitt Clinton Peters served as assistant surgeon in the U.S. Army from 1854 to 1856, and then traveled to Germany in 1857 for further medical study. In June 1860 he was reappointed assistant surgeon and was stationed from 1862 to 1865 at Jarvis Hospital in Baltimore. While there is

no known official record listing the surgeons dispatched to Gettysburg from Washington, Philadelphia, and Baltimore hospitals, a few surgeons are mentioned by name by patients and other caretakers. Captain John Shields, 53rd Pennsylvania, was wounded in the neck and later described how, "Dr. Peters began the operation Dr. Chris Johnson made the incision and finished the job." This is the only mention of Dr. Peters, but Dewitt Clinton Peters fits the profile of skilled surgeons from nearby hospitals who were sent to Gettysburg. Chris Johnson, a civilian doctor from Baltimore, is also mentioned in the memoir of Surgeon William Riddick Whitehead, 44th Virginia. According to family tradition, Peters attended Ford's Theater the night Lincoln was shot. Peters remained in the army, serving at Fort Union, New Mexico, and Nashville, Tennessee, until 1874, when he was placed on disability leave. He died two years later from tuberculosis.

Pascal Alfred Quinan
Surgeon, 150th Pennsylvania
1830–6/30/1889
University of Maryland, 1851
Quinan first studied medicine at Jefferson Medical College and received his degree from the University of Maryland. He was appointed to the medical staff of the U.S. Army in April 1854 and served at Fort Thorn in Apache territory and then at Alcatraz in 1860. He resigned his army commission and was commissioned surgeon of the 150th Pennsylvania in May 1863. The history of the 150th Pennsylvania described him as medically competent, "but a natural or studied cynicism coupled with excessive self-consciousness and a disposition to belittle his superiors in the medical department, failed to commend him to his fellow officers or secure their friendship." Although ordered to rejoin his regiment after the battle of Gettysburg, he petitioned to remain in charge of the 3rd Division hospital at the Catholic church. He was subsequently dismissed in November for absence without authority. He returned to Baltimore to practice medicine and worked as a ship's doctor at one point. Correspondence with the U.S. Department of State asserted his claims of

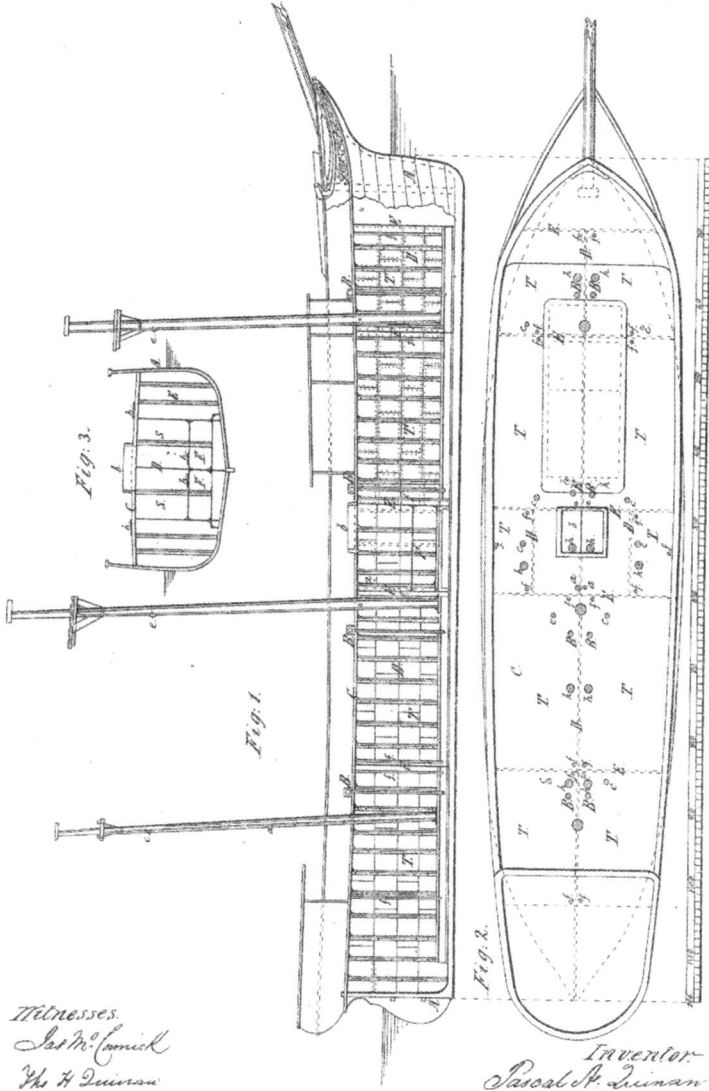

P. A. Quinan.
Vessel for Storing & Transp't'g Oil.
Nº 97442.   Patented Nov. 30. 1869.

Pascal Alfred Quinan, Surgeon, 150th Pennsylvania. Patent No. 97442, November 30, 1869, U.S. Patent Office

discovering guano on Arcos Keys in 1860. In 1869 he received a patent for a sailing vessel designed to carry oil in bulk without barrels.

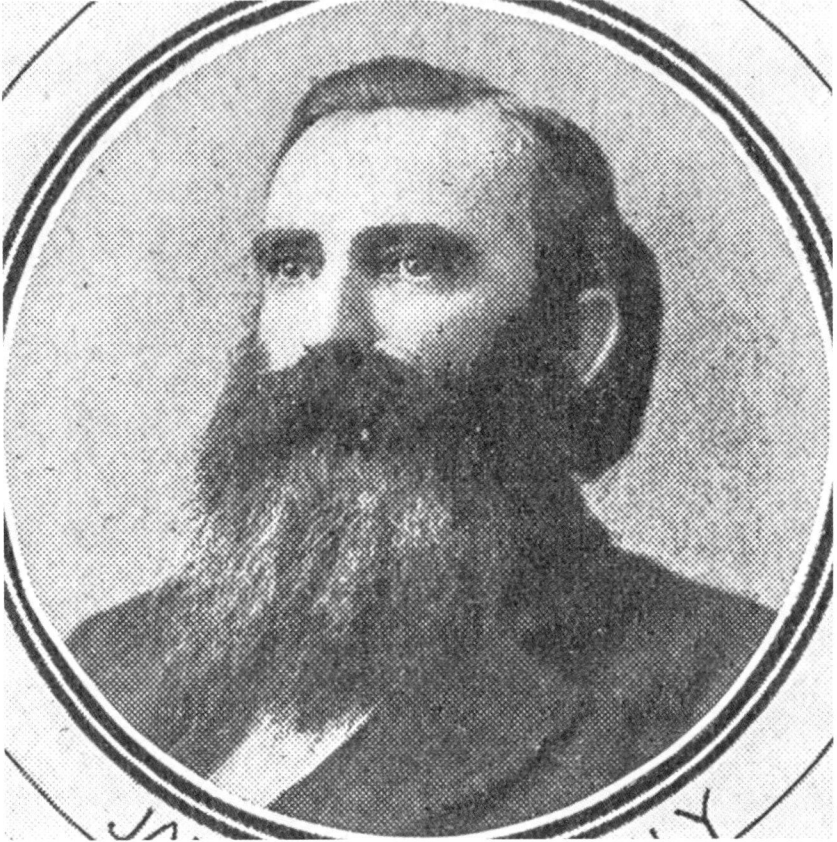

James Ross Reily, U.S. Acting Assistant Surgeon. Daniel S. Lamb, *Medical Society of DC* (1865), 80. Courtesy of Historical Medical Library, The College of Physicians of Philadelphia.

JAMES ROSS REILY
U.S. Acting Assistant Surgeon
3/23/1835–12/12/1904
University of Pennsylvania, 1859

After his father's death in 1844, Reily lived with his uncle, Dr. Luther Reily, of Harrisburg. In 1861 he was commissioned assistant surgeon, 1st Pennsylvania artillery, but was soon promoted to surgeon of the 127th Pennsylvania and then the 179th Pennsylvania. He held positions of acting medical purveyor and acting medical director in the Fourth Corps before mustering out with his regiment at Harrisburg on July 27, 1863. He was among the former regimental surgeons recruited to serve as acting assistant surgeons after the battle of Gettysburg. He was assigned as surgeon in charge of the First Corps hospital at the Seminary. Despite holding positions of authority in the medical corps, his military record was uneven, including letters of complaint for negligence and one court-martial, as well as letters of recommendation. While in charge of the Seminary hospital from August 17 until it closed September 8, one patient described him as "jolly, almost to the point of rowdy and disruptive," while his superiors praised his efficient management of the hospital. He continued his medical career as acting assistant surgeon at the Washington Arsenal, DC, until 1876 and then practiced medicine in the District of Columbia until his death in 1904.

WILLIAM H. RULISON
Surgeon, 9th New York Cavalry
1822–8/29/1864
Albany Medical College, 1855
Born in Herkimer County, New York, Rulison later lived with his family in Oswego County. Before the Civil War he had already pursued several careers. In the 1840s he advertised as a professor of dance and music in Rochester, New York. An accomplished musician, he composed several popular tunes that were widely republished—"Rochester Schottische" and "Good Times Schottische" are still well-known fiddle tunes. He traveled overland to California during the Gold Rush and returned to Oswego County to work as a druggist. In 1855 he graduated from Albany Medical College. By then, he had married Adaline Herbert and was living with her family in Mexico, New York. Five years later, Rulison was living with his older brother Allen in nearby Parish, and Adaline and her parents had moved back to Brooklyn, New York. Rulison was

William H. Rulison, Surgeon, 9th New York Cavalry. "Rochester Schottische," William Hall & Son, New York. From author's collection.

commissioned surgeon of the 9th New York Cavalry in July 1862. At Gettysburg he was in charge of the cavalry hospital at the Presbyterian Church and remained in Gettysburg until mid-August. Agnes Barr, a young Gettysburg resident, remembered that Rulison boarded with her family for about four weeks: "He was a pleasant gentleman made himself very agreeable." A year later, he was fatally shot by a Confederate sharpshooter at Smithfield, Virginia. A general hospital in Annapolis, Maryland, was named in his honor in 1865. You can hear a recording of the "Rochester Schottische" at https://www.loc.gov/item/afcreed000127/.

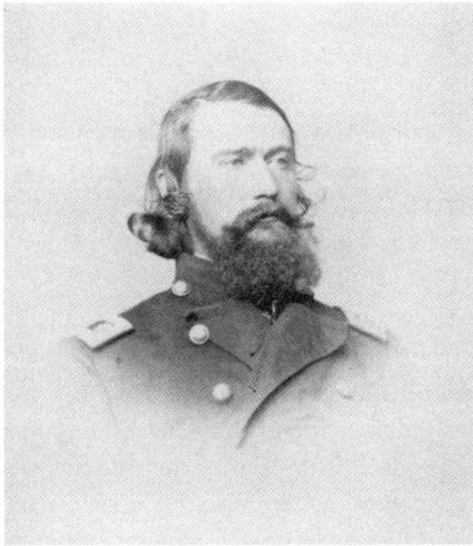

George Suckley, Medical Director, U.S. Eleventh Corps. Courtesy of Douglas Arbittier, MD, MBA, www.medicalantiques.com

GEORGE SUCKLEY
Medical Director, U.S. Eleventh Corps
1830–7/30/1869
College of Physicians and Surgeons, New York, 1851
Born in New York City, George Suckley pursued a lifelong interest in natural history as well as medicine. He studied at the Lyceum of Natural History before graduating from the College of Physicians and Surgeons

(now Columbia University) in 1851. After a year as resident surgeon at New York Hospital, he was appointed assistant surgeon and naturalist to the Pacific Railroad Survey between St. Paul, Minnesota, and Fort Vancouver, Washington Territory. From April to December 1853, his work on the survey included a 1,049-mile, fifty-three-day canoe trip down the Bitter Root, Clark's Fork, and Columbia Rivers to Fort Vancouver and extensive collections of natural history specimens. He joined the U.S. Army as assistant surgeon from December 1853 to 1856 serving in the Washington and Oregon Territories. After resigning from the army to pursue his interest in natural history, he spent the next five years collecting and writing about his findings. Two species of fish are named for him. At the outbreak of the Civil War, he rejoined the army as surgeon. During the battle of Gettysburg, he served as medical director of the Eleventh Corps, responsible for the hospitals at Spangler Farm.

WILLIAM H. TAYLOR
Assistant Surgeon, 19th Virginia
5/17/1835–4/14/1897
Medical College of Virginia, 1856
Quotes from William Taylor on the role of a Confederate assistant surgeon are often misinterpreted by ignoring his biting humor and self-deprecation. Both are evident in his published medical lectures and an account of his travels in Europe after the war. Self-described as slight in stature, he was so near-sighted that he used a magnifying glass to read. During the war he was promoted to surgeon but chose to continue serving as assistant surgeon in the 19th Virginia. At Gettysburg he was on the field with Garnett's Brigade and was wounded during the Confederate charge on July 3rd. After the war, he abandoned medical practice to pursue his interest in chemistry and taught chemistry, toxicology, and medical jurisprudence at the Medical College of Virginia. He was a member of the Richmond Board of Health and served as coroner for twenty-five years from 1872 until his death, reportedly investigating nearly 10,000 cases. He used his knowledge of chemistry to determine cases of criminal poisoning. Newspaper reporters sought him out for his

famous quips. One account described him as a lifelong bachelor who "viewed the ladies with a jaundiced eye."

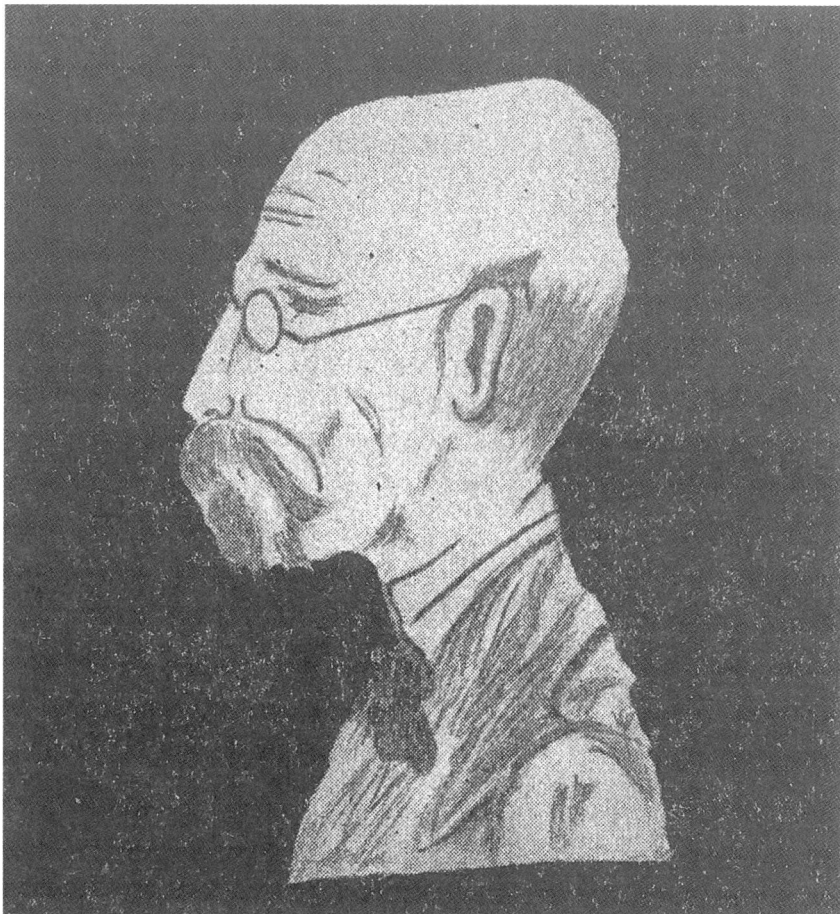

William H. Taylor, Assistant Surgeon, 19th Virginia. *Travels of a Doctor of Physic* (Philadelphia: Lippincott & Company, 1871).

FREDERICK WOLF
Surgeon, 39th New York
1829–11/11/1868
University of Prague, 1853

Fellow surgeons described Frederick Wolf as a "scientific man." Born in Prague, he first pursued an academic education in science and the arts until his father's business failed and the family fortunes changed. Frederick decided to pursue a career in medicine at the University of Prague but left before receiving his diploma to enlist in the Austrian army when war broke out in 1848. After three years as an army surgeon, he completed his medical degree in 1853 and returned to service in the Austrian army until he emigrated to the United States in 1859. His retirement from military life was short lived. In December 1861 he was commissioned surgeon of the 39th New York. Following the battle of Gettysburg, he was among the surgeons who remained at the Second Corps Hospital. In October he was captured at the battle of Bristoe Station, Virginia, and imprisoned at Libby Prison until November 1863. In 1864 he was commissioned assistant surgeon in the U.S. Army and served until June 1865. His examination paper for U.S. assistant surgeon includes detailed anatomical drawings. He died in St. Louis, Missouri, of chronic dysentery.

WILLIAM PROBY YOUNG
Assistant Surgeon, 4th Georgia
1/19/1834–12/9/1912
Jefferson Medical College, 1855
Young grew up in Washington, DC, where his father worked as a clerk. He studied at Rittenhouse Academy and Columbian University (now George Washington University) before graduating from Jefferson Medical College. After graduation he worked first at the newly opened Government Hospital for the Insane in DC and then practiced medicine in Portsmouth, Virginia, and Washington, DC. In June 1860 as an agent of the U.S. government, and as physician for the American Colonization Society, he accompanied a shipload of Africans taken from captured slave ships who were transported to Liberia. When war began in 1861, Young enlisted as a private in the 116th Virginia Militia but a year later was assigned assistant surgeon in the 4th Georgia. At Gettysburg, Young was already a seasoned veteran of battlefield medicine having taken part in major battles, including Antietam. He was assigned to the hospital of Doles's brigade and reportedly served at the Hankey farm. He served

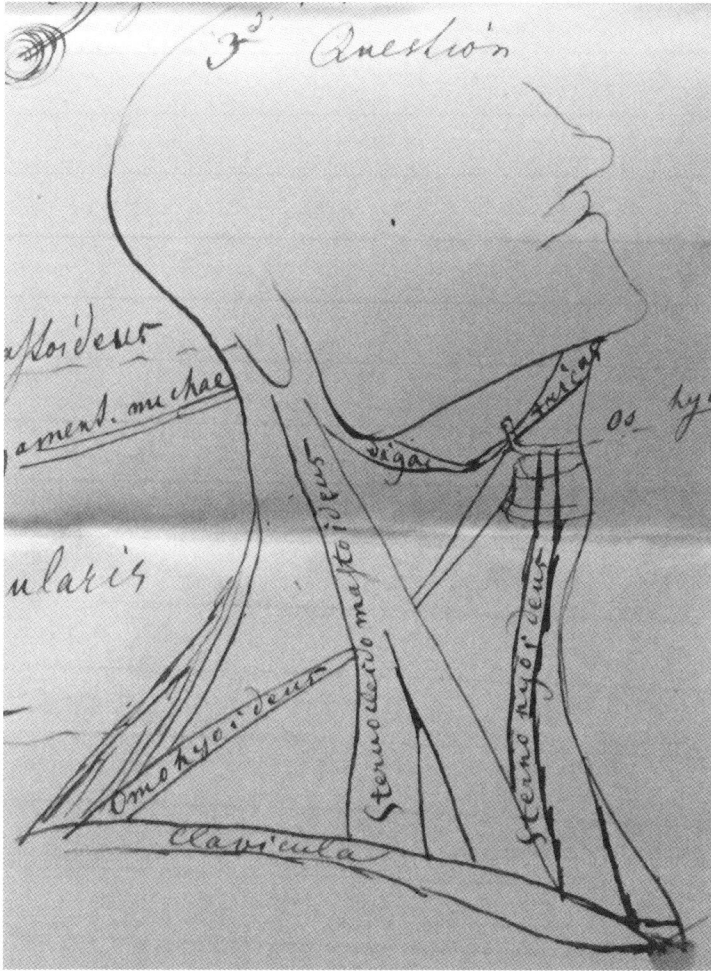

Frederick Wolf, Surgeon, 39th New York. Sketch of nerves in neck in examination for U.S. Assistant Surgeon. Personal papers, National Archives. Author's Photograph.

throughout the war and was paroled at Appomattox. After the war, he returned to Washington where he practiced medicine for the rest of his life. The brigade history described him as "an intelligent and refined gentleman . . . always in good humor with himself and the rest of mankind . . . a truly brave man, and never hesitated to go into the hottest fire on the field of battle in the discharge."

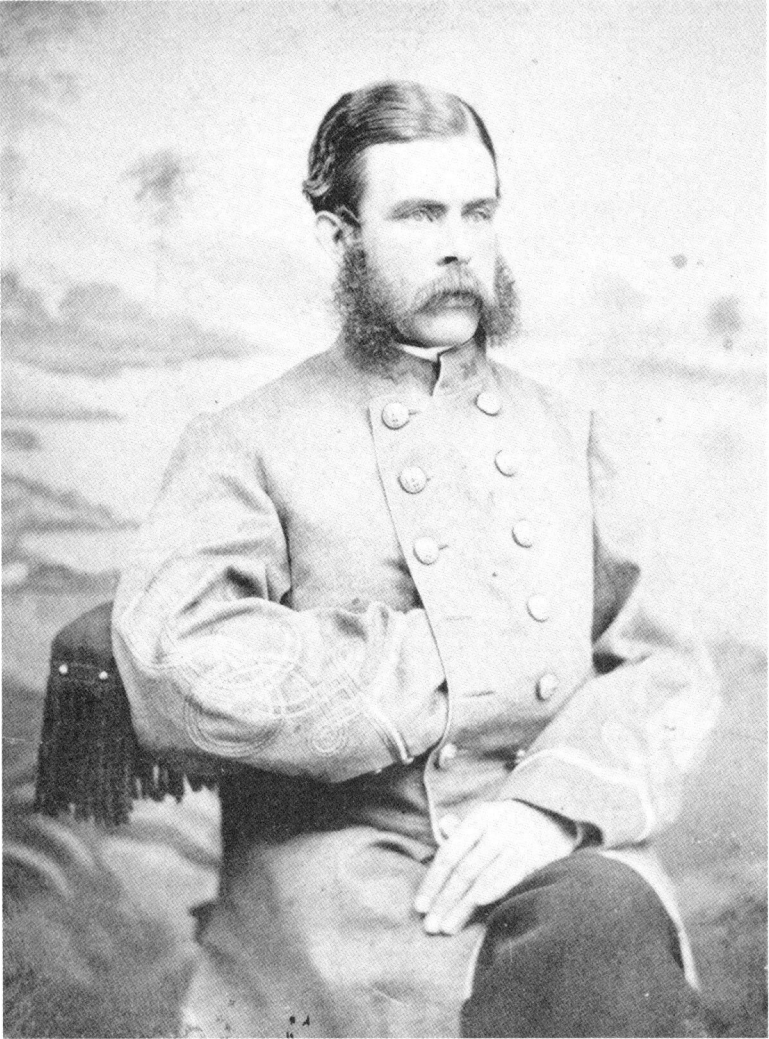

William Proby Young, Assistant Surgeon, 4th Georgia. T. W. Clark & Co., Norfolk, Virginia. Courtesy of Library of Congress, Prints and Photographs Division.

Notes

Preface

1. Katherine S. B. Keats-Rohan, "Biography, Identity and Names: Understanding the Pursuit of the Individual in Prosopography," in *Prosopography Approaches and Applications: A Handbook,* ed. K. S. B. Keats-Rohan (Oxford: Occasional Publications UPR Linacre College, 2007), 146.

2. Joseph Wendel Muffly, *The Story of Our Regiment, a History of the 148th Pennsylvania Volunteers* (Des Moines, IA: Kenyon Printing & Mfg. Co., 1904), 175–76.

Introduction

1. H. Seymour, H. Morford, and H. Cruse Murphy, *Celebration at Tammany Hall, on Saturday, July 4, 1863: Including the Oration, by Hon. Henry C. Murphy, the Poem, by Henry Morford, Esq., the Addresses by Hon. Horatio Seymour and Others* (New York: Baptist & Taylor, Printers, 1863).

2. *Los Angeles Star,* Vol. 13, no. 9, July 4, 1863. Accessed June 2, 2019 at http://digitallibrary.usc.edu/cdm/compoundobject/collection/p15799coll68/id/1047/rec/1.

3. *New York Times,* July 6, 1863.

4. *Richmond Daily Dispatch,* July 4, 1863.

5. *New York Times*, July 8, 1863.

6. *Adams County Compiler,* July 7, 1872, 3.

7. Agnes Barr, Citizen Accounts, Adams County Historical Society (ACHS).

8. Francis Wafer, *A Surgeon in the Army of the Potomac,* ed. Cheryl A. Wells (Montreal: McGill-Queen's University, 2008), 52.

9. J. F. McKenrick, *Reminiscences of the Battle of Gettysburg*, Citizen Accounts, ACHS.

10. Peter Tinsley, unpublished Civil War Diary, Wheaton College, John and Joyce Schmale Civil War Collection, 26–27.

11. J. Franklin Dyer, *The Journal of a Civil War Surgeon*, ed. Michael B. Shesson (Lincoln: University of Nebraska Press, 2009), 216.

12. David Power Conyngham, *The Irish Brigade and Its Campaigns: With Some Account of the Corcoran Legion, and Sketches of the Principal Officers* (Glasgow: Cameron & Ferguson, 1866), 282.

13. Letter to S. Cooper, Adjutant and Inspector General, Richmond from John Work, Atlanta Georgia, May 13, 1864, National Archives and Records Administration (NARA). Accessed November 4, 2019 at https://www.fold3.com/image/271/84505477.

14. Michigan State Medical Society, *Medical History of Michigan* (Bruce Publishing Company, 1930), 299–331.

15. Henry Walter Thomas, *History of the Doles-Cook Brigade* (Atlanta: Franklin Printing and Publishing Company, 1903), 83.

16. Robert D. Hicks, ed., *Civil War Medicine: A Surgeon's Diary* (Bloomington: Indiana University Press, 2019), 85.

17. John B. Linn, "Journal of My Trip to the Battlefield at Gettysburg," Citizen Account, ACHS.

18. Thomas Chamberlin, *History of the One Hundred and Fiftieth Regiment Pennsylvania Volunteers, Second Regiment, Bucktail Brigade* (Philadelphia: J.B. Lippincott, 1895), 97.

19. Mary C. Gillet, *The Army Medical Department 1818–1865* (Washington, DC: Center of Military History, U.S. Army, 1987), 153.

20. Walter Clark, ed., Histories of the Several Regiments and Battalions from North Carolina in the Great War, 1861–1865 (North Carolina, 1901), Vol. IV, 623. Major P. E. Hines described the establishment of North Carolina regiments in 1861.

21. *American Medical Times,* June 1861.

22. H. H. Cunningham, *Doctors in Gray: The Confederate Medical Service* (Baton Rouge: Louisiana State University Press, 1986), 32.

23. NARA. Accessed Fold3 November 4, 2019 at https://www.fold3.com/image/70402751.

24. An 1856 graduate of Jefferson Medical College in Philadelphia, Hickerson strenuously objected to the requirement to go before an examining board invoking his state appointment: "Recognizing the right of NC to say who the medical officers shall be, I most respectfully decline an examination before the Medical Board spoken of in said Circular. Upon this ground I herewith hand you my resignation." Eight days later, Dr. Hickerson submitted a second letter of resignation claiming physical disability due to poor digestion and general debility. This was approved as "Resignation on account of Physical Disability!" Confederate Service Records, NARA. Accessed on November 5, 2019 at https://www.fold3.com/image/51040097.

25. Cunningham, 35.

26. Pennsylvania State Archives, Harrisburg, PA RG19 Surgeon General Records.

27. W. W. Keen, "Surgical Reminiscences of the Civil War," *Transactions of the College of Physicians of Philadelphia* 25 (Philadelphia: 1905), 96.

28. Louis C. Duncan, *The Medical Department of the United States Army in the Civil War* (Washington, DC: Surgeon-General's Office, 1915), 20.

29. Cunningham, 27.

30. Cunningham, 26.

31. Ira M. Rutkow, *Bleeding Blue and Gray: Civil War Surgery and the Evolution of American Medicine* (New York: Random House, 2005), 112.

32. Rutkow, 88, 109.

33. Cunningham, 119.

34. Cunningham, 122.

35. James C. Whorton, *Nature Cures: The History of Alternative Medicine in America* (Oxford and New York: Oxford University Press, 2002), 78.

36. Joseph F. Kett, *The Formation of the American Medical Profession* (New Haven, CT: Yale University Press, 1968), 156.

37. Cunningham, 33.

38. Rutkow, 284.

39. Richard M. Swiderski, *Calomel in America: Mercurial Panacea, War, Song and Ghosts* (Boca Raton, FL: Brown Walker Press, 2008), 159.

40. U.S. Surgeon-General's Office, *The Medical and Surgical History of the War of the Rebellion*, Part I, Volume II, Chapter I, Section II, Miscellaneous Injuries (1870–88), 329.

41. Duncan, 5.

42. Ellerslie Wallace, "Charge to the Graduating Class of Jefferson Medical College," Delivered March 10, 1863 (Philadelphia: Collins Printer, 1863), 6. Accessed July 7, 2019 at https://ia801705.us.archive.org/25/items/9616906.nlm.nih.gov/9616906.pdf.

Chapter 1

1. Patricia Spain Ward, *Simon Baruch: Rebel in the Ranks of Medicine 1840–1921* (Tuscaloosa: University of Alabama Press, 1994), 24.

2. Ward, 34.

3. Fielding H. Garrison, *John Shaw Billings: A Memoir* (New York: G.P. Putnam's Sons, 1913), 12.

4. Max Berman and Michael A. Flannery, *America's Botanico-Medical Movements: Vox Populi* (New York: Haworth Press, 2001), 28.

5. P. M. Hamer, *The Centennial History of the TN State Medical Association* (Nashville, 1930), 19.

6. Unpublished Gettysburg Surgeons Database.

7. Georgia Medical College, *Annual Announcement for 1853*.

8. Unpublished Gettysburg Surgeons Database; Frederick Clayton Waite, *The First Medical College in Vermont: Castleton 1818–1862* (Vermont Historical Society, 1949), 114. It is sometimes difficult to determine whether or not someone graduated with a medical degree since students who attended a school without receiving a degree are often described as alumni.

9. Unpublished Gettysburg Surgeons Database.

10. J. Roberts Deering, "Organization and Personnel of the Medical Department of the Confederacy," in *The Photographic History of the Civil War*, ed. H. Thompson, Vol. 7 (New York: The Review of Reviews, Co., 1911), 351.

11. Waite, 103.

12. Ward, 13.

13. Waite, 102.

14. Unpublished Gettysburg Surgeons Database.

15. Monson Academy, Annual Announcement 1854, Monson, Massachusetts.

16. NARA, F. Wolf Personal Papers 94 561.

17. Caspar C. Henkel correspondence, National Library of Medicine, Bethesda, MD, MS C 291, February 15, 1855 from Caspar Henkel to Dr. Neff.

18. Waite, 117.

19. Ward, 20.

20. Henkel correspondence, February 15, 1855; Caspar Henkel to his father, November 8, 1856.

21. Henkel correspondence, November 19, 1855.

22. Wade, 15.

23. William Osler MD, "Memoir of Alfred Stille MD," read April 2, 1902, *Transactions of the College of Physicians of Philadelphia*, 3rd Ser., Vol. 24 (1902), lxi. Accessed May 6, 2024 at https://babel.hathitrust.org/cgi/pt?id=ien.35558002617310&view=1up&seq=64.

24. Henkel correspondence, November 8, 1856.

25. Henkel correspondence, November 19, 1856.

26. Garrison, 14.

27. The Medical Department of the University of Louisiana, *Annual Circular of the Medical Department of the University of Louisiana, 1859–1860* (New Orleans, 1860), 7.

28. Annual Announcement of Jefferson Medical College of Philadelphia, 1855–56, Philadelphia.

29. Henkel correspondence, November 8, 1856.

30. Henkel correspondence, November 19, 1856.

31. University of Louisiana, *Annual Circular, 1859–1860*, 8.

32. Jefferson Medical College, 1855–56.

33. Jodi L. Koste, "Artifacts and Comingled Skeletal Remains from a Well on the Medical College of Virginia Campus: Anatomical and Surgical Training in Nineteenth-Century Richmond," June 18, 2012, Virginia Commonwealth University. Accessed September 29, 2019 at http://scholarscompass.vcu.edu/arch001/2, 6–7, quoting "An Address to the Public in Regard to the Affairs of Hampden Sidney College" (Richmond: Ritchie and Dunnavant, 1853).

34. Bess Lovejoy, "Meet Grandison Harris, the Grave Robber Enslaved (and Then Employed) by the Georgia Medical College," Smithsonian.com, May 6, 2014. Accessed September 29, 2019 at https://www.smithsonianmag.com/history/meet-grandison-harris-grave-robber-enslaved-and-then-employed-georgia-college-medicine-180951344/; Dolly Stoltze, "Bodies in the Basement: The Hidden Bones of Medical Schools," *Atlas Obscura*, January 22, 2015. Accessed September 29, 2019 at https://www.atlasobscura.com/articles/bodies-in-the-basement-the-forgotten-bones-of-america-s-medical-schools.

35. Koste, 7; Catalogue of the Medical College of Virginia, 1859.

36. Waite, 124–25.

37. Henkel correspondence, February 7, 1857.

38. *A Short Account of the Occurrences Which Led to the Removal of Dr. John Redman Coxe from the Chair of Materia Medica & Pharmacy in the University of Pennsylvania, Philadelphia Jan. 12, 1835.* Accessed November 3, 2019 at https://collections.nlm.nih.gov/bookviewer?PID=nlm:nlmuid-101171718-bk#page/1/mode/2up.

39. Henkel correspondence, February 2, 1857.

40. Henkel correspondence, February 2, 1857.

41. Waite, 132–33. The value of $1 today would be $37.50.

42. Catalogues University of Pennsylvania and Jefferson Medical College, 1847–48.

43. Daniel Kilbride, "Southern Medical Students in Philadelphia, 1800–1861: Science and Sociability in the 'Republic of Medicine,'" *Journal of Southern History* 65, no. 4 (1999): 731.

44. William Riddick Whitehead, *Adventures of an American Surgeon: A 19th Century Memoir*, typescript manuscript copy, National Museum of Civil War Medicine.

45. Whitehead.

46. Whitehead.

47. Garrison, 11.

48. Henkel correspondence, February 7, 1857.

49. Henkel correspondence, March 5, 1857.

50. Henkel correspondence, March 23, 1857.

51. Henkel correspondence, March 9, 1857.

CHAPTER 2

1. Letter from J. N. K. Monmonier to Jefferson Davis, NARA 109 Record Group the Army of the Confederate States, M331, Compiled Service Records. Accessed December 12, 2019 at https://www.fold3.com/image/271/72361390.

2. Letter from J. N. K. Monmonier to Walker, NARA 109 Record Group the Army of the Confederate States, M331, Compiled Service Records, https://www.fold3.com/image/72361511.

3. William W. Potter, *One Surgeon's Private War: Dr. William W. Potter of the 57th NY*, eds. John Michael Priest et al. (Shippensburg, PA: White Mane Publishing Company, 1996), 1. Originally published Buffalo, NY, 1888.

4. Potter, 2.

5. Potter, xii.

6. J. Franklin Dyer, *The Journal of a Civil War Surgeon*, ed. Michael B. Chesson (Lincoln: University of Nebraska Press, 2003), 2.

7. Personal Papers John Tuller Brown, NARA.

8. Theodore Dimon, Diary II April 16, 1861, unpublished transcript, privately owned.

9. Dimon, Diary I April 20, 1862, unpublished transcript, privately owned.

10. Lafayette Guild papers, letter from S. F. Hale to L. P. Walker, March 13, 1861, NARA. Accessed December 12, 2019 at https://www.fold3.com/image/271/70400414.

11. Virginia Martin Brown, *The American Descendants of Dr. Charles Silas (Bigelow) Morton and Mary Lavalette Gilliam Morton*, privately published 1964, 85.

12. Edmund Cody Burnett, "Letters of a Confederate Surgeon: Dr. Abner Embry McGarity, 1862–1865. Part I," *Georgia Historical Quarterly* 29, no. 2 (1945): 76–114.

13. Corydon Ireland, "Saga of a Civil War Surgeon," *Harvard Gazette*, February 13, 2013, Lecture at Countway Medical Library by Mitchell L. Adams. Accessed December 12, 2019 at https://news.harvard.edu/gazette/story/2013/02/saga-of-a-civil-war-surgeon/.

14. *Appletons' Cyclopedia of American Biography* (New York: D. Appleton and Company, 1887–1889), III, 687.

15. Franklin Ellis, *History of Fayette County* (Philadelphia: L H Everts and Company, 1882), 418.

16. *Biographical Souvenir of the States of Georgia and Florida* (Chicago: F.A. Battey & Co., 1889), 267–68.

17. Richard Denny Parker, *Historical Recollections of Robertson County, Texas: With Biographical & Genealogical Notes on the Pioneers & Their Families* (Anson Jones Press, 1955), 181.

18. William Child, *Letters from a Civil War Surgeon* (Solon, ME: Polar Bear and Company, 2001), 291, 25.

19. John S. Richards, Confederate Officers, Letter November 21, 1863, to Secretary of War Seddon from Shelton Leake in Charlottesville expressing need for services of a doctor in their area, NARA.

20. Roland R. Maust, *Grappling with Death: The Union Second Corps Hospital at Gettysburg* (Dayton, OH: Morningside House Inc., 2001), 66.

21. H. H. Cunningham, *Doctors in Gray: The Confederate Medical Service* (Baton Rouge: Louisiana State University Press, 1986), 22.

22. Christopher Loperfido, ed., *Death, Disease, and Life at War: The Civil War Letters of Surgeon James D. Benton, 111th and 98th New York Infantry Regiments 1862–1865* (El Dorado Hills, CA: Savas Beatie, 2018), 7.

23. Child, 80.

24. Benjamin Barr, Personal Papers 94–561, NARA.

25. Charles Taylor Richardson, Confederate Officers papers, NARA.

26. Biography of Charles Taylor Richardson, "Biographies of West Virginia Confederate Soldiers," in *Confederate Military History*, ed. Gen. Clement A. Evans (Atlanta: Confederate Publishing Company, 1899). Accessed May 10, 2024 at https://www.wvgw.net/wvmilitary/confed-all.htm.

27. Donald B. Koonce, ed., *Doctor to the Front: Recollections of Confederate Surgeon Thomas Fanning Wood* (Knoxville: University of Tennessee Press, 2000), 37.

28. Paul B. Kerr, *Civil War Surgeon—Biography of James Langstall Dunn, MD* (Bloomington, IN: Authorhouse, 2005), 27–29.

29. Kerr, 30.

30. John Wilson Letter, NARA, Compiled Service Records of Confederate General and Staff Officers.

31. Francis M. Wafer, *A Surgeon in the Army of the Potomac*, ed. Cheryl A. Wells (Montreal and Kingston: McGill-Queen's University Press, 2008), 6.

32. James Stanislaus Easby-Smith, *Georgetown University in the District of Columbia 1789–1907* (New York: Lewis, 1907), 84–85.

33. David Power Conyngham, *The Irish Brigade with Some Account of the Corcoran Legion, and Sketches of the Principal Officers* (New York: M. McSorley & Co., 1867), 567.

34. George J. Lerski, "Jewish-Polish Amity in Lincoln's America," *Polish Review* 18, no. 4 (1973): 34.

35. Personal Papers Frederick Wolf, NARA.

36. Roster of 119th NY Infantry. Accessed May 10, 2024 at https://dmna.ny.gov/historic/reghist/civil/rosters/Infantry/119th_Infantry_CW_Roster.pdf.

37. Personal Papers Andrew Jackson Ward, NARA.

38. *Columbia Gazette*, Columbia State Historic Park, California. Accessed May 10, 2024 at http://columbiagazette.com/hildreth.htm.

39. Dimon Diary.

40. William F. Liebler, "The United States and the Crimean War 1853–1856" (PhD diss., U. Mass–Amherst, 1972), 7.

41. William Reddick Whitehead, *Adventures of an American Surgeon: A 19th Century Memoir*, typescript manuscript copy, National Museum of Civil War Medicine.

42. Find a Grave, https://www.findagrave.com/memorial/9575166/louis-wernwag -read.

43. Find a Grave, https://www.findagrave.com/memorial/10905414/erwin-j_-eldridge.

44. Conyngham, 559.

45. Kerr, 23.

46. Wafer, 7–8.

47. Koonce, 41.

48. Koonce, 42.

49. Dyer, 2.

50. Loperfido, 18.

51. Loperfido, 28.

52. Child, 19.

53. Kerr, 32.

54. Loperfido, 2.

55. Potter, 10.

56. Paul Fatout, ed., *Letters of a Civil War Surgeon* (West Lafayette, IN: Purdue University Press, 1996), 12–14.

57. George T. Stevens, *Three Years in the Sixth Corps* (Albany, NY: S.R. Gray, 1866), 1.

58. Child, 25.

CHAPTER 3

1. Edmund Cody Burnett, "Letters of a Confederate Surgeon: Dr. Abner Embry McCarity, 1862–1865, Part I," *Georgia Historical Quarterly* 29, no. 2 (1945): 76–114.

2. Donald B. Koonce, ed., *Doctor to the Front: The Recollections of Confederate Surgeon Thomas Fanning Wood 1861–1865* (Knoxville: University of Tennessee Press, 2000), 32.

3. Cyrus Bacon, transcript of unpublished diary, January 8, 1863, Michigan Historical Commission.

4. Paul Fatout, ed., *Letters of a Civil War Surgeon* (West Lafayette, IN: Purdue University Press, 1996), 16.

5. Daniel M. Holt, *A Surgeon's Civil War: The Letters and Diaries of Daniel M. Holt, M.D.*, eds. James M. Greiner, Janet L Coryell, and James R. Smither (Kent, OH: Kent State University Press, 1994), 36, 48.

6. Fielding H. Garrison, *John Shaw Billings: A Memoir* (New York: G.P. Putnam's Sons, 1913), 33. Letter to his wife, April 8, 1863.

7. Holt, 23–24.

8. Holt, 30.

9. William W. Potter, *One Surgeon's Private War: Dr. William W. Potter of the 57th NY*, eds. John Michael Priest et al. (Shippensburg, PA: White Mane Publishing Company, 1996), 10.

10. Fatout, 33.

11. Fatout, 50.

12. Fatout, 69–70.

13. Spencer Glasgow Welch, *A Confederate Surgeon's Letters to his Wife* (New York and Washington: Neale Publishing Company, 1911), 58, 60.

14. Welch, 76, 87.

15. Samuel Morrison letter to his wife, August 9, 1863, Virginia Historical Society, Mss1 M8347 a 1–17.

16. Morrison letter to his wife.

17. Clayton Glanville Coleman, letter August 26, 1863, Virginia Historical Society, Mss 2 C6772 b (CMLS).

18. Glen L. McMullen, ed., *A Surgeon with Stonewall Jackson: The Civil War Letters of Dr. Harvey Black* (Baltimore: Butternut and Blue, 1995), 41.

19. Fatout, 23.

20. Fatout, 80.

21. Holt, 61.

22. Holt, 77.

23. William Child, *Letters from a Civil War Surgeon* (Solon, ME: Polar Bear and Company, 2001), 215.

24. Potter, 37, 39.

25. Paul B. Kerr, *Civil War Surgeon—Biography of James Langstall Dunn, MD* (Bloomington, IN: Authorhouse, 2005), 115.

26. *Lansdale* (PA) *Reporter*, April 6, 1905.

27. James M. Paradis, *African Americans and the Gettysburg Campaign* (Lanham, MD: Scarecrow Press, 2005), 55.

28. Holt, 31–32.

29. Bacon, January 8, 1863.

30. William H. Taylor, "Some Experiences of a Confederate Asst. Surgeon," *Transactions of the College of Physicians of Philadelphia*, Ser. 3, Vol. 28 (Philadelphia, 1906): 100.

31. Bacon, February 21, March 2, 1863; Child, 86; Potter, 61.

32. John D. Billings, *Hardtack and Coffee*, reprinted from original edition published in 1887 (Lincoln: University of Nebraska Press, 1993), 173.

33. Fatout, 59.

34. Fatout, 104.

35. Gilbert Adams Hays, *Under the Red Patch. Story of the 63rd Regiment, Pennsylvania Volunteers 1861–1864* (Pittsburgh: Sixty-third Pennsylvania Volunteers Regimental Association, 1908), 70–71.

36. *Bellows Falls* (VT) *Times*, October 23, 1863.

37. Koonce, 54–55.

38. Holt, 37.

39. Holt, 36.

40. Thomas P. Lowry and Terry Reimer, *Bad Doctors: Military Justice Proceedings Against 622 Civil War Surgeons* (Frederick, MD: National Museum of Civil War Medicine (NMCWM) Press, 2010), 100.

41. Thomas Harold Wilson Upshur, Confederate Officers papers, NARA.

42. Lowry and Reimer, 32, 40; NY Civil War Muster Roll extracts, Adj General's Office, August 7, 1863.

43. Bacon, 24.

44. Bacon, 47, 78. An 1862 graduate of Cincinnati Medical College, Colton died at the age of twenty-six in 1864 of gastroenteritis.

45. Lowry and Reimer, 13.

46. Taylor, 105.

47. Taylor, 101.

48. Henkel Family Correspondence, 1786–1940, History of Medicine Division, National Library of Medicine, Bethesda, Maryland, MS C 291, Caspar C. Henkel correspondence, February 23, 1863 to Samuel Godfrey Henkel.

49. Matthew Ridd et al., "The Patient-Doctor Relationship: A Synthesis of the Qualitative Literature on Patients' Perspectives," *British Journal of General Practice*, April 2009. Accessed May 10, 2024 at https://bjgp.org/content/bjgp/59/561/e116.full.pdf.

50. Holt, 89, April 10, 1863. Reference to "medicine not killing them" reflects his more eclectic approach. At another point he refers to cold water baths and water as the best cure suggesting his familiarity with hydropathic treatments, 112.

51. Julian John Chisolm, *A Manual of Military Surgery, for the Use of Surgeons in the Confederate Army; with an Appendix of the Rules and Regulations of the Medical Department of the Confederate Army* (Richmond, VA: West & Johnson, 1861), 11.

52. Taylor, 105–6.

53. Christopher E. Loperfido, ed., *Death, Disease, and Life at War: The Civil War Letters of Surgeon James D. Benton* (El Dorado Hills, CA: Savas Beatie, 2018), 49.

54. Joseph Wendel Muffly, *The Story of Our Regiment, a History of the 148th Pennsylvania Volunteers* (Des Moines, IA: Kenyon Printing & Mfg. Co., 1904), 167.

55. Muffly.

56. Holt, 71.

57. Bacon, June 20, 1862.

58. Joseph Janvier Woodward, *Outline of the Chief Camp Diseases of the United States Armies* (Philadelphia; J.B. Lippincott & Co., 1863).

59. Theodore Dimon, unpublished transcript, Diary II, July 30–August 1, 186, 113–14.

60. Dimon Diary. In 1849, he went to California following the Gold Rush and practiced medicine for about three years in San Francisco, becoming the first president of the first Medical Society organized in California.

61. J. Franklin Dyer, *The Journal of a Civil War Surgeon,* ed. Michael B. Chesson (Lincoln: University of Nebraska Press, 2003), 24.

62. Isaac Scott Tanner Ledgers, Virginia Historical Society, copy of circular dated March 28, 1863, Ms1 T1578 a 1–24; 25–30.

63. McMullen, 67.

64. Chisolm, 103.

65. Taylor, 104.

66. Bacon, March 10, 1863.

67. Dyer, 11.

68. Fatout, 101.

69. Potter, 13, 28.

70. Tanner papers, Virginia Historical Society.

71. Koonce, 92.

72. Koonce, 93.

73. Garrison, 49–50.

74. Garrison, 53.

75. Robert D. Hicks, ed., *Civil War Medicine: A Surgeon's Diary* (Bloomington: Indiana University Press, 2019), 76.

CHAPTER 4

1. George T. Stevens, *Three Years in the Sixth Corps* (Albany, NY: S.R. Gray, Publishers, 1866), 223.

2. Edward Ayers, *The Thin Light of Freedom* (New York: W. W. Norton & Co., 2017), 48.

3. Spencer Glasgow Welch, *A Confederate Surgeon's Letters to His Wife* (New York and Washington: Neale Publishing Company, 1911), 57.

4. Jonathan Letterman, *Medical Recollections of the Army of the Potomac* (Bedford, MA: Applewood Books, originally printed 1866), 153.

5. Fielding H. Garrison, *John Shaw Billings: A Memoir* (New York: G.P. Putnam's Sons, 1913), 60.

6. Garrison, 56.

7. David T. Hedrick and Gordon Barry Davis Jr., *I'm Surrounded by Methodists . . . Diary of John H.W. Stuckenberg, Chaplain of the 145th Pennsylvania Volunteer Infantry* (Gettysburg, PA: Thomas Publications, 1995), 70.

8. Donald B. Koonce, ed., *Doctor to the Front: The Recollections of Confederate Surgeon Thomas Fanning Wood 1861–1865* (Knoxville: University of Tennessee Press, 2000), 94.

9. George T. Stevens, *Three Years in the Sixth Corps* (Albany, NY: S.R. Gray, Publishers, 1866), 226, 239, 241. The number of 38 miles is probably overstated. Most scholars estimate that the distance was probably 32 miles.

10. J. Franklin Dyer, *The Journal of a Civil War Surgeon*, ed. Michael B. Chesson (Lincoln: University of Nebraska Press, 2003), 90. Gen. John Gibbon commanded the Second Corps, 2nd Division.

11. Joseph Wendel Muffly, *The Story of Our Regiment, a History of the 148th Pennsylvania Volunteers* (Des Moines, IA: Kenyon Printing & Mfg. Co., 1904), 170–71.

12. H. P. Moyer, *History of 17th Pennsylvania Volunteer Cavalry* (Lebanon, PA: Sowers Printing Co., 1911), 61.

13. Welch, 63, 67. The site of the hospital was near the Samuel Lohr Farm along the Chambersburg Pike. Other surgeons reported working at this location were Dr. Ward, 11th Mississippi, Dr. Green, 55th North Carolina, Dr. Wilson, 42nd Mississippi, Dr. Warren, 26th North Carolina, Dr. Hubbard, 2nd Mississippi. Gregory A. Coco, *A Vast Sea of Misery* (Gettysburg, PA: Thomas Publications, 1988), 135–37.

14. Robert D. Hicks, ed., *Civil War Medicine: A Surgeon's Diary* (Bloomington: Indiana University Press, 2019), 103–6.

15. George New Letter, Gettysburg National Military Park (GNMP); Coco, 23.

16. Abner Hard, *A Surgeon of the Eighth Cavalry Regiment Illinois Volunteers*, originally published 1868 (Big Byte Books, 2014), 202.

17. Agnes Barr Account, Gettysburg Citizen Accounts, ACHS.

18. "Penned Up in Gettysburg" by Richard M. Bache, *Gettysburg Compiler,* March 2, 1897, reprinted from the *Philadelphia Times.* Richard Bache was Thomas Hewson Bache's brother.

19. Hicks, 106; Coco, 18.

20. Jacob Ebersole, "Incidents of Field Hospital Life with the Army of the Potomac," in *Sketches of War History 1861–1865, Papers Read Before the Ohio Commandery of the Military Order of the Loyal Legion of the United States*, W. H. Chamberlin ed., Vol. 4 (Cincinnati: R. Clarke & Co., 1896), 328.

21. Rufus R. Dawes, *Service with the Sixth Wisconsin Volunteers* (Marietta, OH: E.R. Alderman & Sons, 1890), 179; Coco, 4.

22. Algernon S. Coe, "The 14th N. Y. Zouaves," *National Tribune*, August 13, 1885. Accessed April 11, 2020 at https://www.newyorkroots.org/oswego/military/147thnypt1.html.

23. Coco, 20.

24. *Philadelphia Inquirer*, July 8, 1863, 4.

25. Coco, 20.

26. William F. Osborn, unpublished diary and letters, private owner, https://www.jloakleyauthor.com/contact/; Coco, 35.

27. Henry C. Bradsby, *History of Bradford County, Pennsylvania* (Bradford, PA: S.B. Nelson, 1891), 1237.

28. John D. Vautier, *History of the 88th Pennsylvania Volunteers* (Philadelphia: J.B. Lippincott & Company, 1894), 113.

29. Frank Moore, *Women of the War: Their Heroism and Self-Sacrifice* (Hartford, CT: S.S. Scranton & Co., 1866), 242–43.

30. Asa Sleath Hardman, "As a Union Prisoner Saw the Battle of Gettysburg," *Civil War Times Illustrated* (July 1962): 49.

31. *Maine at Gettysburg. Report of Maine Commissioners* (Portland, ME: Lakeside Press, 1898), 51, 5.

32. John Tullar Brown, Personal Papers, NARA.

33. D. G. Brinton Thomson, "From Chancellorsville to Gettysburg, A Doctor's Diary," *Pennsylvania Magazine of History and Biography* LXXXIX (1965): 292–315; 313.

34. Carolyn Ivanoff, *We Fought at Gettysburg: Firsthand Accounts by the Survivors of the 17th Connecticut Volunteer Infantry* (Gettysburg, PA: Gettysburg Publishing, 2023), 83, 88.

35. William R. Kiefer, *History of the 153rd Regiment Pennsylvania Volunteer Infantry* (Easton, PA: Press of the Chemical Publishing Co., 1909), 131.

36. Kiefer, 216.

37. Ivanoff, 140.

38 Francis Huebschmann Papers, Milwaukee County Historical Society.

39. Dawes, 179.

40. Welch, 67.

41. Augustus D. Dickert, *History of Kershaw's Brigade* (Newberry, SC: Elbert H. Aull Co., 1899), 231–32.

42. Wharton J. Green, *Recollections and Reflections, An Auto of Half a Century and More* (Raleigh, NC: Edwards and Broughton Publishing Company, 1906), 176, 262. Accessed April 22, 2020 at https://docsouth.unc.edu/fpn/green/green.html.

43. George C. Underwood, *History of the 26th Regiment of NC Troops* (Goldsboro, NC: Nash Bros., 1901), 111.

44. Interview with Tim Smith, Licensed Battlefield Guide, American Battlefield Trust. Accessed February 18, 2024 at https://www.battlefields.org/learn/articles/first-day -gettysburg-then-now.

CHAPTER 5

1. Harriet Bayly, Civilian Accounts, ACHS.

2. Carolyn Ivanoff, *We Fought at Gettysburg: Firsthand Accounts by the Survivors of the 17th Connecticut Volunteer Infantry* (Gettysburg, PA: Gettysburg Publishing, 2003), 207. John H. Benedict, 17th Connecticut, who had his wound dressed by two Union surgeons at the Alms House on July 3rd, also described a German surgeon who handled him "very carefully and tenderly."

3. Michael Dreese, *The Hospital on Seminary Ridge* (Jefferson, NC: McFarland & Co., 2002), 91.

4. Gregory A. Coco, *A Vast Sea of Misery* (Gettysburg, PA: Thomas Publications, 1988), 20.

5. Robert D. Hicks, ed., *Civil War Medicine: A Surgeon's Diary* (Bloomington: Indiana University Press, 2019), 126.

6. *Alumni Register of the University of Pennsylvania*, Vol. 15 (Philadelphia: General Alumni Society, 1912), 61.

7. J. H. Brinton, *Personal Memoirs of John H. Brinton: Civil War Surgeon, 1861–1865* (Carbondale: Southern Illinois University Press, 1996), 246.

8. Fielding H. Garrison, *John Shaw Billings: A Memoir* (New York: G.P. Putnam's Sons, 1913), 61.

9. William F. Breakey, "Recollections and Incidents of Military Service," Read February 4, 1897, in *War Papers Read Before the Michigan Commandery of the Military Order of the Loyal Legion of the United States* (Detroit: James H. Stone & Co., 1898), 139–41.

10. Breakey.

11. Roland R. Maust, *Grappling with Death: The Union Second Corps Hospital at Gettysburg* (Dayton, OH: Morningside House Inc., 2001), 193.

12. William W. Potter, *One Surgeon's Private War: Dr. William W. Potter of the 57th NY*, eds. John Michael Priest et al. (Shippensburg, PA: White Mane Publishing Company, 1996), 72.

13. D. Augustus Dickert, *History of Kershaw's Brigade* (Newberry, SC: Elbert H. Aull Co., 1899), 246.

14. Garrison, 61.

15. Garrison, 61.

16. Garrison, 61. The Autenrieth Wagon, developed by Jonathan Letterman and used by the Army of the Potomac at Gettysburg, was specially outfitted to transport medicines and other surgical and medical supplies needed in the field.

17. Maust, 86, 106.

18. Cyrus Bacon, July 2, 1863, transcript of unpublished diary, Michigan Historical Commission, 91–92.

19. Breakey, 141–42.

20. Joseph Wendel Muffly, *The Story of Our Regiment, a History of the 148th Pennsylvania Volunteers* (Des Moines, IA: Kenyon Printing & Mfg. Co., 1904), 325.

21. Donald B. Koonce, ed., *Doctor to the Front: The Recollections of Confederate Surgeon Thomas Fanning Wood 1861–1865* (Knoxville: University of Tennessee Press, 2000), 104, 107. Dr. Coke was Lucius C. Coke, Confederate States of America (CSA) Assistant Surgeon, 1st North Carolina. The farm was probably Christian Benner Farm.

22. U.S. War Department, *The War of Rebellion: A Compilation of the Official Records of the Union and Confederate Armies*, XXV, part 1 (Washington, DC: Government Printing Office, 1880–1901), 503. Report of Col. Hiram Berdan, 1st U.S. Sharpshooters, commanding Third Brigade, on the Battle of Chancellorsville.

23. Francis M. Wafer, *A Surgeon in the Army of the Potomac*, ed. Cheryl A. Wells (Montreal and Kingston: McGill-Queen's University Press, 2008), 44.

24. Maust, 134.

25. J. B. Clifton Diary. July 2, 1863, original diary transcript, NMCWM, Frederick, Maryland.

26. George A. Bruce, *The Twentieth Regiment of Massachusetts Volunteer Infantry, 1861–1865* (Boston: Houghton, Mifflin and Company, 1906), 283–284.

27. Simon Baruch, "A Surgeon's Story of Battle and Capture," *Confederate Veteran* 22 (1914): 545–48.

28. J. Franklin Dyer, *The Journal of a Civil War Surgeon*, ed. Michael B. Chesson (Lincoln: University of Nebraska Press, 2003), 97.

29. Dyer, 91–92.

30. Clifton Diary, July 3, 1863.

31. Wafer, 44.

32. Ronald D. Kirkwood, *"Too Much for Human Endurance:" The George Spangler Farm Hospitals and the Battle of Gettysburg* (El Dorado Hills, CA: Savas Beatie, 2021), 24–26.

33. Garrison, 62.

34. Maust, 164.

35. Hicks, 123.

36. Wafer, 50. Coco identifies as Peter Frey Farm.

37. Wafer, 50.

38. Wafer, 51.

39. Potter, 74.

40. Henrietta Stratton Jaquette, ed., *South After Gettysburg: Letters of Cornelia Hancock 1863–1868* (New York: Thomas Y. Crowell Company, 1956), 41.

41. Samuel Toombs, *New Jersey Troops in the Gettysburg Campaign from June 5 to July 31, 1863* (Orange, NJ: Evening Mail Publishing House, 1888), 326–27.

42. William H. Taylor, "Some Experiences of a Confederate Assistant Surgeon," *Transactions of the College of Physicians of Philadelphia*, Ser. 3, Vol. 28 (Philadelphia: 1906), 114, 117–18.

43. Peter Tinsley, *Civil War Diary*, unpublished manuscript, Wheaton College, John and Joyce Schmale Civil War Collection, 24–25.

44. Asa Sleath Hardman, "As a Union Prisoner Saw the Battle of Gettysburg," Civil War Times (August 2012), 49.

CHAPTER 6

1. William Child, *Letters from a Civil War Surgeon* (Solon, ME: Polar Bear and Company, 2001), 60.

2. Thomas Francis Galwey, *The Valiant Hours: Narrative of "Captain Brevet," an Irish-American in the Army of the Potomac* (Harrisburg, PA: Stackpole Books, 1961), 120.

3. Henry Janes, "Why Is the Profession of Killing More Generally Honored Than That of Saving Life?," Transactions of the Vermont State Medical Society (Burlington, VT: Burlington Free Press Association 1903), 187.

4. Decimus et Ultimus Barziza, *The Adventures of a Prisoner of War 1863–1864*, R. Henderson Shuffler, ed. (Austin: University of Texas, 1964), 54–55.

5. Louis C. Duncan, *The Medical Department of the United States Army in the Civil War* (Washington, DC: Surgeon General's Office, c. 1917), 262; Kent Masterson Brown, *Retreat from Gettysburg* (Chapel Hill: University of North Carolina, 2005), 384; American Battlefield Trust, accessed on February 19, 2024 at https://www.battlefields.org/learn/civil-war/battles/gettysburg. Duncan estimated 14,491 Union wounded and cited a Confederate report of 12,706 as the number of their wounded but thought that the Confederate number was certainly higher.

6. Donald B. Koonce, ed., *Doctor to the Front: Recollections of Confederate Surgeon Thomas Fanning Wood* (Knoxville: University of Tennessee Press, 2000), 108.

7. Koonce, 108.

8. Isaac Tanner Ledgers, Virginia Historical Society Collection.

9. Edmund Cody Burnett, "Letters of a Confederate Surgeon: Dr. Abner Embry McGarity, 1862–1865, Part I," *Georgia Historical Quarterly* 29, no. 2 (1945): 76–114; Confederate Service Records, NARA; Brown, 100, 128, 142. Surgeon Louis E. Gott, 49th Virginia, was left in charge, along with Surgeon Judson A. Butts, 31st Georgia; Surgeon William Lewis Reese, 6th North Carolina; and Assistant Surgeon William Mayberry Strickler, 5th Louisiana. Several surgeons of Rodes's Division were among those captured en route to Williamsport: Surgeon William T. Brewer, 43rd North Carolina, accompanying wounded Colonel Kenon of his regiment; Assistant Surgeon John Elisha Blocker, 4th Georgia; Assistant Surgeon John Henry Hicks, 20th North Carolina, and Surgeon Lauriston H. Hill, 53rd North Carolina.

10. Beverly Clifton unpublished diary, July 4, 1863, North Carolina Department of Archives and History.

11. Clifton Diary, July 5, 1863.

12. Erwin James Eldridge, Confederate Officers, NARA.

13. Unpublished Gettysburg Surgeons Database. Additional Confederate surgeons were taken prisoner at various points in the campaign, during the retreat and at other hospital locations.

14. William Riddick Whitehead, *Adventures of an American Surgeon: A 19th Century Memoir*, typescript manuscript copy, NMCWM.

15. Whitehead memoir. Taney and Whitehead knew each other from their medical studies in Paris and worked together at the division hospital, located at the Montfort House. The other surgeons of Johnson's Division who remained with the wounded were: Surgeon Dabney Herndon, 15th Louisiana; Acting Assistant Surgeon Augustus B. Sholars, 2nd Louisiana; and Surgeon Samuel Rush Sayers, 27th Virginia. Herndon and Sholars stayed with the wounded at Benner Depot; John Herbert Roper, *Repairing the March of Mars: The Civil War Diaries of John Samuel Apperson* (Macon, GA: Mercer University Press, 2002), 289–90. Note that Sayers was wounded and taken prisoner at Gettysburg (Duncan, 265). Duncan estimated that 446 of the 1,300 wounded in Johnson's Division were left at Gettysburg.

16. Duncan, 265. He estimated that 259 of the 806 wounded of Early's Division were ordered to remain in the division hospitals.

17. Assistant Surgeon Isaac Godwin, 2nd North Carolina Battalion, and Assistant Surgeon Anthony Benning Johns, 45th North Carolina, remained at the Jacob Plank Farm; Surgeon Isaac Pearson, 5th North Carolina, and John H. Purefoy, Assistant Surgeon 23rd North Carolina, remained at the Hankey Farm. At the Schriver Farm, John Moore Hayes, Surgeon 26th Alabama, was left in charge of the division hospitals along with Assistant Surgeon Robert Gordon Southall, 6th Alabama.

18. Assistant Surgeon John Tyler McLean, 33rd North Carolina; Assistant Surgeon William Miller Scarborough, 14th South Carolina; Surgeon Paul Gervais Robinson, 22nd North Carolina; and Assistant Surgeon William P. Hill, 35th Georgia.

19. Surgeon Aurelius Grigsby Emory and Assistant Surgeon Thomas Jefferson Norfleet, both of 14th Tennessee; Surgeon Benjamin Thorp Green and Assistant Surgeon Thornton Parker, both of 55th North Carolina; Hospital Steward/Assistant Surgeon William Green McCreight, 42nd Mississippi; Surgeon James Henry Southall, 55th Virginia; and Assistant Surgeon James Parks McCombs, 11th North Carolina. Llewellyn Powell Warren, Brigade Surgeon 26th North Carolina, reportedly took care of his wounded brother at Gettysburg, but his military records indicate he was captured at Williamsport on July 5th. Edward Warren, *A Doctor's Experiences on Three Continents* (Baltimore: Cushings & Bailey, 1885), 15–21.

20. Acting Assistant Surgeon Daniel Blythewood Baker and Assistant Surgeon Thomas Jefferson Vance, of the 12th Virginia; Assistant Surgeon William F. Richardson and Acting Assistant Surgeon W. F. Nance, both of 2nd Florida; Surgeon Henry Augustine Minor, 9th Alabama; Assistant Surgeon Daniel Parker, 8th Alabama; and Acting Assistant Surgeon James Robie Wood, 2nd Georgia Infantry Battalion.

21. Duncan, 259–62. U.S. reports placed the number higher at 700 wounded.

22. Remaining with him were eight other surgeons: Assistant Surgeon William Hinson Cole, 8th Georgia; Assistant Surgeon Thomas Cloman Pugh, 9th Georgia; Surgeon

William Bartleman Gregory, 2nd Georgia, Surgeon Solomon Secord, 20th Georgia; Acting Assistant Surgeon Alexander G. Carswell, 20th Georgia; Assistant Surgeon Fabius Haywood Seawell, 1st North Carolina Artillery; Assistant Surgeon Alexander Rives, 15th Alabama; and Acting Assistant Surgeon William Pentecost Powell, 5th Texas.

23. Simon Baruch, "A Surgeon's Story of Battle and Capture," *Confederate Veteran* 22 (1914): 545. Left behind with Baruch from Kershaw's Brigade were Surgeon James Furman Pearce, 8th South Carolina, and Assistant Surgeon Henry Junius Nott, 2nd South Carolina. Assistant Surgeon Thomas Young Aby serving with Alexander's Artillery Reserve also remained with the wounded at Black Horse Tavern.

24. Peter Tinsley, *Civil War Diary*, Wheaton College, John and Joyce Schmale Civil War Collection, 28, July 4, 1863. Surgeons Edward C. Rives, 28th Virginia; Alexander Spottswood Grigsby, 1st Virginia; Theodorick P. Mayo, 3rd Virginia; and John Mutius Gaines, 18th Virginia remained. Assistant surgeons remaining in Pickett's Division were Burleigh Cunningham Harrison, 56th Virginia, and William S. Nowlin, 38th Virginia. The remaining thirty-one surgeons and assistant surgeons retreated with the Army of Northern Virginia.

25. Tinsley, *Diary*, 31–32, July 5, 1863.

26. Benjamin Rohrer, unpublished diary, NMCWM.

27. Cyrus Bacon, transcript of unpublished diary, Michigan Historical Commission, July 4, 1863, 92. Although "tiffed" usually refers to a minor quarrel, Bacon is probably using it instead of "tiffled," meaning inebriated. Bacon mentions Colton's excessive drinking on several occasions in his diary.

28. Alfred Thornley Hamilton, diary, GNMP Library.

29. D. G. Brinton Thompson, "From Chancellorsville to Gettysburg, A Doctor's Diary," *Pennsylvania Magazine of History and Biography* 89, no. 3 (July 1965): 313.

30. J. W. Lyman, "Extract from a Report with Regard to the Battle of Gettysburg," in *Medical and Surgical History of the War of the Rebellion*, CXXXVI, appendix to Part I (Washington, DC: 1870), 147.

31. W. F. Breakey, "Recollections and Incidents of Medical Military Service," *War Papers Read Before the Michigan Commandery of the Military Order of the Loyal Legion of the United States*, vol. 2 (Detroit: James H. Stone & Co., 1898), 145.

32. Jonathan Letterman, "Report on the Operations of the Medical Department during the Battle of Gettysburg," October 3, 1863, in *Medical and Surgical History of the War of the Rebellion*, CXXXVI, appendix to Part I (Washington, DC: 1870), 141.

33. Francis M. Wafer, *A Surgeon in the Army of the Potomac*, ed. Cheryl A. Wells (Montreal and Kingston: McGill-Queen's University Press, 2008), 50.

34. William B. Chambers, personal papers, NARA.

35. *The War of the Rebellion: A Compilation of the Official Records of the Union and Confederate Armies* (Washington, D.C: Government Printing Office, 1880–1905), Ser. I, Vol. XXVIII, 114–19.

36. Galwey, 121.

37. Letterman, "Report," 141.

38. Duncan, 254.

39. Fielding H. Garrison, *John Shaw Billings: A Memoir* (New York: G.P. Putnam's Sons, 1913), 62, 63. Surgeon Brinton is Jeremiah Bernard Brinton, Assistant Surgeon, U.S. Volunteers, Medical Purveyor. Arrived July 4th with supplies.

40. Duncan, 235.

41. Justin Dwinelle, Manuscript Medical Report of the Second Corps hospital MSC 129, National Library of Medicine, Bethesda, Maryland, CXXXVI, quoted in Roland R. Maust, *Grappling with Death: The Union Second Corps Hospital at Gettysburg* (Dayton, OH: Morningside House Inc., 2001), 299.

42. Coco Collection GNMP Archives.

43. Garrison, 65.

44. Lyman, "Extract from a Report," 147.

45. Daniel J. Hoisington, *Gettysburg and the Christian Commission* (Minnesota: Edinborough Press, 2002), 12.

46. Ladies' Aid Society of Philadelphia, *Fifth Semi-Annual Report of the Ladies' Aid Society of Philadelphia* (Philadelphia: C. Sherman Son & Co., 1863).

47. *Portland* (ME) *Daily Press*, August 5, 1863, 2, letter dated July 27, 1863.

48. "Generous Citizens," *Philadelphia Inquirer*, July 8, 1863, 4.

49. Mary Cadwell Fisher, "A Week on Gettysburg Field," *Philadelphia Times*, December 23, 1882.

50. Andrew B. Cross, "Battle of Gettysburg and the Christian Commission," in *The War and the Christian Commission*, 1865, 7. Another wagon of supplies from York arrived on July 5th with William Latimer Small, a hardware merchant.

51. Fisher.

52. At the 1st Division hospital Surgeon George New, 7th Indiana, and Assistant Surgeon Charles A. Hamilton, 76th New York, remained. Ferdinand DeWilton Ward, Chaplain 104th New York, wrote home on July 15 describing the 2nd Division hospital staffed by Surgeon Enos Chase and Assistant Surgeon Charles Herbert Richmond, both of the 104th New York; Surgeon William B. Chambers, 97th New York; Assistant Surgeon Edmund Gaines Derby, 94th New York; and Assistant Surgeon Charles Augustus Wheeler, 12th Massachusetts. At the 3rd Division hospital Assistant Surgeon Howard Eugene Gates, 80th New York, and Assistant Surgeon Lucretius Dewey Ross, 14th Vermont, remained.

53. At the Second Corps 1st Division hospital, Surgeon Charles Squire Wood, 66th New York, was left in charge along with Surgeon Uriah Q. Davis, 148th Pennsylvania, and four Assistant Surgeons: William W. Sharp, 140th Pennsylvania; Charles T. Kelsey, 64th New York; Charles Smart, 63rd New York; and William P. Bush, 61st New York. At the 2nd Division hospital, three surgeons, Frederick, F. Burrmeister, 69th Pennsylvania, Nathan Hayward, 20th Massachusetts, and William Josiah Burr, 42nd New York, were joined by three assistant surgeons: Theodore Osgood Cornish, 15th Massachusetts, Henry Coombs Levansaler, 19th Maine, and Abraham Stokes Jones, 72nd Pennsylvania. In addition to Surgeon Henry McKindree McAbee, 4th Ohio, medical staff left at the 3rd Division hospital included Surgeon Frederick Wolf, 39th New York, Assistant Surgeon Joseph McCullough, 1st Delaware, and Assistant Surgeon Washington Akin, 125th New York. Maust, 334–35, 453.

54. Christopher E. Loperfido, ed., *Death, Disease, and Life at War: The Civil War Letters of Surgeon James D. Benton* (El Dorado Hills, CA: Savas Beatie, 2018), 8. Benton's account conflicts with a letter of Hospital Steward Merrick who wrote on July 6th that Dr. J. L. Brenton was ordered to the Regiment that morning. He may not have left immediately. Maust, 368.

55. Third Corps 1st Division surgeons were Assistant Surgeon James Davis Watson, 3rd Maine, Surgeon William Watson, 105th Pennsylvania, Surgeon David Sterent Hays, 110th Pennsylvania. Surgeons from the 2nd Division included Surgeon Edward Andem Whitson, 1st Massachusetts, Assistant Surgeon Thomas Crozier Jr., 16th Massachusetts, Assistant Surgeon Sylvanus Bunton, 2nd New Hampshire, Assistant Surgeon Charles W. Hunt, 12th New Hampshire, and Surgeon DeWitt Clinton Hough, 7th New Jersey,

56. Staff for the 1st Division included Surgeon Zabdiel Boylston Jr., 32nd Massachusetts, Assistant Surgeon William Fleming Breakey, 16th Michigan, and Surgeon Joseph Thomas, 118th Pennsylvania. Some surgeons succumbed to exhaustion and/or disease. Boylston, for example, was relieved on July 7th due to temporary blindness. Assistant Surgeon Cyrus Bacon, 2nd U.S. Volunteers, recorded in his diary that six surgeons were left at the Fifth Corps 2nd Division hospital, including himself, Assistant Surgeon John Billings, 7th U.S., Surgeon Joseph A. E. Reed, 155th Pennsylvania, and Surgeon Thomas M. Flandreau, 146th New York. Assistant Surgeon Edward Breneman, 12th U.S., soon rejoined his regiment, while Assistant Surgeon Edward Thomas Whittingham, 3rd U.S., and Assistant Surgeon William R. Ramsey, 1st U.S., remained until August. The staff of the 3rd Division hospital included Surgeon Joseph Augustus Phillips, 9th Pennsylvania; Surgeon Benjamin Rohrer, 10th Pennsylvania; Assistant Surgeon Evan Owen Jackson, 2nd Pennsylvania; and Assistant Surgeon Henry A. Grim, 12th Pennsylvania. Bacon Diary, Michigan Historical Commission.

57. At the 1st Division hospital, Surgeon Lewis Williams Oakley, 2nd New Jersey, and Surgeon Joseph Davis Osborne, 4th New Jersey, remained on duty. Surgeon Charles Marcellus Chandler, 6th Vermont, remained with the 2nd Division. Surgeons from the 3rd Division included Surgeon Louis Manly Emmanuel, 82nd Pennsylvania, Assistant Surgeon John Phillips Richardson, 82nd Pennsylvania, Assistant Surgeon Samuel Burton Sturdevant, 139th Pennsylvania, and Assistant Surgeon Franklin Grube, U.S. Battery.

58. Medical staff at 11th Corps hospitals included Surgeon Jacob Young Cantwell, 82nd Ohio; Assistant Surgeon William Henry Ginkinger, 27th Pennsylvania; Assistant Surgeon John Mortimer Crawe, 157th New York; Assistant Surgeon William Augusta Barry, 75th Pennsylvania; Surgeon Robert Hubbard, 17th Connecticut; Assistant Surgeon Dwight Washington Day, 154th New York; Assistant Surgeon Daniel Graffus Caldwell, 74th Pennsylvania; Surgeon Henry Kauffman Neff, 153rd Pennsylvania; Assistant Surgeon Amos Shaw Jr., 41st New York. Assistant Surgeon Abraham Stout, 153rd Pennsylvania, remained on duty at the Public School in Gettysburg.

59. Assistant Surgeon Henry Clay May, 145th New York, and Assistant Surgeon Joseph Addison Freeman, 13th New Jersey, remained with the 1st Division. Surgeon Joseph Adam Smith, 29th Pennsylvania, and Assistant Surgeon David M. Brubaker, 109th Pennsylvania, remained with the 2nd Division.

60. *Journal of the Michigan State Medical Society* 4, (1905): 227. Surgeon John P. Wilson, 5th Michigan Cavalry, was with wounded at Hanover but was stricken with typhoid fever and remained ill at Gettysburg until he was removed to Annapolis for medical treatment. He was one of the many surgeons and caregivers who became ill from the contaminated water and unhealthy conditions in the aftermath of the battle.

61. William W. Potter, *One Surgeon's Private War: Dr. William W. Potter of the 57th NY*, eds. John Michael Priest et al. (Shippensburg, PA: White Mane Publishing Company, 1996), 74.

62. Daniel Holt, *A Surgeon's Civil War: The Letters and Diaries of Daniel M. Holt, M.D*, eds. James M. Greiner, Janet L Coryell, and James R. Smither (Kent, OH: Kent State University Press, 1994), 124.

CHAPTER 7

1. Sophronia Bucklin, *In Hospital and Camp* (Philadelphia: J.E. Potter & Company, 1869), 79.

2. *Philadelphia Inquirer,* July 10, 1863, 1. "Colonel Smith" is Capt. Wilbur Smith who was acting provost marshal between July 7 and 9. Quartermaster General Montgomery Meigs sent him to Gettysburg from Washington to oversee the recovery of battlefield arms and equipment.

3. *Lewistown Gazette*, July 22, 1863, G. R. Frysinger letter dated July 17, 1863.

4. Henrietta Stratton Jaquette, *South After Gettysburg, Letters of Cornelia Hancock* (New York: Thomas Y. Crowell Company, 1956), 7–8.

5. Jonathan Letterman, "Report on the Operations of the Medical Department during the Battle of Gettysburg," October 3, 1863, in *Medical and Surgical History of the War of the Rebellion,* appendix to part I, CXXX (Washington, DC: U.S. Surgeon General's Office, 1870–1888), 140.

6. Bennett A. Clements, *Memoir of Jonathan Letterman Reprinted from the Journal of the Military Service Institution* IV, no. 15 (September 1883) (New York: G.P. Putnam's Sons 1883), 13, 17.

7. J. H. Douglas, Document No. 71, "Report on the Operations of the Sanitary Commission During and After the Battle at Gettysburg," August 15, 1863, in *Documents of the US Sanitary Commission*, Vol. 2 (New York: 1866), 20, 208, 210.

8. Bushrod Washington James, *Echoes of Battle* (Philadelphia: T. Coates & Co., 1895), 101–4.

9. Gerard A. Patterson, *Debris of Battle: The Wounded of Gettysburg* (Mechanicsburg, PA: Stackpole Books, 1997), 211, letter of resignation to U.S. Secretary of War Stanton.

10. Cyrus Bacon transcript of unpublished diary, July 6, July 8, 1863, Michigan Historical Commission.

11. Bacon transcript, July 12, July 20, 1863. In addition to Bacon, the following surgeons were on duty at the Fifth Corps 2nd Division hospital: Surgeon Thomas M. Flandreau, 146th New York and surgeon in charge of 2nd Division; Surgeon Joseph A. E. Reed, 155th Pennsylvania; Assistant Surgeon Edward Thomas Whittingham, 3rd U.S.; Assistant Surgeon John Shaw Billings, 7th U.S.; Assistant Surgeon William R. Ramsey, 11th U.S.

12. Paul Fatout, ed., *Letters of a Civil War Surgeon* (West Lafayette, IN: Purdue University Press, 1996), 109–10. Five surgeons have been identified from the 2nd Division, but Watson may be referring to the total number of operators from the 3rd Corps. Altogether the Corps estimated about 2,500 wounded in 1st and 2nd Divisions.

13. Simon Baruch, "A Surgeon's Story of Battle and Capture," *Confederate Veteran* 22 (1914): 546.

14. Douglas, "Report on Gettysburg," dated July 22, 1863, in *Documents of Sanitary Commission*, 171.

15. John Y. Foster, "Four Days at Gettysburg," *Harper's New Monthly Magazine* 28, no. 165 (February 1864): 381–88.

16. Letterman, Gettysburg Report.

17. The following were dispatched to Gettysburg: Medical Inspectors John Mack Cuyler and Edward Perry Vollum; Surgeons John H. Brinton and Dewitt Clinton Peters; and Assistant Surgeons William Williams Keen, Park Holland Loring, and William Norris. Acting assistant surgeons included: Thomas Forrest Betton, Benjamin F. Butcher, Charles Fuller, Edward Francis Guth, Henry Hartshorne, Hugh Lenox Hodge, John B. McCaffrey, Silas Weir Mitchell, James Cheston Morris, John H. Packard, James Knight Shivers, A. B. Stonelake, William Henry True, Charles H. Von Tagen, T. H. Walker, George Mason Ward, and William Miller Welch.

18. U.S. War Department, *The War of Rebellion: A Compilation of the Official Records of the Union and Confederate Armies* (OR) 27, part 1 (Washington, DC: Government Printing Office, 1880–1901), 26; Roland R. Maust, *Grappling with Death: The Union Second Corps Hospital at Gettysburg* (Dayton, OH: Morningside House Inc., 2001), 440.

19. Maust, 539; OR 27 part 1, 27.

20. John Hill Brinton, *Personal Memoirs of John H. Brinton: Civil War Surgeon*, 1861–1865, (Carbondale: Southern Illinois University Press, 1996), 240, 246.

21. William Fisher Norris, manuscript letters, Gettysburg July 11, 1863, College of Physicians and Surgeons, Philadelphia, Cage 10a463.

22. Norris letter, July 15, 1863.

23. W. W. Keen, *Transactions of the College of Physicians of Philadelphia* 25 (1905), 87–113; 108–9.

24. OR 27, part 1, 24–25.

25. Maust, 503. Quote from John Dooley Diary, 121.

26. Justin Dwinelle, "Manuscript Report of the Second Corps hospital during the Battle of Gettysburg," National Library of Medicine, Bethesda, Maryland, MSC 129. Quoted in Maust, 401. J. H or T. H. Walker, Acting Assistant Surgeon; James Cheston Morris, Acting Assistant Surgeon. Identity of Norris not confirmed, but possibly William Fisher Norris. A large contingent of civilian surgeons arrived from Pittsburgh and Philadelphia soon after the battle.

27. Letterman, Gettysburg Report.

28. Maust, 420; Dwinelle hospital report.

29. Maust, 504; OR 27 part 1, 25.

30. Charles J. Stille, *History of the United States Sanitary Commission* (Philadelphia: J.B. Lippincott & Co., 1866), 168. USSC Relief Department was in operation by

September 1861 with depots in New York, Boston, Philadelphia, Washington, Cincinnati, and Wheeling.

31. Stille, 151, 189.

32. George G. Edgerly; Samuel Bacon Jr.; Nicholas Murray; John G. Bowers; J. Warner Johnson; James Gall Jr.; Franklin Enoch Paige. Henry P. Dechert took charge of the storehouse assisted by agents Hoag, Edgerly, Bacon, Murray, Bowers, Johnson, Gall, and Paige.

33. Frederick Law Olmsted, "Preliminary Report: Operations of the Sanitary Commission with the Army of the Potomac, Jul 23, 1863," in *Documents of the U.S. Sanitary Commission*, Vol. 2 (New York: 1866).

34. USSC, *Sanitary Commission of the United States Army: A Succinct Narrative of Its Works and Purposes* (New York: U.S. Sanitary Commission, 1864), 152–55. Dr. Robert William Hooper of Boston was assisted by Joshua Boylston Clar of New Hampshire; David R. Hawkins of Media, Pennsylvania; Joseph Shippen of Pittsburgh; and Oliver Crosby Bullard of Baltimore, as well as Mr. Murray, Edmund Mills Barton, and two unnamed Germans from Washington, DC, who volunteered to cook.

35. Georgeanna Woolsey, *Three Weeks at Gettysburg* (New York: Anson D.F. Randolph, 1863), 4.

36. USSC, *A Succinct Narrative of Its Works and Purposes*, 155–56.

37. Other women who worked closely with the Sanitary Commission at various locations included Sophronia Bucklin, Rebecca Caldwell, Helen Louise Gilson, Jane Kirby Senseny, and Sarah E. Hooper. Many like Georgeanna Woolsey were veterans of the Sanitary Commission transport ships in 1862 or had served as nurses after other battles.

38. USSC, *A Succinct Narrative of Its Works and Purposes*, 157. Mr. Dooley from the Directory Office was assisted by Charles Stille, William Struthers, James Wright Hazlehurst, possibly William Dulles, David Beitler Tracy from Philadelphia, and Hosford, Myers, and Braman from New York.

39. U.S. Christian Commission, *2nd Annual Report for 1863*, April 1864, 17.

40. Daniel J. Hoisington, *Gettysburg and the Christian Commission* (Minnesota: Edinborough Press, 2002), 9.

41. USCC, *2nd Annual Report for 1863*, 17; Chamberlain account, 67.

42. Clarissa Jones pension file, NARA; Maust, 411.

43. Andrew B. Cross, "Battle of Gettysburg and the Christian Commission," in *The War and the Christian Commission* (1865), 27.

44. Baruch, 545–48. The Howard party consisted of Ann Harrison Howard, her cousin, Alice Key Howard, and their chaperone Mary Lewis. The Howard family were staunch Confederate supporters. Charles Howard and his son Frank Key Howard were imprisoned at Fort McHenry in 1862, and Charles Ridgely Howard, Ann Howard's brother, was one of the founders of the pro-slavery Memorial Episcopal Church. Baltimore sisters Melissa Baker and Olivia Baker Warfield and their niece Jane B. Converse were described as "refined, cultivated, elegant women," who "ministered unto the wounded prisoners" of Hood's division at the Plank farm.

45. See Edward Steers, *The Trial: The Assassination of President Lincoln and the Trial of the Conspirators* (University Press of Kentucky, 2003); and Edward Steers Jr. *Blood on*

the Moon: The Assassination of Abraham Lincoln (University Press of Kentucky, 2001) for information on Lincoln assassination conspirators. W. C. Ward, "Incidents and Personal Experiences on the Battlefield at Gettysburg," *Confederate Veteran* 8 (1900): 349.

46. *United States Christian Commission Second Report of the Committee of Maryland September 1, 1863* (Baltimore: Sherwood & Co. 1863), 48.

47. U.S. Christian Commission Second Report, iv, 81. Christian Commission staff included field agent Frederic Eichelberger Shearer Esq.; assistant field agent and field inspector Rev. Edward Franklin Williams; and disbursing agent James Russell Miller. Receiving agent Robert Grier McCreary Esq. of Gettysburg led a local volunteer committee of the Christian Commission in Gettysburg that was active before, during, and after the battle. Members of Gettysburg's Christian Commission included: R. G. McCreary, Robert F. P. Bucher, Martin Luther Stoever, John Lawrence Schick, Abraham Essick, Henry Graham Finney, James Fahnestock, and Miss Patten among others.

48. U.S. Christian Commission Second Report, 80.

49. U.S. Christian Commission Second Report, 69. Muller and his squad were all from Baltimore: James E. Swindell was a glassblower; Edward Woodward and his son James F. Woodward were gunsmiths.

50. *Baltimore Sun*, July 6, 1863; *Pittsburgh Daily Post*, July 14, 1863; *Philadelphia Inquirer*, July 17, 1863, 1; The Adams Express Company, 150 years, accessed on May 18, 2024 at https://www.adamsfunds.com/wp-content/uploads/adams_history.pdf.

51. *Baltimore Sun*, July 10, 1863. Assisting Herring were Baltimore doctors Edwin Thomas, John A. Doyle, and Dewitt Clinton Morgan. John M. Smith, Thomas Norris, W. Harris, and W. H. Horner were also mentioned for their work with the Adams Express Company Ambulance Corps.

52. John Shaw Billings, "Medical Reminiscences of the Civil War," *Transactions of the College of Physicians of Philadelphia*, Ser. 3, Vol. 27 (1905), 119.

53. *Documentary Journal of the General Assembly of the State of Indiana,* (Indiana: State Printer, 1865), 293; Obituary, *Presbyterian Banner*, November 20, 1902, 29; Charlotte McKay, *Stories of Hospital and Camp* (Philadelphia: Claxton, Remsen & Haffelfinger, 1876), 50.

54. Mike Pride, *No Place for a Woman: Harriet Dame's Civil War* (Kent, OH: Kent State University Press, 2022), 126–27.

55. *Detroit Free Press*, July 13, 1; July 18, 3. James Buchanan Shearer, William Jenison Jr., Dr. James A. Brown, and Dr. Louis C. Davenport. Two nurses, Harriet Jane Barnard and Elmira Maria Brainard.

56. Jane Augusta Gunn, *Memorial Sketches of Dr. Moses Gunn* (Chicago: WT Keener, 1889), 167–68; *Detroit Free Press*, July 18, 1863, 1; Mayor William C. Duncan, aldermen Joseph Hoek and James McGonegal, and several members of the Detroit Board of Trade reportedly visited the battlefield.

57. *New York Tribune*, July 15, 1863, 2.

58. Hazard Arnold Potter resigned as surgeon of 50th Engineers in 1862, "Volunteered his services at battle of Gettysburg where he treated a large number of cases and accompanied many sick and wounded to the NY City Hospital." *An Elaborate History and Geneaology of Ballous in America,* ed. Adin Ballou (E. L. Freeman & Son, 1888),

511. Theodore Dimon (transcript of report on Gettysburg and Civil War diaries, Private Collection and GNMP).

59. Maust, 648. Dimon diary, "From Auburn to Antietam," transcript GNMP. The supervising surgeon, James L. Farley, surgeon of the 84th New York, known as the "Fighting 14th" after its original designation as the 14th Militia, was popular with his men, but shared their fondness for alcohol. Dimon stepped in and went to work for several days at the hotel to improve conditions until it was consolidated with another facility.

60. Theodore Dimon Report to John Seymour, August 1, transcript, GNMP.

61. *New York Herald*, July 6, 1863, 10, "The wounded in the Recent Battles" Letter to Surgeon General Hammond dated July 5, Harrisburg, from Governor R. G. Curtin.

62. Maust, 332; NARA Record Group 112, Vol. 35, July 5, 1863; *Pittsburgh Post-Gazette*, July 7, 1863, 3.

63. Names of Pittsburgh surgeons included: Joseph Abel; Alexander W. Alcorn; Addison and Biddle Arthurs; Tristram Brown; John Campbell; Henry Tarring Coffey; Daniel Cornman; Marcus S. Hulings; William D. Kearns; Alexander Guy McCandless; George and George Latimer McCook; Nesbit McDonald; Robert B. Mowry; Andrew Patrick; John Perchment; Charles E. Poe; Benjamin Wiley Preston; Thomas Wilson Shaw; William M. Simcox; Ferdinand Venn; Albert Gustav Walter; John Wilson; Barnett A. Wolfe; Hugh Wright. *Pittsburgh Gazette*, July 6, 1863, 3. Also mentioned: John and John H. Dickson; Thomas J. Gallaher in *Under the Maltese Cross, Antietam to Appomattox: The Loyal Uprising in Western Pennsylvania, 1861–1865* (Pittsburgh: 155th Regimental Association 1910), 19.

64. Military Dispatches, PHMC Archives, 1861–1867. Series 19.181. July 9–31, 1863.

65. Local Gettysburg physicians included Dr. Henry S. Huber, Drs. Robert and Charles Horner, Dr. John W. C. O'Neal, Dr. James Cress, and Dr. D. William Taylor.

66. The group from Phoenixville included Rebecca Lane Pennypacker Price, Eliza Hinkle Spear, Martha M. Jones, Elizabeth Buckwalter Pennypacker, Esther Buckwalter, Catherine K. Ashenfelter, Anne S. White, Melissa Pennypacker. Historical Society of Pennsylvania, *Newsletter,* September 1993.

67. *Philadelphia Inquirer,* July 6, 1863, 4.

68. Mrs. Edmund A. Souder, *Leaves from the Battle-field of Gettysburg* (Philadelphia: Caxton Press of C. Sherman, Son & Co., 1864), 7.

69. Souder left Philadelphia on July 13th with Julia Stevens Raymond (Mrs. James L.) Claghorn, Miss Anna Raymond, Mrs. Claghorn's sister, and Martha Reeve (Mrs. Joseph H.) Campion. They were accompanied by Rev. George Bringhurst, a Philadelphia delegate of the Christian Commission. Mrs. Curtis who earlier traveled with John W. Claghorn was Souder's sister-in-law.

70. Theresa Kaminski, *Dr. Mary Walker's Civil War* (Guilford, CT: Lyons Press, 2020), 89–91. Esther Kersey Painter traveled with her husband Joseph Painter, of the 7th New Jersey. Dr. Walker and the Painters were traveling together on the way to Gettysburg in June 1863. Farnham, Painter, and Walker had all studied medicine and were active in the nineteenth-century health movement to reform women's dress by abandoning corsets and adopting the so-called "Bloomer" outfit.

71. Peter Tinsley, unpublished diary, July 10, 1863, Wheaton College, John and Joyce Schmale Civil War Collection. Tinsley was on his way to the Second Corps Hospital to visit Confederate wounded and the "She Doctor" he described walking ahead of him was almost certainly nurse Cornelia Hancock.

72. Frederick Law Olmsted to Edward Lawrence Godkin, Frederick, Maryland, July 15, 1863, manuscript letter, Houghton Library, Harvard.

73. Scott Hartwig, "Eliza W. Farnham–An Unsung Heroine of Gettysburg," March 2, 2012, GNMP. Accessed May 18, 2024 at https://npsgnmp.wordpress.com/2012/03/02/eliza-w-farnham-an-unsung-heroine-of-gettysburg/.

74. Jaquette, 16.

75. *Baltimore Sun*, July 24, 1863, 2, letter dated July 22, 1863, to G. S. Griffith, Christian Commission, from I. O. Sloan.

CHAPTER 8

1. Letters and diaries at first refer to the hospital simply as the "General Hospital." Cornelia Hancock's letters are written from "General Hospital" until August 17 when she first uses "Camp Letterman, General Hospital."

2. U.S. War Department, *The War of Rebellion: A Compilation of the Official Records of the Union and Confederate Armies* (Washington, DC: Government Printing Office, 1880–1901), OR Series I, 27 (1): 27.

3. Dr. Theodore Dimon's report to John F. Seymour of New York, transcript, GNHP, 11–13.

4. Dimon Report, 5–7.

5. Mrs. Edmund A. Souder, *Leaves from the Battle-field of Gettysburg* (Philadelphia: Caxton Press of C. Sherman, Son & Co., 1864), 56.

6. Souder, 57.

7. George Gordon Meade, ed., *The Life and Letters of George Gordon Meade, Major-General United States Army*, Vol. II (New York: Charles Scribner's Sons, 1913), 120.

8. OR Series I, 27(1): 620.

9. OR Series I, 27(1): 700.

10. OR Series I, 27(1): 706.

11. A graduate of the Vermont Medical College in 1850, Chamberlain served with the 10th Massachusetts Infantry from 1861 until he was commissioned as an officer in the U.S. Volunteers Medical Staff in May 1863. Dr. Theodore Dimon's report to John F. Seymour of New York notes that the site is under construction on July 16th. Dimon Report, 9–11.

12. Andrew B. Cross, "Battle of Gettysburg and the Christian Commission," in *The War and the Christian Commission* (1865), 19.

13. Henrietta Stratton Jaquette, ed., *South After Gettysburg: Letters of Cornelia Hancock 1863–1868* (New York: Thomas Y. Crowell Company, 1956), 20.

14. William F. Norris Letters, College of Physicians and Surgeons, Philadelphia, Norris to his father, Gettysburg, July 26, 1863.

15. Dr. William F. Breakey, "Recollections and Incidents of Military Service," in *War Papers Read Before the Michigan Commandery of the Military Order of the Loyal Legion of the United States* (Detroit: James H. Stone & Co., 1898), 147.

16. Gettysburg Battlefield guide, Phil Letchak tour of Camp Letterman recorded in 2008, https://www.gettysburgdaily.com/camp-letterman-part-1/; *United States Christian Commission Second Report of the Committee of Maryland September 1, 1863* (Baltimore: Sherwood & Co., 1863), 27. Some division surgeons, like Breakey, may have doubled as both division and ward surgeons.

17. Breakey, 147.

18. Sophronia Bucklin, *In Hospital and Camp* (Philadelphia: J.E. Potter & Company, 1869), 80–81. Bucklin overstates the number of tents. Other accounts are considerably lower, but she may be referring to the number of single tents.

19. Norris Letters, William F. Norris to his father, Gettysburg, July 26, 1863.

20. Norris Letters, July 26, 1863.

21. Souder, 61.

22. Souder, 61–62.

23. Dimon Report, 17.

24. Gregory A. Coco, *A Vast Sea of Misery* (Gettysburg, PA: Thomas Publications, 1988), 168; Quote from Jacob Shenkel diary; Cyrus Bacon transcript of unpublished diary, Michigan Historical Commission, July 31, 1863.

25. Souder, 61.

26. Clarissa Jones, manuscript letters, NMCWM, Frederick, Maryland, August 5, 1863.

27. Jaquette, 19.

28. Norris Letters, July 27, 1863. Confederate patient Lt. Elisha S. Wildman (1828–1879) of the 28th Virginia was wounded July 3rd and had his right leg amputated July 7th by James Fulton Grove, Surgeon 3rd Michigan, at 3rd Corps Hosp; transferred to Letterman July 27; received West's Building Baltimore October 22; sent to Point Lookout January 23, 1864; exchanged April 27, 1864. NARA Confederate records.

29. Peter Tinsley Civil War Diary, Wheaton College, John and Joyce Schmale Civil War Collection, July 24, 1863. Theodore Thompson Tate (1831–1915), Surgeon 3rd Pennsylvania Cavalry, was left in charge of Confederate wounded at the Public School. A group of physicians from Pittsburgh arrived in Gettysburg July 7th. Among them were Dr. George L. McCook, affiliated with the Sanitary Commission, and Drs. John and Joseph Dickson representing the Christian Commission.

30. S. Weir Mitchell Scrapbook, College of Physicians of Philadelphia. His list of Letterman surgeons included nine Confederate surgeons: Daniel Baker, 12th Virginia; J. M. Hays, 26th Alabama; F. A. Means, 11th Georgia [Thomas Alexander Means]; H. A. Minor, 8th Alabama [9th Alabama]; W. F. Nance, 2nd Florida; D. H. Parker; W. F. Richardson, 9th Alabama [2nd Florida]; R. G. Sethall [Robert Gordon Southall, 6th Alabama]; F. J. Vance, 12th Virginia.

31. Decimus et Ultimus Barziza, *The Adventures of A Prisoner of War 1863–1864*, R. Henderson Shuffler, ed. (Austin: University of Texas, 1964), 57.

32. Tricia Runzel, "Gettysburg College: A Memorial Landmark," *Gettysburg Compiler*, December 11, 2012. Accessed May 21, 2024 at https://gettysburgcompiler.org/2012/12/11/gettysburg-college-a-memorial-landmark/.

33. Frederick Pratt Letters, August 4, 1863, private collection.

34. Pratt Letters, August 8, 1863.

35. Coco Collection, GNMP Box 14, Henry Janes letter, August 17, 1863.

36. *Adams Sentinel*, August 18, 1863, 2; Gregory A. Coco, *A Strange and Blighted Land: Gettysburg the Aftermath of a Battle* (El Dorado Hills, CA: Savas Beatie, 2017), 228. Coco describes 200 patients at the Seminary, including one hundred Confederates, thirty at the Railroad "express office," and seventy at the Union Schoolhouse.

37. William R. Kiefer, *History of the One Hundred and Fifty-third Regiment Pennsylvania Volunteers Infantry* (Easton, PA: Press of the Chemical Publishing Co., 1909), 131–32. Assistant Surgeon Abraham Clemens Stout was in charge of Union wounded at the Public School for three weeks until they were removed to Harrisburg around July 24. Surgeon John Henry Beech, 24th Michigan, remained at the Express Office Hospital until August 19th.

38. Jonathan Letterman, "Report on the Operations of the Medical Department during the Battle of Gettysburg," October 3, 1863, *Medical History of the War of the Rebellion*, appendix to part I, CXXX, 140.

39. King began his military career in 1837 after graduating from the University of Pennsylvania in 1833. He served in the Mexican War as an assistant surgeon and held various posts in the West prior to the Civil War. In 1861 he became medical director of the Army of Northeastern Virginia, overseeing the disastrous medical response at the battle of Bull Run. He served as medical director of the Department of the Susquehanna from June to October 1863, and continued in the Army until his retirement in 1882.

40. J. R. Smith to W. S. King, July 18, 1863, Office of the Surgeon General, Letters and Endorsements Sent to Medical Officers, Vol. 4, Record Group 112, NARA; Gerard A. Patterson, *Debris of Battle: The Wounded of Gettysburg* (Mechanicsburg, PA: Stackpole Books, 1997), 160–61.

41. Personal Papers of Robert Horner and Henry Huber, NARA Records.

42. E. S. [Edward S.] Dunster to W. S. King, July 28, 1863, Office of the Surgeon General, Letters and Endorsements Sent to Medical Officers, Vol. 4, Record Group 112, NARA; Patterson, 160–61.

43. Neff's role at Gettysburg remains unclear. In Neff's explanation, he was at the battle of Gettysburg as surgeon of the 153rd Pennsylvania and assigned to the 11th Corps hospital by Medical Director Jonathan Letterman. But the account of his assistant surgeon, Abraham Stout, indicates that after being taken prisoner at Chancellorsville, sent to Libby prison, and released, Neff was recuperating at home in Huntingdon, Pennsylvania, and did not rejoin the regiment. It is quite possible that Neff arrived in Gettysburg soon after the battle and was assigned to the 11th Corps hospital until July 18th. Kiefer, 131–32; Henry K. Neff Personal Papers NARA, letter December 3, 1863.

44. James Ross Reily, Personal Papers, NARA.

45. Coco Collection, GNMP, King to Janes, August 29, 1863.

46. Jaquette, 22.

47. Coco Collection, GNMP, King to Janes, August 5, 1863.

48. Coco Collection, GNMP, Janes correspondence August 18, 1863. Surgeons remaining were: C. N. Chamberlin, U.S. Volunteers; L. W. Oakley, 2nd New Jersey; W. H. Rulison, 9th New York Cavalry; J. Osborn, 4th New Jersey. Assistant surgeons remaining were William Brakey [Breakey], 16th Michigan; H. C. Macy [May], 145th New York; L. B. Sturdevant, 139th Pennsylvania; and J. B. Brinton, U.S. Army.

49. Coco Collection, GNMP, Janes to King, August 17, 1863.

50. Coco Collection, GNMP, King to Janes, August 11, 1863.

51. Coco Collection, GNMP Letter from Janes October 15, 1863. James Brayton Carpenter (1819–1895) graduated from Castleton Medical School in 1847 and served as assistant surgeon in the 35th and 73rd New York.

52. Contract surgeons assigned to Seminary hospital included: James R. Reily (July 27–September 8); John B. McCaffrey (July 11–September 8); Charles Horner (July 23–September 8); Robert Horner (July 24–October 23), Henry S. Huber (July 23–September 8); Henry Leaman (August 1–September 5), John Nice Jacobs (July 26–September 5), W. M. Welch (?–November), and Charles Fuller (unknown dates). Robert Horner, Leaman, and Welch later served at Letterman.

53. Breakey, 147.

54. Christian Commission Second Report of the Committee of Maryland, 27, 32, https://archive.org/details/repo2unit.

55. Coco, *Strange and Blighted Land*, 228. Although Coco states that the nine Confederate surgeons were under Surgeon L. H. Hill of Daniel's Brigade, the military records of Lauristin Hardin Hill, Surgeon 53rd North Carolina, show that he was received at Fort Monroe from Baltimore on August 6th. NARA. The Confederate surgeons on duty at Letterman from August until October included three surgeons (John Moore Hayes, 26th Alabama; Thomas Alexander Means, 11th Georgia; and Henry Augustine Minor, 9th Alabama), four assistant surgeons (Daniel Parker, 8th Alabama; William F. Richardson, 2nd Florida; Robert Gordon Southall, 6th Alabama; and Thomas Jefferson Vance, 12th Virginia), and two acting assistant surgeons (Daniel Blythewood Baker, 12th Virginia, and W. F. Nance, 2nd Florida). Six of them were from Anderson's Division of the Confederate Third Corps, two from the Second Corps, and one from the First Corps. Unpublished Gettysburg Surgeons Database.

56. Union surgeons at Letterman included Louis Manly Emanuel, 82nd Pennsylvania; Lewis Williams Oakley, 2nd New Jersey; Joseph Davis Osborne, 4th New Jersey—all of the 6th Corps—and Henry Kauffman Neff, formerly Surgeon 155th Pennsylvania; they all served as division surgeons at Letterman. Assistant surgeons included: David M. Brubaker, 109th Pennsylvania; William Fleming Breakey, 16th Michigan; Charles Alexander Hamilton, 76th New York; Henry Clay May, 145th New York; Samuel Burton Sturdevant, 139th Pennsylvania; Hiram Dana Vosburgh, 8th New York Cavalry; and James Davis Watson, 3rd Maine. Unpublished Gettysburg Surgeons Database.

57. Documented acting assistant surgeons included George Washington Boughman, Benjamin F. Butcher, James Brayton Carpenter, Charles Stockton Gauntt, Alfred Seymour Gibbs, Daniel R. Good, Edward F. Guth, Michael Abbott Hanley, William L. Hays, Robert Horner, William B. Jones, John J. Kelly, Egon A. Koerper, Henry

Leaman, John Thorn Laning, Peter Schindel Leisenring, Edwin G. Martin, John Alexander McArthur, Alex McWilliams, Henry K. Neff, James K. Newcombe, John Rowand, Abraham B. Shekell, James K. Shivers, Thomas Tucker Smiley, Francis Gurney Smith, Thomas Smith, Albert B. Stonelake, H. H. Sutton, Ellis P. Townsend, Thomas H. Walker, Ralph Suckett Lee Walsh, George Mason Ward, William M. Welch, James Henry Wilson, Francis Wyncoop. Unpublished Gettysburg Surgeons Database.

58. Jaquette, 19.

59. USSC, *The United States Sanitary Commission: A Sketch of Its Purposes and Its Work* (Boston: Little, Brown and Company, 1863), 145. The 300 tents may be an overstatement or refer to 150 double tents.

60. Breakey, 148.

61. Henry Janes Register, University of Vermont Special Collections, 289.

62. Janes Register, 100.

63. Jaquette, 23.

64. Bucklin, 83.

65. *Adams Sentinel*, July 21, 1863, 2.

66. Souder, 59; Cyrus Bacon Diary, August 4, 1863.

67. *Adams Sentinel*, August 18, 1863.

68. Jaquette, 20, letter dated August 6, 1863.

69. Pratt, August 28, 1863.

70. Letter from Col. William Hoffman, Commissary General of Prisoners, to Henry Janes August 27, 1863. University of Virginia, Small Collection.

71. Henry Janes Collection, University of Vermont Special Collections.

72. Henry Janes letter, December 5, 1863, Cowans Auctions, privately owned.

73. USSC, *Documents of the U.S. Sanitary Commission*, Vol. 2 (New York: 1866), 160.

74. USSC, *The United States Sanitary Commission: A Sketch of Its Purposes and Its Work* (Boston: Little, Brown and Company, 1863), 146.

75. *United States Christian Commission 2nd Annual Report for 1863*, April 1864, 85. Christian Commission delegates who remained at Letterman included Superintendent Matthias Evans Willing, Andrew Boyd Cross, James Peter Ludlow, and Charles H. Keener. The Reverend George Junkin, father-in-law of Stonewall Jackson, remained for nineteen days. Isaac Oliver Sloan, one of the first Christian Commission delegates to arrive immediately after the battle, continued at the Seminary Hospital until the end of August.

76. Cross, 20.

77. Bucklin, 101.

78. Jaquette, 24; Bucklin, 98.

79. Jaquette, 21.

80. Bucklin, 81.

81. Jaquette, 21, 26.

82. Bucklin, 102.

83. Henry Janes Papers, University of Virginia.

84. Jaquette, 26.

85. Bucklin, 100.

86. Franklin Jacob Fogel Schantz, "Recollections of Visitations at Gettysburg after the Great Battle in July 1863," *Lebanon County Historical Society* XIII, no. 6 (1963): 275–303.

87. Michael Dreese, *The Hospital on Seminary Ridge at the Battle of Gettysburg* (Jefferson, NC: McFarland & Co., 2002), 142.

88. Breakey, 149.

89. Anna Morris Ellis Holstein, *Three Years in Field Hospitals of the Army of the Potomac* (Philadelphia: J.B. Lippincott and Co., 1867), 50.

90. Holstein, 50; *Adams Sentinel*, September 22, 1863, 2.

91. Holstein, 51–52; *Adams Sentinel*, November 3, 1863. Holstein provided an excellent description of the flag event: "To two of the ladies most active in procuring it, was given the pleasure of conveying it to Gettysburg. Many of the wounded knew when it arrived, and the arrangements being made to receive it; at their request, the flag (twenty-five feet in length) was carried through the streets of the hospital, then taken to 'Round Top.' All who could leave the hospital, officers, ladies, and soldiers—joined the procession. A large concourse of persons manifested, by their presence, the pleasure they felt in the event. Appropriate and eloquent addresses were delivered by David Wills, Esq. of Gettysburg; J.T. Seymour of New York; and Surgeon H.C. May of the 145th New York Vols."

92. Holstein, 53.

93. *Adams Sentinel*, November 10, 1863, 2.

94. Breakey's account confirms that while he was ill with fever, he was injured by a fall when he rushed "in the night to a case of secondary hemorrhage, and was disabled for weeks after, being confined to my bed with serious illness. I rejoined my regiment on its return to the State to re-enlist and re-organize, leaving Washington the night of the cold New Year's of 1864."

95. USSC, *Documents*, 161.

96. Bucklin, 115.

97. Holstein, 54.

98. Coco Collection, GNMP.

99. *Adams Sentinel*, November 10, 1863.

Chapter 9

1. S. Weir Mitchell, "Some Personal Recollections of the Civil War," *Transactions of the College of Physicians of Philadelphia*, Third Ser., Vol. 25 (1905): 87–94.

2. Harvey Ellicott Brown, *Medical Department of the United States Army from 1775 to 1873* (U.S. Surgeon-General's Office, 1873), 220.

3. Louis C. Duncan, "Bull Run," *The Medical Department of the United States Army in the Civil War* (Washington, DC: Surgeon-General's Office, c. 1915), 18–19.

4. William Spencer, *Seven Months in Libby Prison: From the Diary of a Recently Released United States Army Surgeon,* transcript of unpublished manuscript, 1863–1864. White County Historical Society, Monticello, Indiana, 44.

5. George H. Weaver, "Surgeons As Prisoners of War," *Bulletin of the Society of Medical History* IV, no. 3 (January 1933).

6. Weaver. Copy made by Assistant Surgeon Philip Adolphus of agreement between D. Hunter McGuire, Medical Director of Army of the Valley of the CSA, and seven

Union surgeons who were prisoners at Winchester, Virginia, on May 31, 1862. McGuire is often credited with initiating the practice at Winchester, and he continued to advocate for appropriate treatment of surgeons. Serving as General Ewell's medical director at Gettysburg, he may have been partially responsible for allowing the Union surgeons held as prisoners in town during the battle to continue their work and then releasing them without parole when Ewell's Corps retreated.

7. OR Series II, Vol. 3, 654.

8. OR Series II, Vol. 4, 45.

9. OR Series II, Vol. 4, 101, letter from H. W. Halleck to Edwin Stanton, June 29, 1862.

10. OR Series II, Vol. 3, 618, June 1, 1862. Also see Charles W. Sanders Jr., *While in the Hands of the Enemy: Military Prisons of the Civil War (*Baton Rouge: Louisiana State University Press, 2005), 15–20.

11. https://www.battlefields.org/learn/primary-sources/cartel-exchange-prisoners-war. Accessed June 14, 2024.

12. OR Series II, Vol. 4, 266–68, text of Dix-Hill Cartel; Sanders, 116–17.

13. Judge Robert Ould was CSA agent for the duration of the war. Agents for the U.S. Army were, in sequence: Gen. Lorenzo Thomas; Col. William Hardy Ludlow; Gen. Sullivan A. Meredith; Gen. Benjamin F. Butler; at the end of the war General Grant handled exchanges directly.

14. OR Series III, Vol. 3, 154.

15. OR Series II, Vol. 3, 27–28 and 154; Brown, 233. For a full explanation of retaliation see Lorien Foote, *Rituals of Retaliation* (Chapel Hill: University of North Carolina Press, 2021).

16. Michael P. Rucker, *Bridge Burner* (Charleston WV: Quarrier Press, 2014), 72; OR Series II, Vol. 5, 212, Ludlow to Hitchcock, January 25, 1863.

17. OR Series II, Vol. 5, 217. James Colquhoun Green, the first Confederate surgeon held hostage, left the University of Virginia Medical College when the war began but left school to enlist as a private and completed his medical training after the war at New York University. In October 1862, he was appointed Assistant Surgeon, 5th Virginia Cavalry at the age of twenty-four and captured at Dumfries, Virginia, December 1862.

18. William Spencer, Assistant Surgeon, 73rd Indiana; William W. Myers, Surgeon, U.S. Navy; and Thomas F. Morgan, Assistant Surgeon, 10th Missouri were imprisoned as hostages in retaliation against the imprisonment of Confederate surgeon Green.

19. OR Series II, Vol. 6, 96, General Meade to General Halleck.

20. Unpublished Gettysburg Surgeons Database. Charles Alexander and William W. Eaton of 16th Maine, Horace Babcock, 2nd Wisconsin, and George P. Tracy, 90th Pennsylvania, were paroled.

21. Charles E. Humphrey was captured at the Lutheran Seminary when it was occupied by Confederates on July 1st. According to the *Pennsylvania College Book 1832–1882* (Philadelphia: Lutheran Publication Society, 1882), he was "Stationed during Battle of Gettysburg in Seminary Building Hospital; Prisoner of war Libby Prison 1863." Daniel Bishop Wren was captured at Gettysburg, on July 1st with retreating 11th Corps troops. The roster for the 75th Ohio notes he was captured July 1863 at Gettysburg and

returned to regiment December 1863. Lewis Applegate of 12th Corps was captured July 2, 1863. *Ohio Medical and Surgical Journal* (November 1863): 537–38.

22. "Michigan Surgeons Captured," *Weekly Michigan Argus*, July 17, 1863.

23. "'Richmond Prisons' Report of Dr. McDonald," *Sanitary Commission Bulletin* 1 no. 2 (November 15, 1863): 35–41. Dr. Alexander McDonald of Charlestown, Massachusetts, worked at the Massachusetts School for Idiotic and Feeble-Minded Youth before becoming an inspector for the Sanitary Commission. Rev. William George Scandlin (1828–1871) of Grafton was an agent for the Sanitary Commission. Both were released September 22, 1863.

24. *Gettysburg Times*, November 17, 1994, Vol. 92, no. 217, 1 and 10a; OR Series II, Vol. 6, 28. On June 19, Agent W. H. Ludlow wrote to William Hoffman, Commissary General of Prisoners, "One of the objects of the present raid into Maryland and Pennsylvania is to capture citizens and take or send them as prisoners to Richmond in retaliation, as the rebels say, for our arrests of non-combatants and then after collecting a very large number they hope to dictate terms which we now deem absurd and inadmissible." The Gettysburg citizens were held until 1865. Robert Ould, CSA Agent for Exchange, reported later that more than fifty civilians from Pennsylvania and Maryland were captured during the Gettysburg campaign. *The Annals of the Civil War Written by Leading Participants North and South*, Alexander Kelly McClure, ed. (Philadelphia: Times Publishing Company, 1879), 50.

25. Spencer, 27–28.

26. OR Series II, Vol. 6, 335, From B. Bragg, General commanding to General S. Cooper Adj. and Inspector General, Chickamauga, October 1, 1863.

27. OR Series II, Vol. 6, 335, To Brig General L. Thomas Adj General US Army Washington from General Rosecrans, Chattanooga, Tennessee, October 2, 1863.

28. OR Series II, Vol. 6, 381. Letter to General Rosecrans from General Bragg, October 15, 1863.

29. OR Series II, Vol. 6, 382. Rosecrans forwarded Bragg's letter to Maj. Gen. H. W. Halleck, U.S. General-in-Chief.

30. OR Series II, Vol. 6, 544, Report of Isaac Carrington to General Winder on hospitals in Richmond, November 18, 1863.

31. OR Series II, Vol. 6, 572. At a meeting of the surgeons of the U.S. Army and Navy lately confined in prison in Richmond, Virginia, on board Steamer *Adelaide*, Chesapeake Bay, November 26, 1863.

32. Spencer, 36, 44.

33. OR Series II, Vol. 6, 572.

34. Spencer, 30; Statement of Robert S. Northcott, November 1867, Clarksburg, West Virginia in Committee Report of House of Representatives on "Treatment of Prisoners of War by Rebel Authorities" (Washington, DC: Government Printing Office, 1869), 1104. The two surgeons shot at were Frederick H. Patten, Assistant Surgeon, U.S. 12th Virginia, and W. F. Bowes, Assistant Surgeon, 12th Pennsylvania Cavalry.

35. Federico F. Cavada, *Libby Life: Experiences of a Prisoner of War in Richmond, VA, 1863–64* (Philadelphia: King & Baird, 1864), 36–37.

36. Spencer, 28.

37. Spencer, 44.

38. Simon Baruch, "A Surgeon's Story of Battle and Capture," *Confederate Veteran* 22 (1914): 545–48.

39. Baruch.

40. Richard Clem, "Country Doctor Aids Both Sides," *Washington Times*, March 3, 2006 (Boonsboro, Washington County, Maryland).

41. Henry de Saussure Fraser, Records of Confederate Officers, NARA.

42. *Baltimore Sun*, July 25, 1863, 1. Benjamin Franklin Ward, Surgeon, 11th Mississippi; James Henry Southall, Surgeon, 55th Virginia; Benjamin Thorp Green, Surgeon, 55th North Carolina; William Thornton Parker, Assistant Surgeon, 55th North Carolina; William Green McCreight, Assistant Surgeon, 42nd Mississippi; James M. Stokes, Chaplain, 48th Georgia; J. Osgood A. Cook, Chaplain, 2nd Georgia; Aurelius Gregory Emory, Surgeon, 14th Tennessee, were not released as expected and instead remained at Fort Norfolk until early August when they joined other Confederate surgeons from Gettysburg at Fort McHenry.

43. William Riddick Whitehead, *Adventures of an American Surgeon: A 19th Century Memoir*, typescript of manuscript, NMCWM.

44. Peter Tinsley, *Civil War Diary*, 28th Virginia Chaplain, Wheaton College, John and Joyce Schmale Civil War Collection, August 7, 1863.

45. Tinsley, August 10, 1863.

46. Tinsley, August 10, 1863.

47. Witherspoon, "Prison Life at Fort McHenry," *Southern Historical Society Papers* VIII, no. 2 (February 1880): 82.

48. Baruch, 547.

49. Life at Fort McHenry is described in accounts by Chaplains Tinsley and Witherspoon. Surgeons Baruch and Whitehead also left accounts of their experiences as prisoners.

50. Baruch, 548. Dr. DeG is Assistant Surgeon Edwin F. DeGraffenried, 4th Alabama and Dr. N. is Assistant Surgeon Henry Junius Nott, 2nd South Carolina.

51. Tinsley, September 1, 1863.

52. Tinsley, September 14, 1863. Dr. Loyd is Assistant Surgeon J. P. Loyd, 24th Mississippi. captured Elk River Tennessee, July 1, 1863 and held at various prisons, in Louisville, Cincinnati, and Johnson's Island before transfer to Fort McHenry on August 14. Contri is Assistant Surgeon Giuseppe Contri, 34th Virginia Cavalry, captured June 12, 1863, Hagerstown, Maryland. Confederate Files, NARA.

53. Baruch, 547. Also mentioned by Tinsley, September 19, 1863. Dr. H. is probably Surgeon Shered Pierce Hobgood, 53rd Georgia.

54. Six other surgeons who escaped included Assistant Surgeon Thomas Cloman Pugh, 9th Georgia; Assistant Surgeon Alexander Rives Jr., 15th Alabama; Surgeon Solomon Secord, 20th Georgia; and Assistant Surgeon Thomas Young Aby, Louisiana Washington Artillery—all captured at Gettysburg—and two surgeons not at Gettysburg, Surgeon James Guild Jr., 1st Alabama, and Assistant Surgeon Louis Giuseppe Contri, 34th Virginia Cavalry Battalion.

55. Tinsley, September 14, 1863; Baruch, 543; Whitehead.

56. OR Series II, Vol. 6, 474, Letter to Hoffman from Surgeon Suckley, Office of Medical Director, Baltimore, Maryland, November 6, 1863.

57. OR Series II, Vol. 6, 492, Letter from W. Hoffman to Surg. George Suckley, November 9, 1863.

58. Spencer, 54, 56.

59. OR Series II, Vol. 6, 543, To Col. Hoffman from P. A. Porter, Commanding Fort McHenry, November 21, 1863.

60. Spencer, 57.

61. OR Series II, Vol. 6., 572, steamer *Adelaide*, Chesapeake Bay, report dated November 26, 1863.

62. "Exchange of Prisoners," Judge Robert Ould, 35 and "Union View of the Exchange of Prisoners," Roberts S. Northcott, 189, in Alexander Kelly McClure, ed., *The Annals of the Civil War Written by Leading Participants North and South* (Philadelphia: Times Publishing Company, 1879).

63. R. Randolph Stevenson, *The Southern Side; or Andersonville Prison. Compiled Official Documents . . . Together with an Examination of the Wirz Trial; a Comparison of the Mortality in Northern and Southern Prisons; Remarks on the Exchange Bureau, etc.* (Baltimore: Turnbull Brothers, 1876), 5.

CHAPTER 10

1. William H. Taylor, *De Quibus* (Richmond, VA: Bell Book and Stationery Co., 1908), 325.

2. William G. Nine and Ronald G. Wilson, *The Appomattox Paroles April 9–15, 1865* (Lynchburg, VA: H.E. Howard, Inc., 1989), 4th ed.

3. Unpublished Gettysburg Surgeons Database.

4. John Herbert Roper, *Repairing the March of Mars: The Civil War Diaries of John Samuel Apperson* (Macon, GA: Mercer University Press, 2002), 611. Other surgeons mentioned include John Stevens, 2nd Louisiana; Harvey Black, 4th Virginia; Caspar Henkel, 37th Virginia; Samuel Sayers, 27th Virginia.

5. Roper, 612.

6. F. T. Hambrecht & J. L. Koste, *Biographical Register of Physicians Who Served the Confederacy in a Medical Capacity.* Unpublished database.

7. At least eighteen surgeons were paroled in North Carolina locations and in Georgia. In Georgia: Henry William Waters, 1st Texas, paroled May 19, 1865; and Elisha James Roach, 5th Texas, July 1865.

8. Surrender documents accessed May 24, 2024 at https://www.nps.gov/apco/learn/historyculture/surrender-documents.htm.

9. Confederate Records, NARA.

10. James Stanislaus Easby-Smith, *Georgetown University in the District of Columbia, 1789–1907: Its Founders, Benefactors* (Georgetown: 1907), 84–85.

11. Emerging Civil War, "Dr. Henry A. Minor's Account of General Lee's Surrender at Appomattox from Macon (MS) Beacon, April 1914," posted July 27, 2016. Accessed May 4, 2024 at https://emergingcivilwar.com/2016/07/27/dr-henry-a-minors-account-of-lees-surrender-at-appomattox/.

12. *Biographical Souvenir of the States of Georgia and Florida* (Chicago: F.A. Battey & Co., 1889), 267–68.

13. Moses Thurston Runnels, *Memorial Sketches and History of the Class of 1853, Dartmouth College* (Dartmouth College, Class of 1853, Barton & Wheeler, 1895), 112–16.

The Reconstruction troubles referred to the elections of 1876 when white Southerners attempted to take back control of state government. Democratic Military Clubs disrupted Republican political meetings and used violence to intimidate Black voters. Moore probably fled to avoid arrest after federal troops were sent in to maintain order.

14. Daniel M. Holt, *A Surgeon's Civil War: The Letters and Diaries of Daniel M. Holt, M.D.*, eds. James M. Greiner, Janet L Coryell, and James R. Smither (Kent, OH: Kent State University Press, 1994), 269–70.

15. Paul B. Kerr, *Civil War Surgeon—Biography of James Langstall Dunn, MD* (Bloomington, IN: Authorhouse, 2005), 207.

16. William Child, *Letters from a Civil War Surgeon* (Solon, ME: Polar Bear and Company, 2001), 359.

17. Paul Fatout, ed., *Letters of a Civil War Surgeon* (West Lafayette, IN: Purdue University Press, 1996), 151.

18. Unpublished Gettysburg Surgeons Database.

19. At least six Gettysburg surgeons later served with USCT: William Craig, 26th Pennsylvania appointed to USCT July 15, 1865–February 1867; Arthur Cowdrey, 7th Massachusetts, USCT 1863–1865; Ai Waterhouse, 7th Maine, USCT 1864–December 1865; James Uglow, 43rd New York, USCT 1864 until death in Beaufort, South Carolina in 1865; Carl Uterhart, 119th New York, USCT 1864–1865; Herman Niedermeyer, 107th Ohio, USCT 1864–1865. Unpublished Gettysburg Surgeons Database.

20. *Biographical Souvenir of the States of Georgia and Florida*, 758.

21. *Annual Report of the Surgeon General 1885* (Washington, DC: Marine Hospital Services), 28.

22. Fielding H. Garrison, *John Shaw Billings: A Memoir* (New York: G.P. Putnam's Sons, 1915).

23. *The Army Medical Bulletin*, No. 48 (April 1939). Accessed May 24, 2024 at https://achh.army.mil/history/biography-smart.

24. Michael Robert Patterson, "William Henry Forwood—Brigadier General United States Army," Arlington National Cemetery. Accessed May 24, 2024 at www.arlingtoncemetery.net/whforwood.htm.

25. *Confederate Veteran* 11, no. 10 (October 1903): 467.

26. William M. Edwards, "Why He Watched the Doves," *Forest and Stream*, Vol. 28 (May 5, 1887): 324.

27. Hambrecht Database.

28. William Riddick Whitehead, *Adventures of an American Surgeon: A 19th Century Memoir*, typescript manuscript copy, NMCWM.

29. Find a Grave, https://www.findagrave.com/memorial/18348717/william-maberry-strickler.

30. *Biographical and Historical Memoirs of Story County, Iowa* (Chicago: Goodspeed Publishing Co., 1890), 434.

31. Child, 363.

32. S. Weir Mitchell, "Some Personal Recollections of the Civil War," *Transactions of the College of Physicians of Philadelphia*, Third Ser., Vol. 25 (1905): 87–94.

33. Don D. Grout, MD, *Vermont Medicine, The Official Organ of the Vermont State Medical Society*, Vol. 1, no., 1 (January 1916): 25–26.

34. Taylor, *De Quibus*, 283–84; 276.

35. Kemp Plummer Battle, *History of the University of North Carolina* (Raleigh, NC: Edwards & Broughton Printing Company, 1912), 780. Hospital renamed Cherry Hospital in 1959.

36. *Transactions of the Medical Society of the State of North Carolina* (Raleigh, NC: Edwards & Broughton Printing Company, 1906), 159.

37. Joseph L. Fetterman and Jack Horrocks, "Psychiatric Progress in Ohio in the Twentieth Century," *Ohio History Journal* 58, no. 4 (October 1949): 381–82.

38. "A Fatal Dose of Poison," *Daily Review*, Decatur, Illinois, December 10, 1878.

39. Patricia Spain Ward, *Simon Baruch: Rebel in the Ranks of Medicine 1840–1921* (Tuscaloosa: University of Alabama Press, 1994), 208.

40. Rockbridge Historical Society, *What Mean These Stones*, filmed by Bernard Bangle, 1976. Accessed May 24, 2024 at https://www.youtube.com/watch?v=R66TU5ZdOdw.

41. Confederate Military Officers records, NARA; *Journal of the American Medical Association* 5 (1885): 279.

42. Carolyn Ivanoff, *We Fought at Gettysburg: Firsthand Accounts by the Survivors of the 17th Connecticut Volunteer Infantry* (Gettysburg, PA: Gettysburg Publishing, 2023), 201.

43. William S. Tilden, *History of the Town of Medfield Massachusetts—1650–1886* (Boston: Geo. H. Ellis, Publisher, 1887), 290.

44. George F. Adams, *Turkish Bath Hand Book* (St. Louis: Little & Becker, 1881), 6. Accessed May 24, 2024 at https://www.google.com/books/edition/Turkish_Bath_Hand_Book/fqnuASwqWSoC?hl=en&gbpv=1&printsec=frontcover.

45. Mark Aldrich, "Train Wrecks to Typhoid Fever: The Development of Railroad Medicine Organizations, 1850 to World War I," *Bulletin of the History of Medicine* 75, no. 2 (Summer 2001): 254–89.

46. Hambrecht Database.

47. *Virginia Medical Semi-Monthly* 17 (1913): 468.

48. Obituary, *Sioux City Journal*, December 6, 1895.

49. *Escanaba* (MI) *Daily Press*, August 29, 1977, 7.

50. *Confederate Veteran* 25 (August 1917): 374.

51. See Douglas Blackmon, *Slavery by Another Name*, 2008, for more information about Black convict labor in post–Civil War America.

52. John Witherspoon DuBose, *Jefferson County and Birmingham Alabama Historical and Biographical* (Birmingham, AL: Teeple and Smith Publishers, 1887), 594–95.

53. Shauna Devine, *Learning from the Wounded: The Civil War and the Rise of American Medical Science* (Chapel Hill: University of North Carolina Press, 2014), 138–50.

54. Howard A. Kelly and Walter L. Burrage, *American Medical Biographies* (Baltimore: Norman Remington Co., 1920), 39.

55. Robert T. Coleman, Confederate chief surgeon for Johnson's Division, became professor of obstetrics and diseases of women at the Medical College of Virginia in 1874; Joseph J. Holt, Assistant Surgeon, 2nd Mississippi, appointed a professor of obstetrics at the New Orleans School of Medicine; Adrian T. Woodward, Surgeon 14th Vermont, made a specialty of surgical diseases of women.

56. *The Medical Bulletin: A Monthly Journal of Medicine and Surgery* 26 (1904): 22.

57. "New England Heroes of Land and Sea," *Boston Globe*, February 4, 1918, 9.

58. William Biddle Atkinson, *The Physicians and Surgeons of the United States* (Philadelphia: Charles Robson, 1878), 325–26.

59. William Riddick Whitehead, "Autobiography of a Western Surgeon," *Magazine of Western History* XI (1890): 197–206.

60. Taylor, *De Quibus*, 135.

61. Stephen R. Doty, "History of Weather Observations, Aiken South Carolina 1851–2005," NOAA (Asheville, NC: Information Manufacturing Corporation, Rocket Center, WV, August 2005), 10, 24–25.

62. Greenly Woollen obituary and biography. Accessed May 24, 2024 at https://www.findagrave.com/memorial/28579526/greenly-vinton-woollen.

63. Boyd Crumrine, *History of Washington County, Pennsylvania with Biographical Sketches of Many of Its Pioneers and Prominent Men* (Philadelphia: L. H. Leverts & Co., 1882), 958–59.

64. William N. Grafton, "History of Botany in West Virginia." Accessed June 18, 2023 at https://static1.squarespace.com/static/617ef2725f1b09518b9b1256/t/62e18c8f5b940072a7c82547/1658948751776/HISTORY+OF+BOTANY+IN+WEST+VIRGINIA.pdf.

65. Everhart biography. Accessed June 18, 2023 at http://www.everhart-museum.org/About/Everhart.htm.

66. "Biographical Sketch of Dr. J. Bernard Brinton," *Bulletin of the Torrey Botanical Club* 22, no. 3 (March 27, 1895): 93–97.

67. *American Journal of Numismatics* 34, no. 1 (July 1899): 29.

68. Thomas Horrocks, "The College of Physicians of Philadelphia: 'Not for Oneself, But for All,'" *Pennsylvania Heritage* (Winter 1987). Accessed May 24, 2024 at http://paheritage.wpengine.com/article/college-physicians-philadelphia/.

69. Granville P. Conn, *History of New Hampshire Surgeons in the War of Rebellion* (Concord, NH: Order of the New Hampshire Association of Military Surgeons, Ira C. Evans Co. Printers, 1906), 72.

70. *History of Texas Together with Biographical History of Tarrant and Parker Counties* (Chicago: Lewis Publishing Company, 1895), 611–13.

71. Gazetteer and Business Directory of Franklin and Grand Isle Counties, Vt., for 1882–83 (Syracuse, NY: 1883).

72. *Biographical and Historical Record of Greene and Carroll Counties, Iowa* (Chicago: Lewis Publishing Company, 1887), 379.

73. *New York Times*, February 3, 1877, 1.

74. *Medical Record: A Weekly Journal of Medicine and Surgery* 69, no. 19 (May 12, 1906): 760.

75. Hambrecht Database.

76. Hambrecht Database.

77. Find a Grave, https://www.findagrave.com/memorial/87298631/james-w.-anawalt; Military Pension Records for James W. Anawalt, NARA; *Historical Register of National Homes for Disabled Volunteer Soldiers, 1866–1938*; Series M1749, NARA.

78. Find a Grave, https://www.findagrave.com/memorial/58669150/louis-evans -atkinson; Veteran Schedule of the U.S. Census, 1890, NARA, Series Number M123; Record Group Title: Records of the Department of Veterans Affairs; Record Group Number: 15; Census Year: 1890.

79. William A. Ellis, *Norwich University, Her History, Her Graduates, Her Roll of Honor* (Norwich University, 1898), 374. Parker's paintings are on display in Massachusetts at Cary Memorial Library, Lexington; Faneuil Hall, Boston; and Memorial Hall Library, Andover.

80. Confederate Officers Records, NARA.

81. Peyton F. Carter III, *Hitherto Above Reproach: The Life of Dr. Thomas Harold Wilson Upshur* (Salem, MA: Higginson Book Company, 2003). Information included from letters sent to Dr. Jordan in the University of Pennsylvania archives.

82. Spencer Glasgow Welch, *A Confederate Surgeon's Letters to His Wife* (New York: Neale Publishing Company, 1911), 91.

83. *Eastern Medical Journal*, Vol. 5 (February 15, 1886): 70.

8485. Grenville P. Conn, *History of the New Hampshire Surgeons in the War of Rebellion* (Concord, NH: Ira C. Evans Printer, 1906), 66.

85. Conn, 69.

86. Conn, 69.

CHAPTER 11

1. Andrew B. Cross, "Battle of Gettysburg and the Christian Commission," *The War and the Christian Commission* (1865), 26.

2. Drew Gilpin Faust, *This Republic of Suffering* (New York: Vintage Books, 2009), 17.

3. Anna Holstein, *Three Years in the Field Hospitals of the Army of the Potomac* (Philadelphia: J.B. Lippincott and Co., 1867), 47.

4. Samuel Brown Morrison Papers, Virginia Historical Society, letter to his wife, August 5, 1863, Headquarters Early's Division, Mss1 M8347 a 1–1.

5. U.S. Surgeon General's Office, *The Medical and Surgical History of the War of the Rebellion (1861–65), 1870–1888.*

6. Henry Janes, Hospital Notes, manuscript volume, University of Vermont Special Collections Library.

7. William H. Taylor, "Science and the Soul," in *De Quibus* (Richmond, VA: Bell Book and Stationery Co., 1908), 12.

8. Taylor, "Reply to Criticisms," in *De Quibus*, 54.

9. William Maberry Strickler, "Relation of Ethics and Religion," in *Essays on Human Nature* (Colorado Springs, CO: Prompt Printery, 1906), 22. George Herbert Palmer was a professor at Harvard University from 1889 to 1913.

10. Henrietta Stratton Jaquette, *South After Gettysburg: Letters of Cornelia Hancock 1863–1868* (New York: Thomas Y. Crowell Company, 1956), 21, 67. Dr. Dudley refers to Surgeon Frederick A. Dudley, 14th Connecticut.

11. John H. Brinton, *Personal Memoirs of John H. Brinton, Civil War Surgeon 1861–1865* (Carbondale: Southern Illinois University Press, 1996), 180.

12. Brinton, 187.

13. Shauna Devine, "Producing Knowledge: Civil War Bodies and the Development of Scientific Medicine in Nineteenth Century America," Thesis, School of Graduate and Postdoctoral Studies, University of Western Ontario, Canada, 2010, 68.

14. Janes, Hospital Notes, 239.

15. Janes, Hospital Notes, 42.

16. John W. Elarton, *Andersonville* (1913). Accessed May 28, 2024 at https://digicom .bpl.lib.me.us/books_pubs/6.

17. *Philadelphia Inquirer*, July 25, 1863.

18. Coco Collection, GNMP Box 14, letter from Henry Janes, August 17, 1863.

19. Carolyn Ivanoff, *We Fought at Gettysburg: Firsthand Accounts by the Survivors of the 17th Connecticut Volunteer Infantry* (Gettysburg, PA: Gettysburg Publishing, 2023), 303–6.

20. Reported Union casualties include: John T. Heard, Edgar Parker, Charles Alexander, and William Winslow Eaton of First Corps on July 1; Frederick Dudley, Second Corps on July 3; Joseph Dunton Stewart, July 2, and John Weston Brennan, Third Corps; Jacob Laubly on July 1 and William S. Moore and Edward B. Heckel of Eleventh Corps on July 3; John Stevenson, Twelfth Corps, July 2; William Notson, 6th U.S. Cavalry. Confirmed Confederate wounded include William H. Taylor and Robert Herbert Warrington, both in Pickett's Division on July 3; on July 2nd Matthew Butler, 37th Virginia, was wounded and James Aston Groves, 16th Mississippi, died of his wounds.

21. Strickler, 278.

22. Strickler, 278.

23. *Medical Record*, eds. George Frederick Shrady and Thomas Lathrop Stedman, 74 (November 21, 1908): 886.

24. "Death of Coroner," *Richmond Times Dispatch*, April 15, 1917, 1.

25. "Death of Coroner."

26. *Akron Beacon Journal*, June 9, 1890, 1.

27. Historical Register of National Homes for Disabled Volunteer Soldiers, 1866–1938; Series: M1749, 1760, NARA.

28. *Philadelphia Times*, October 22, 1899, 45; Will dated January 24, 1906, Pennsylvania Wills and Probate Records, accessed May 28. 2024 at https://www.ancestry.com/discoveryui-content/view/2202799:8802.

29. *Batavia* (NY) *Daily News*, March 18, 1902.

30. Will of John McNulty, Webster County Iowa Probate Records Vol. 2–5, 1895–1911, 328 no. 3 (filmstrip image #215).

31. Will of John McNulty.

32. Edgar Allan Poe, "The Premature Burial," *Philadelphia Dollar Newspaper*, 1844; *Akron Beacon Journal*, "An Entranced Man Carelessly Buried Alive," June 10, 1890,

1. Patents for "safety" coffins provided for bells, flags, air tubes, and other methods for those buried alive to communicate.

33. Holstein, 41.

34. Records of Lishur White, 20th Massachusetts, NARA. Lishur G. White is also listed among wounded at Gettysburg in George A. Bruce, *The Twentieth Regiment of Massachusetts Volunteer Infantry, 1861–1865* (Boston: Houghton, Mifflin, and Company, 1906).

35. The Gettysburg Surgeons unpublished database includes 255 Union, 202 Confederate, and 54 contract and volunteer surgeons who survived into the twentieth century.

36. Henry Janes, "Why Is the Profession of Killing More Generally Honored Than That of Saving Life?," Transactions of the Vermont State Medical Society, 1903 (Burlington Free Press Association, 1903), 190–191, 200.

37. Silas Weir Mitchell, Scrapbook, Philadelphia College of Physicians and Surgeons.

38. Silas Weir Mitchell, "Some Personal Recollections of the Civil War," *Transactions of the College of Physicians of Philadelphia*, Third Ser., Vol. 25 (1905): 87–94.

BIBLIOGRAPHY

Unpublished Letters, Diaries, etc.

Atkinson, Archibald. Memoir. 1890, Virginia Tech MS 1994–022.

Bacon, Cyrus. Transcript of unpublished diary. Michigan Historical Commission.

Clifton, James Beverly. Unpublished diary. North Carolina Department of Archives and History. Transcript, National Museum of Civil War Medicine, Frederick, Maryland.

Dimon, Theodore. Report on Gettysburg and Civil War diaries. Private collection.

Hamilton, Alfred Thorley. Manuscript diary. Gettysburg National Historic Park Library.

Harris, Isaac. Diary June 12–July 18, 1863. Transcript, Dickinson College Archives.

Henkel Family Correspondence 1786–1940. MS C 291, History of Medicine Division, National Library of Medicine, Bethesda, Maryland.

Janes, Henry. Hospital register and notes. University of Vermont, Burlington, Vermont.

Jones, Clarissa Fellowes (Dye). Manuscript letters. National Museum of Civil War Medicine, Frederick, Maryland.

Mitchell, S. Weir. Scrapbook. College of Physicians, Philadelphia.

Myers, Robert Pooler. Manuscript diary. Mss5:5 M99277:1, Virginia Historical Society.

Norris, William F. Manuscript letters. College of Physicians, Philadelphia, and Adams County Historical Society.

Powell, John Walker, *C.S.A. Hosp. Dept. Surgical Notes*. Virginia Historical Society.

Pratt, Frederick. Manuscript letters. Private collection.

Rohrer, Benjamin. Manuscript papers. National Museum of Civil War Medicine.

Samuel Adams Papers. NMAH.AC.1310, Archives Center, National Museum of American History.

Scott, Isaac Tanner. Ledgers. Virginia Historical Society Collection.

Spencer, William. *Seven Months in Libby Prison: From the Diary of a Recently Released United States Army Surgeon.* Transcript of unpublished manuscript. White County Historical Society, Monticello, Indiana.

Tinsley, Peter. Diary. Wheaton College, John and Joyce Schmale Civil War Collection.

Whitehead, William Riddick. *Adventures of an American Surgeon: A 19th Century Memoir.* Typescript copy, National Museum of Civil War Medicine.

Published Letters, Diaries, Addresses, Contemporary Accounts

Bacon, Georgeanna Woolsey, and Eliza Woolsey Howland. *My Heart Toward Home: Letters of a Family During the Civil War*. Daniel John Hoisington, ed. Minnesota: Edinborough Press, 2001.

Baruch, Simon. "A Surgeon's Story of Battle and Capture." *Confederate Veteran* 22 (1914): 545–48.

Barziza, Decimus et Ultimus. *The Adventures of a Prisoner of War 1863–1864*. R. Henderson Shuffler, ed.. Austin: University of Texas, 1964.

Billings, John Shaw. "Medical Reminiscences of the Civil War." *Transactions of the College of Physicians of Philadelphia*. Ser. 3, Vol. 27 (1905): 119.

Breakey, Dr. William F. "Recollections and Incidents of Military Service." In *War Papers Read Before the Michigan Commandery of the Military Order of the Loyal Legion of the United States*. Detroit: James H. Stone & Co., 1898, 120–52.

Brinton, John Hill. *Personal Memoirs of John H. Brinton: Civil War Surgeon, 1861–1865*. Carbondale: Southern Illinois University Press, 1996.

Broadhead, Sarah. *The Diary of a Lady of Gettysburg, Pennsylvania: From June 15 to July 15, 1863*. Philadelphia: 1864.

Bucklin, Sophronia. *In Hospital and Camp*. Philadelphia: J.E. Potter & Company, 1869.

Burnett, Edmund Cody. "Letters of a Confederate Surgeon: Dr. Abner Embry McGarity, 1862–1865. Part I." *Georgia Historical Quarterly* 29, no. 2 (1945): 76–114.

Cavada, Federico F. *Libby Life: Experiences of a Prisoner of War in Richmond, VA, 1863–64*. Philadelphia: King & Baird, 1864.

Child, William. *Letters from a Civil War Surgeon*. Solon, ME: Polar Bear and Company, 2001.

Chisolm, Julian John. *A Manual of Military Surgery, for the Use of Surgeons in the Confederate Army; with an Appendix of the Rules and Regulations of the Medical Department of the Confederate Army*. Richmond, VA: West & Johnson, 1861.

Cross, Andrew B. "Battle of Gettysburg and the Christian Commission." In *The War and the Christian Commission*, 1865.

Dyer, J. Franklin. *The Journal of a Civil War Surgeon*. Michael B. Chesson, ed. Lincoln: University of Nebraska Press, 2003.

Ebersole, Jacob. "Incidents of Field Hospital Life with the Army of the Potomac." In *Sketches of War History 1861–1865, Papers Read Before the Ohio Commandery of the Military Order of the Loyal Legion of the United States*. W. H. Chamberlin, ed. Vol. 4. Cincinnati: R. Clarke & Co., 1896, 327–33.

Fatout, Paul, ed. *Letters of a Civil War Surgeon*. West Lafayette, IN: Purdue University Press, 1996.

Fisher, Mary Caldwell. "A Week on Gettysburg Field." *Philadelphia Times*, December 23, 1883.

Galwey, Thomas Francis. *The Valiant Hours: Narrative of "Captain Brevet," an Irish-American in the Army of the Potomac*. Harrisburg, PA: Stackpole, 1961.

Garrison, Fielding H. *John Shaw Billings: A Memoir*. New York: G.P. Putnam's Sons, 1913.

Gunn, Jane Augusta, *Memorial Sketches of Dr. Moses Gunn*. Chicago: WT Keener, 1889.

Hard, Abner. *A Surgeon of the Eighth Cavalry Regiment Illinois Volunteers.* Big Byte Books, 2014.

Hardman, Asa Sleath. "As a Union Prisoner Saw the Battle of Gettysburg." Civil War Times (August 2012).

Haupt, Herman. Reminiscences of General Herman Haupt. Milwaukee, WI: Wright & Joys Co., 1901.

Hedrick, David T., and Gordon Barry Davis Jr. *I'm Surrounded by Methodists . . . Diary of John H.W. Stuckenberg Chaplain of the 145th Pennsylvania Volunteer Infantry.* Gettysburg, PA: Thomas Publications, 1995.

Hicks, Robert D., ed. *Civil War Medicine: A Surgeon's Diary.* Bloomington: Indiana University Press, 2019.

Holmes, Oliver Wendell. "Currents And Counter-Currents in Medical Science." An Address delivered before the Massachusetts Medical Society, at the Annual Meeting, May 30, 1860. Accessed June 3, 2024 at http://www.online-literature.com/oliver-holmes/medical-essays/3/.

Holstein, Anna Morris Ellis. *Three Years in Field Hospitals of the Army of the Potomac.* Philadelphia: J.B. Lippincott and Co., 1867.

Holt, Daniel M. *A Surgeon's Civil War: The Letters and Diaries of Daniel M. Holt, M.D.* James M. Greiner, Janet L Coryell, and James R. Smither, eds. Kent, OH: Kent State University Press, 1994.

Howard, Benjamin. *Prisoners of Russia.* New York: D. Appleton & Co., 1902.

Jaquette, Henrietta Stratton, ed. *South After Gettysburg: Letters of Cornelia Hancock 1863–1868.* New York: Thomas Y. Crowell Company, 1956.

James, Bushrod Washington. *Echoes of Battle.* Philadelphia: Henry T. Coates & Co., 1895.

Janes, Henry. "Why Is the Profession of Killing More Generally Honored Than That of Saving Life?" Transactions of the Vermont State Medical Society (1903): 186–206.

Keen, W. W. *Transactions of the College of Physicians of Philadelphia* 25 (1905): 87–113.

Kerr, Paul B. *Civil War Surgeon—Biography of James Langstall Dunn, MD.* Bloomington, IN: Authorhouse, 2005.

Koonce, Donald B., ed. *Doctor to the Front: The Recollections of Confederate Surgeon Thomas Fanning Wood 1861–1865.* Knoxville: University of Tennessee Press, 2000.

Ladies' Aid Society of Philadelphia. *Fifth Semi-Annual Report of the Ladies' Aid Society of Philadelphia.* Philadelphia: C. Sherman Son & Co., 1863.

Loperfido, Christopher E., ed. *Death, Disease, and Life at War: The Civil War Letters of Surgeon James D. Bento.* El Dorado Hills, CA: Savas Beatie, 2018.

McKay, Charlotte Elizabeth. *Stories of Hospital and Camp.* Philadelphia: Claxton, Remsen & Haffelfinger, 1876.

McMullen, Glen L., ed. *A Surgeon with Stonewall Jackson: The Civil War Letters of Dr. Harvey Black.* Baltimore: Butternut and Blue, 1995.

Meade, George. *The Life and Letters of George Gordon Meade, Major-General United States Army.* Vol II. New York: Charles Scribner's Sons, 1913.

Mitchell, S. Weir. "Some Personal Recollections of the Civil War." *Transactions of the College of Physicians of Philadelphia.* Third Ser., 25 (1905): 87–94.

Patriot Daughters of Lancaster. *Hospital Scenes After the Battle of Gettysburg, July 1863*. Daily Inquirer Steam Job Print, 1864.

Pierce, Matilda J. (Mrs. M. J. "Tillie" Alleman). *At Gettysburg; What a Girl Saw and Heard at the Battle*. New York: 1889.

Potter, William W. *One Surgeon's Private War: Dr. William W. Potter of the 57th NY*. John Michael Priest et al., eds. Shippensburg, PA: White Mane Publishing Company, 1996.

Roper, John Herbert. *Repairing the March of Mars: The Civil War Diaries of John Samuel Apperson*. Macon, GA: Mercer University Press, 2002.

Schantz, Franklin Jacob Fogel. "Recollections of Visitations at Gettysburg After the Great Battle in July 1863." *Lebanon County Historical Society* XIII, no. 6 (1963): 275–303.

Smith, Edward Parmelee. *Incidents of the United States Christian Commission*. Philadelphia: J. B. Lippincott & Company, 1871.

Souder, Mrs. Edmund A. *Leaves from the Battle-field of Gettysburg*. Philadelphia: Caxton Press of C. Sherman, Son & Co., 1864.

Stevens, George T. *Three Years in the Sixth Corps*. Albany, NY: S.R. Gray, Publishers, 1866.

Stevenson, R. Randolph. *The Southern Side; or, Andersonville Prison. Compiled from Official Documents . . . Together with an Examination of the Wirz Trial; a Comparison of the Mortality in Northern and Southern Prisons; Remarks on the Exchange Bureau, etc.* Baltimore: Turnbull Brothers, 1876.

Stille, Charles J. *History of the United States Sanitary Commission*. Philadelphia: J. B. Lippincott & Co., 1866.

Strickler, William Maberry. *Essays on Human Nature*. Colorado Springs, CO: Prompt Printer, 1906. Reprint from collection of University of Michigan Library.

Taylor, William H. *De Quibus*. Richmond, VA: Bell Book and Stationery Co., 1908.

Taylor, William H. "Some Experiences of a Confederate Asst. Surgeon." *Transactions of the College of Physicians of Philadelphia*. Ser. 3, Vol. 28 (1906): 91–121.

Taylor, William H. *Travels of a Doctor of Physic*. Philadelphia: J.B. Lippincott & Company, 1871.

Thomson, D. G. Brinton. "From Chancellorsville to Gettysburg, A Doctor's Diary." *Pennsylvania Magazine of History and Biography* 89, no. 3 (1965): 292–315.

U.S. Christian Commission Second Report of the Committee of Maryland September 1, 1863. Baltimore: Sherwood & Co., 1863.

U.S. Christian Commission 2nd Annual Report for 1863. April 1864.

U.S. Sanitary Commission. *Bulletin*. Vol. 1 (1863).

U.S. Sanitary Commission. *Documents of the U.S. Sanitary Commission*. Vol. 2. New York: 1866.

U.S. Sanitary Commission. *Sanitary Commission of the United States Army: A Succinct Narrative of Its Works and Purposes*. New York: 1864.

U.S. Sanitary Commission. *The United States Sanitary Commission: A Sketch of Its Purposes and Its Work*. Boston: Little, Brown and Company, 1863.

U.S. Surgeon-General's Office. *The Medical and Surgical History of the War of the Rebellion (1861–65)*. Washington, DC: 1870–1888.

U.S. War Department. *The War of Rebellion: A Compilation of the Official Records of the Union and Confederate Armies.* Washington, DC: Government Printing Office, 1880–1901.

Wafer, Francis M. *A Surgeon in the Army of the Potomac.* Cheryl A. Wells, ed. Montreal and Kingston: McGill-Queen's University Press, 2008.

Welch, Spencer Glasgow. *A Confederate Surgeon's Letters to His Wife.* New York and Washington: Neale Publishing Company, 1911.

Whitehead, William Riddick. "Autobiography of a Western Surgeon." *Magazine of Western History* XI (November 1889–April 1890): 197–206.

Witherspoon, T. D. "Prison Life at Fort McHenry." *Southern Historical Society Papers* VIII, no. 2 (February 1880): 77.

Wood, Thomas Fanning. *Doctor to the Front: Recollections of Confederate Surgeon Thomas Fanning Wood.* Donald B. Koonce, ed. Knoxville: University of Tennessee Press, 2000.

Woodward, Joseph Janvier. *Outline of the Chief Camp Diseases of the United States Armies.* Philadelphia: J.B. Lippincott & Co., 1863.

Woolsey, Georgeanna Muirson. *Three Weeks at Gettysburg.* New York: Anson D.F. Randolph, 1863.

REGIMENTAL HISTORIES, MEMOIRS, ETC.

Annual Circular of the Medical Department of the University of Louisiana, 1859–1860. New Orleans: 1860.

Bartlett, A. W. *History of the Twelfth New Hampshire Volunteers in the War of the Rebellion.* Concord, NH: Ira C. Evans, 1897.

Brown, Harvey Ellicott. *Medical Department of the United States Army from 1775 to 1873.* U.S. Surgeon-General's Office, 1873.

Bruce, George A. *The Twentieth Regiment of Massachusetts Volunteer Infantry, 1861–1865.* Boston: Houghton, Mifflin and Company, 1906.

Chamberlin, Thomas. *History of the One Hundred and Fiftieth Regiment Pennsylvania Volunteers, Second Regiment, Bucktail Brigade.* Philadelphia: J. B. Lippincott, 1895.

Clark, Walter. Histories of the Several Regiments and Battalions from North Carolina in the Great War, 1861–1865. State of North Carolina, 1901.

Clements, Bennett A. *Memoir of Jonathan Letterman Reprinted from the Journal of the Military Service Institution.* Vol. iv, no. 15 (September 1883). New York: G.P. Putnam's Sons, 1883.

Coe, Algernon S. "The 14th N. Y. Zouaves." *National Tribune*, August 13, 1885, 3.

Conn, Grenville P. *History of the New Hampshire Surgeons in the War of Rebellion.* Concord, NH: Ira C. Evans, 1906.

Conyngham, David Power. *The Irish Brigade with Some Account of the Corcoran Legion, and Sketches of the Principal Officers.* New York: McSorley & Co., 1867.

Curtis. Orson B. *History of the Twenty-Fourth Michigan of the Iron Brigade.* Detroit: Winn & Hammond, 1891.

Dawes, Rufus R. *Service with the Sixth Wisconsin Volunteers.* Marietta, OH: E.R. Alderman & Sons, 1890.

Dickert, D. Augustus. *History of Kershaw's Brigade*. Newberry, SC: Elbert H. Aull Co, 1899.

Garrison, Fielding H. *John Shaw Billings: A Memoir*. New York: G.P. Putnam's Sons, 1915.

Green, Wharton J. *Recollections and Reflections, An Auto of Half a Century and More*. Edwards and Broughton Publishing Company, 1906.

Hays, Gilbert Adams. *Under the Red Patch. Story of the 63rd Regiment, Pennsylvania Volunteers 1861–1864*. Pittsburgh: Sixty-Third Pennsylvania Volunteers Regimental Association, 1908.

Henry, Guy Vernor. *Military Record of Civilian Appointments in the United States Army*. New York: Van Nostrand, 1873.

Hussey, George A., and William Todd. *History of the Ninth Regiment N.Y.S.M. 83rd N.Y. Volunteers*. New York: Oglivie, 1889.

Ivanoff, Carolyn. *We Fought at Gettysburg: Firsthand Accounts by the Survivors of the 17th Connecticut Volunteer Infantry*. Gettysburg, PA: Gettysburg Publishing, 2023.

Kepler, William. *History of the Three Months' and Three Years' Service from April 16th, 1861, to June 22d, 1864, of the Fourth Regiment Ohio Volunteer Infantry in the War for the Union*. Cleveland: Cleveland Leader Printing Co, 1886.

Kiefer, William R. *History of the One Hundred and Fifty-third Regiment Pennsylvania Volunteers Infantry*. Easton, PA: Press of the Chemical Publishing Co., 1909.

Kulp, George B. *Families of the Wyoming Valley: Sketches of the Bench and Bar*. Vol. 1. Wilkes Barre, PA: 1885.

Letterman, Jonathan. *Medical Recollections of the Army of the Potomac*. Bedford, MA: Applewood Books, 1866.

List of Staff Officers of the Confederate States Army, 1861–1865. Washington, DC: Government Printing Office, 1891.

Maine at Gettysburg. Report of Maine Commissioners. Portland, ME: Lakeside Press, 1898.

McClure, Alexander Kelly, ed. *The Annals of the Civil War Written by Leading Participants North and South*. Philadelphia: Times Publishing Company, 1879.

Medical and Surgical Directory of the United States. Polk & Company, 1886.

Moyer, H. P. *History of 17th Pennsylvania Volunteer Cavalry*. Lebanon, PA: Sowers Printing Co., 1911.

Muffly, Joseph Wendel. *The Story of Our Regiment, a History of the 148th Pennsylvania Volunteers*. Des Moines, IA: Kenyon Printing & Mfg. Co., 1904.

Phisterer, Frederick. *New York in the War of the Rebellion 1861–1865*. Albany, NY: 1912.

Potter, W. W. "Reminiscences of Field-Hospital Service with the Army of the Potomac." *Buffalo Medical and Surgical Journal* XXIX, no. 3 (October 1889), 137–47. Accessed 11/5/2024 at https://pubmed.ncbi.nlm.nih.gov/36667110/.

Quint, Alonzo H. *The Record of the Second Massachusetts Infantry 1861–65*. Boston: James P. Walker, 1867.

Small, Abner Ralph. *The Sixteenth Maine Regiment in the War of the Rebellion, 1861–1865*. Portland, ME: Published for the Regimental Association by B. Thurston & Co, 1886.

Stevens, Charles Augustus. *Berdan's Sharpshooters in the Army of the Potomac 1861–1865*. St. Paul, MN: Price-McGill Company, 1892.

Strait, N. A. *Roster of All Regimental Surgeons and Assistant Surgeons.* Washington, DC: U.S. Pension Office, 1882.

Under the Maltese Cross, Antietam to Appomattox: The Loyal Uprising in Western Pennsylvania, 1861–1865. Pittsburgh: 155th Regimental Association, 1910.

Underwood, George. *History of the 26th Regiment of NC Troops.* Goldsboro, NC: Nash Bros, 1901.

U.S. Department of War. *War of the Rebellion: A Compilation of the Official Records of the Union and Confederate Armies.* Washington, DC: Government Printing Office, 1880–1901.

U.S. Surgeon's General Office. *The Medical and Surgical History of the War of the Rebellion.* Washington, DC: 1870–1888.

University of Pennsylvania. *General Alumni Catalogue of the University of Pennsylvania, 1917.* Philadelphia.

Vautier, John D. *History of the 88th Pennsylvania Volunteers in the War for the Union 1861–1865.* Philadelphia: J.B. Lippincott Company, 1894.

Warren, Edward. *A Doctor's Experiences on Three Continents.* Baltimore: Cushings & Bailey, 1885.

SECONDARY SOURCES

Abrahams, Harold J. *Extinct Medical Schools of Nineteenth-Century Philadelphia.* Philadelphia: University of Pennsylvania Press, 1966.

Ayers, Edward L. *The Thin Light of Freedom: The Civil War and Emancipation in the Heart of America.* New York: WW Norton & Company, 2017.

Berman, Max, and Michael A. Flannery. *America's Botanico-Medical Movements: Vox Populi.* New York: Haworth Press, 2001.

Bollet, Alfred Jay. "An Analysis of Medical Problems of the Civil War." *Transactions of the American and Climatological Association,* Vol. 103 (1992): 128–41.

Breeden, James O. "The Winchester Accord: The Confederacy and the Humane Treatment of Captive Medical Officers." *Military Medicine* 158 (1993): 689–92.

Brown, Kent Masterson. *Retreat from Gettysburg.* Chapel Hill: University of North Carolina Press, 2005.

Carter, Peyton F. *Hitherto Above Reproach: The Life of Dr. Thomas Harold Wilson Upshur.* Salem, MA: Higginson Book Company, 2003.

Christie, Jeanne Marie. *The Women of City Point, Virginia, 1864–1865.* Jefferson, NC: McFarland & Co., 2020.

Cimbala, Paul A. *Veterans North and South: The Transition from Soldier to Civilian After the American Civil War.* Santa Barbara, CA: Praeger, 2015.

Coco, Gregory A. *A Strange and Blighted Land: Gettysburg, the Aftermath of a Battle.* El Dorado Hills, CA: Savas Beatie, 2017.

Coco, Gregory A. *A Vast Sea of Misery.* Gettysburg, PA: Thomas Publications, 1988.

Coddington, Ronald S. *Faces of Civil War Nurses.* Baltimore: Johns Hopkins University Press, 2020.

Conklin, Eileen F. *Women at Gettysburg 1863 Revisited.* Gettysburg, PA: Americana Souvenirs and Gifts, 2013.

Cunningham, H. H. *Doctors in Gray: The Confederate Medical Service.* Baton Rouge: Louisiana State University Press, 1986.

Devine, Shauna. *Learning from the Wounded: The Civil War and the Rise of American Medical Science.* Chapel Hill: University of North Carolina Press, 2014.

Devine, Shauna. "Producing Knowledge: Civil War Bodies and the Development of Scientific Medicine in Nineteenth Century America." School of Graduate and Postdoctoral Studies, University of Western Ontario, Canada, 2010.

Dreese. Michael. *The Hospital on Seminary Ridge at the Battle of Gettysburg.* Jefferson, NC: McFarland & Co., 2002.

Duncan, Louis C. "The Greatest Battle of the War—Gettysburg." *Military Surgeon* 33, no. 5 (1913).

Duncan, Louis C. *The Medical Department of the United States Army in the Civil War.* 1917.

Dunglison, Robley. *Medical Lexicon: A Dictionary of Medical Science.* Philadelphia: Blanchard and Lea, 1865.

Faust, Drew Gilpin. *This Republic of Suffering: Death and the American Civil War.* New York: Vintage Books, 2009.

Foote, Lorien. "Prisoners of War." *The Cambridge History of the American Civil War.* Vol. II. Cambridge: Cambridge University Press, 2019.

Foote, Lorien. *Rites of Retaliation.* Chapel Hill: University of North Carolina Press, 2021.

Frassanito, William A. *Early Photography at Gettysburg.* Gettysburg: Thomas Publications, 1995.

Frassanito, William A. *Gettysburg: A Journey in Time.* New York: Charles Scribner's Sons, 1975.

Giesburg, Judith Ann. *Civil War Sisterhood: The US Sanitary Commission and Women's Politics in Transition.* Boston: Northeastern University Press, 2000.

Gillett, Mary C. *The Army Medical Department 1818–1865.* Washington, DC: Center of Military History United States Army, 1987.

Gindlesperger, James. *Bullets & Bandages: The Aid Stations and Field Hospitals at Gettysburg.* Durham, NC: Blair/Carolina Wren Press, 2020.

Graf, Mercedes. *A Woman of Honor: Dr. Mary E. Walker and the Civil War.* Gettysburg, PA: Thomas Publications, 2001.

Hamilton, Marsha J. "Mercury and Water: Two Civil War Surgeons of the 148th Pennsylvania Volunteers." *Pennsylvania History: A Journal of Mid-Atlantic Studies* 75, no. 4 (2008): 467–504.

Hasegawa, Guy R. *Matchless Organization: The Confederate Army Medical Department.* Carbondale: Southern Illinois University Press, 2021.

Hoisington, Daniel J. *Gettysburg and the Christian Commission.* Minnesota: Edinborough Press, 2002.

Hoke, Thelma Vaine. *The First 125 Years of the Medical College of Virginia.* Richmond: Medical College of Virginia, 1963.

Jordan, Brian Matthew. *Marching Home: Union Veterans and Their Unending Civil War.* New York: Liveright Publishing Corporation, 2014.

Jordan, Brian Matthew, and Evan C. Rothera, eds. *The War Went On: Reconsidering the Lives of Civil War Veterans.* Baton Rouge: Louisiana State University Press, 2020.

Kaminski, Theresa, *Dr. Mary Walker's Civil War*. Guilford, CT: Lyons Press, 2020.

Kett, Joseph F. *The Formation of the American Medical Profession*. New Haven, CT: Yale University Press, 1968.

Kilbride, Daniel. "Southern Medical Students in Philadelphia, 1800–1861: Science and Sociability in the 'Republic of Medicine.'" *Journal of Southern History* 65, no. 4 (1999), 697–732.

Kirkwood, Ronald D. *"Too Much for Human Endurance:" The George Spangler Farm Hospitals and the Battle of Gettysburg*. El Dorado Hills, CA: Savas Beatie, 2021.

Koste, Jodi L. "Artifacts and Comingled Skeletal Remains from a Well on the Medical College of Virginia Campus: Anatomical and Surgical Training in Nineteenth-Century Richmond." June 18, 2012, Virginia Commonwealth University. Accessed September 29, 2019 at http://scholarscompass.vcu.edu/arch001/2.

Liebler, William F. "The United States and the Crimean War 1853–1856." PhD dissertation, University of Massachusetts–Amherst, 1972.

Logan, Mrs. John A. (Mary Simmerson Cunningham Logan). *The Part Taken by Women in American History*. Wilmington, DE: Perry-Nalle Publishing Co., 1912.

Lovejoy, Bess, "Meet Grandison Harris, the Grave Robber Enslaved (and Then Employed) by the Georgia Medical College." May 6, 2014. Accessed September 29, 2019 at https://www.smithsonianmag.com/history/meet-grandison-harris-grave-robber-enslaved-and-then-employed-georgia-college-medicine-180951344/.

Lowry, Thomas P., and Terry Reimer. *Bad Doctors: Military Justice Proceedings Against 622 Civil War Surgeons*. Frederick, MD: National Museum of Civil War Medicine Press, 2010.

Lowry, Thomas P., and Jack D. Welsh. *Tarnished Scalpels: The Court-Martials of Fifty Union Surgeons*. Mechanicsburg, PA: Stackpole Books, 2000.

MacKay, Winnifred K. "Philadelphia During the Civil War, 1861–1865." *Pennsylvania Magazine of History and Biography* 70, no. 1 (1946): 3–51.

Marten, James. *Sing Not War: The Lives of Union & Confederate Veterans in Gilded Age America*. Chapel Hill: University of North Carolina Press, 2011.

Maust, Roland R. *Grappling with Death: The Union Second Corps Hospital at Gettysburg*. Dayton, OH: Morningside House Inc., 2001.

McGaugh, Scott. *Surgeon in Blue: Jonathan Letterman, the Civil War Doctor Who Pioneered Battlefield Care*. New York: Arcade Publishing, 2013.

Mingus, Scott, "Lancaster County and Civil War Medicine: Civilian Physicians Turned Military Surgeons." *Journal of Lancaster County's Historical Society* 117, no. 4 (Fall/Winter 2016–2017): 199–211.

Moore, Frank. *Women of the War: Their Heroism and Self-Sacrifice*. Hartford, CT: S.S. Scranton & Co., 1866.

Mugridge, Donald H. "The United States Sanitary Commission in Washington, 1861–1865." *Records of the Columbia Historical Society, Washington, D.C.* 60/62 (1960): 134–49.

Paradis, James M. *African Americans and the Gettysburg Campaign*. Lanham, MD: Scarecrow Press, 2005.

Patterson, Gerard A. *Debris of Battle: The Wounded of Gettysburg*. Mechanicsburg, PA: Stackpole Books, 1997.

Pride, Mike. *No Place for a Woman: Harriet Dame's Civil War*. Kent, OH: Kent State University Press, 2022.

Rothstein, William G. *American Physicians in the 19th Century: From Sects to Science*. Baltimore: Johns Hopkins University Press, 1985.

Rucker, Michael P. *Bridge Burner*. Charleston, WV: Quarrier Press, 2014.

Rutkow, Ira M. *Bleeding Blue and Gray: Civil War Surgery and the Evolution of American Medicine*. New York: Random House, 2005.

Sanders, Charles W., Jr. *While in the Hands of the Enemy: Military Prisons of the Civil War*. Baton Rouge: Louisiana State University Press, 2005.

Savitt, Todd L. "The Use of Blacks for Medical Experimentation and Demonstration in the Old South." *Journal of Southern History* 48, no. 3 (1982): 331–48.

Schlaifer, Charles, and Lucy Freeman. *Heart's Work: Civil War Heroine and Champion of the Mentally Ill Dorothea Lunde Dix*. New York: Paragon House, 1991.

Schultz, Jane E. "The Inhospitable Hospital: Gender and Professionalism in Civil War Medicine." *Signs* 17, no. 2 (1992): 363–92. Accessed May 13, 2021 at www.jstor.org/stable/3174468.

Schultz, Jane E. *Women at the Front: Hospital Workers in Civil War America*. Chapel Hill: University of North Carolina Press, 2004.

Slawson, R. G. "Medical Training in the United States Prior to the Civil War." *Journal of Evidence-Based Complementary & Alternative Medicine* 17, no.1 (2012): 11–27.

Starr, Paul. *The Social Transformation of American Medicine: The Rise of a Sovereign Profession & the Making of a Vast Industry*. New York: Basic Books, 1982.

Stoltze, Dolly. "Bodies in the Basement: The Hidden Bones of Medical Schools." *Atlas Obscura*, January 22, 2015. Accessed September 29, 2019 at https://www.atlasobscura.com/articles/bodies-in-the-basement-the-forgotten-bones-of-america-s-medical-schools.

Waite, Frederick Clayton. *The First Medical College in Vermont: Castleton 1818–1862*. Vermont Historical Society, 1949.

Ward, Patricia Spain. *Simon Baruch: Rebel in the Ranks of Medicine 1840–1921*. Tuscaloosa: University of Alabama Press, 1994.

Whorton, James C. *Nature Cures: The History of Alternative Medicine in America*. Oxford and New York: Oxford University Press, 2002.

NEWSPAPERS

Baltimore Sun, Baltimore, Maryland.
Detroit Free Press, Detroit, Michigan.
Indiana State Sentinel, Indianapolis, Indiana.
Medical and Surgical Reporter, Philadelphia, Pennsylvania. https://catalog.hathitrust.org/Record/000054252
New York Tribune, New York City, New York.
Philadelphia Inquirer, Philadelphia, Pennsylvania.
Pittsburgh Daily Post, Pittsburgh, Pennsylvania.

New York Times, New York City, New York.

ARCHIVAL COLLECTIONS
Adams County Historical Society, Gettysburg, Pennsylvania.
Gettysburg National Military Park, Gettysburg, Pennsylvania.
National Archives and Records Administration (NARA), Washington, DC.
Pennsylvania State Archives, Harrisburg, Pennsylvania.
University of Vermont Special Collections, Burlington, Vermont.
U.S. Army Heritage and Education Center, Carlisle, Pennsylvania.
Virginia Historical Society, Richmond, Virginia.

.

INDEX

Page numbers for illustrations and charts are italicized.

About the Author

Barbara Franco has extensive experience in public history as a museum director, curator, and exhibition developer, including as assistant director for museums at the Minnesota Historical Society, executive director of the Pennsylvania Historical and Museum Commission, and founding director of the Gettysburg Seminary Ridge Museum. She has written numerous articles on museum practice and historical interpretation, and currently works as an independent scholar and museum consultant. She serves as president of the Advent Historical Society, preserving and interpreting a historic 1849 Millerite chapel in Centre County, Pennsylvania. Her broad interest in the social, cultural, and intellectual history of the nineteenth century has included the decorative and fine arts, communal societies, fraternal organizations, the role of religion, and the Civil War era. In addition to numerous exhibition catalogs and articles, she co-edited *Ideas and Images: Developing Interpretive History Exhibits* (1992) and *Interpreting Religion at Museums and Historic Sites* (2018). She is a graduate of Bryn Mawr College and the Cooperstown Graduate Program in Museum Studies.